PAINTING SHARP FOCUS STILL LIFES

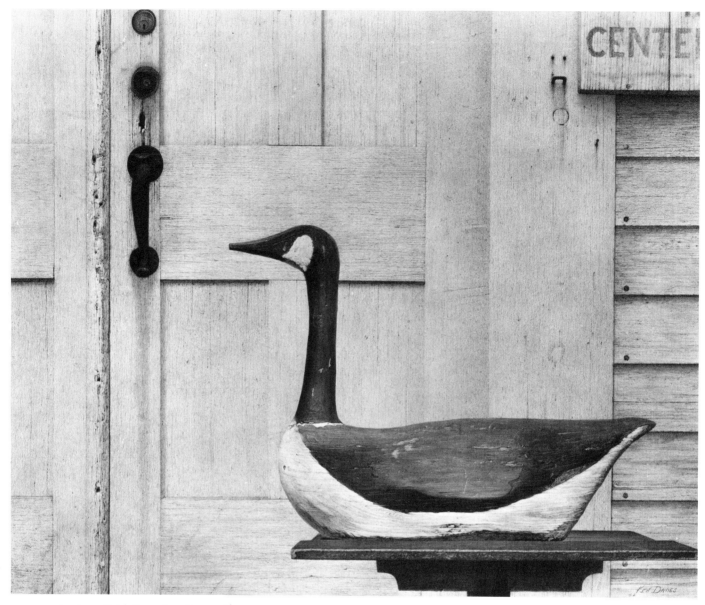

Antique Sale, Canadian Goose Decoy

PAINTING SHARP FOCUS STILL LIFES

TROMPE L'OEIL OIL TECHNIQUES

BY KEN DAVIES AND ELLYE BLOOM

WATSON-GUPTILL PUBLICATIONS/NEW YORK

PITMAN PUBLISHING/LONDON

First published 1975 in the United States and Canada by Watson-Guptill Publications
a division of Billboard Publications, Inc.
One Astor Plaza, New York, N.Y. 10036

Library of Congress Cataloging in Publication Data
Davies, Ken, 1926–
    Painting sharp focus still lifes.
    Includes index.
    1. Still-life painting—Technique. 2. Trompe l'oeil
painting. I. Bloom, Ellye, 1929–   joint author.
II. Title.
ND1390.D35 1975   758'.4   75-20196
ISBN 0-8230-3856-4

Published in Great Britain by Sir Isaac Pitman & Sons Ltd.
39 Parker Street, London WC2B 5PB
ISBN 0-273-00091-8

Manufactured in U.S.A.

First Printing, 1975
Second Printing, 1976

To Fox and Norman

CONTENTS

ACKNOWLEDGMENTS

The authors wish to express their appreciation to Adele and Edward Paier for their patience and cooperation during the writing of This book; to Don Holden, who initially believed in our project; to our editor, Sarah Bodine, for the skill and diplomacy with which she coordinated the book's content and brought it to completion. Thanks also to Dan Becker, who masterfully processed all black and white photographic material.

INTRODUCTION

In this book I hope to provide logical, step-by-step information that will enable the reader to paint sharp focus realistic still life paintings. The information is intended for the serious student or the experienced painter who is willing to devote many hours of hard work to practicing the essentials. It is not for the hobbyist or the casual "Sunday painter." To avoid misunderstanding, please let me hasten to add that I intend no snobbery. It is simply a fact that sharp focus realism needs more time, practice, hard work, and endurance than the average hobbyist is probably willing or able to devote. The arduous steps involved can be tremendously exciting and rewarding to the student who is interested in sharp focus realism. To those who are not, it can be a colossal bore! I know this is true from my first-hand experience of 25 years spent in teaching. During this time I've watched art students react and respond (positively and negatively) to the same information that you're about to be faced with.

The first two parts of this book contain a detailed series of projects and exercises that I developed for the first- and second-year drawing and painting courses at the Paier School of Art in Hamden, Connecticut. These lessons are still being taught at the school. In fact, many of the illustrations included here have been done by Paier students who have followed this course. Both these parts are in-tended to provide the technical "know-how" needed to produce exhibit-worthy paintings. However, your total work output during this time should be regarded as strictly practice pieces—not finished paintings. Their only purpose is to teach how to see and record ac-curately *shapes, values,* and *colors*! If you per-sist and conscientiously develop the ability to accomplish those three very important things, I promise that eventually you'll have the ability to represent on canvas or panel a highly accurate reproduction of any object or group of objects you choose. My instructions will often seem dogmatic, and some of the time limits set for completing paintings might seem oppressively short, but bear with me. I know it works. Have faith, and remember, upon "graduation" from the last exercise *you* can make the rules.

The demonstrations in Part Three welcome the reader into my studio where I'll "think aloud" during the painting of four pictures. I'll try to describe in detail the how and why of the evolution of a painting by my own methods. I'll let you share some of the labor pains, too. In addition, in the portfolio of paintings that I have done over the years each reproduction is accompanied by some of my thoughts about it.

I hope that I've aroused your interest and your sense of challenge. If I've succeeded, let's get to work.

MATERIALS AND EQUIPMENT

During my 25 years of teaching and painting experience, I've naturally developed preferences for certain kinds of materials that I think give me the best performance. For the purposes of this book I've extracted a basic list, but you may want to add to it as you become more familiar with your own painting needs. With few exceptions, the supplies can be easily found in any art supply store.

In tallying up the cost of everything you'll need, with the exception of an easel, I can fairly well predict that your initial outlay will be around $100. I haven't included the cost of an easel simply because the prices vary as widely as their quality and sturdiness.

Don't feel that it's necessary to buy all the supplies in the beginning. The first two projects deal with line drawing and perspective, so if you wish you can postpone buying paints and brushes until the third project, on black and white oil painting.

DRAWING SUPPLIES

Keep the following supplies close by during the drawing projects. It saves time and frustration to know that something you may need is within easy reach.

Bond Pad. You'll find that the paper of the bond pad is smooth and will give you a precise pencil line as you draw on it, whereas a rough or textured paper would give a quality that's undesirable in precise still life painting. Further, the bond pad comes in convenient sizes (9" x 12", 11" x 14", 14" x 17"), which you can hold in your lap or on the table with equal ease.

Tracing Pad. Tracing paper (14" x 17") is both convenient and necessary, especially for drawing in correct perspective. The tracing pad does not need to be of the finest quality; a thin, inexpensive onionskin should do nicely.

White and Gray Charcoal Paper. Any kind of white and gray charcoal paper will do and can be bought either in the form of a pad or in separate sheets, usually 19" x 25".

Drafting Pencil. Through experience I have found that a mechanical drawing pencil is a great convenience. The leads are replaceable and can be retracted and ejected at will. The 2H, HB, and 2B leads are of varying degrees of hardness (the 2H being the hardest). They will produce a thin, pure line on the bond paper, especially when the point is sharpened on a sandpaper block.

Charcoal Pencils. In general for making line drawings on charcoal paper you'll need charcoal pencils 2B, 4B, and 6B. They are soft pencils that respond easily to the surface texture of the charcoal paper. The 2B pencil will be needed for shading light values. I'd like to stress the importance of keeping long, sharp points on all the pencils you use. If you let your pencil points get stubby, you'll end up with messy, smudged lines.

White Conté Pencil. As you'll see, the white Conté pencil is absolutely essential for shading procedures on gray charcoal paper. Again, keep the point long and sharp.

Sandpaper Block and Single-edged Razor Blade. With these two important tools you can keep your pencil points in great shape. Use the razor blade to sharpen the pencils to elongated points, and keep rubbing the tip of the point on the sandpaper block as you draw to keep the points very sharp.

Kneaded Eraser. Nobody's perfect; we all make mistakes in drawing no matter how careful we are. This soft, gummy type of eraser can be kneaded into the shape you want and can be manipulated very easily to delete lines with a minimum of smudging.

Plumb Bob. You can fashion your own plumb bob from a large nut or bolt, a heavy fishing weight, or any other weighted object. Tie the weight to a piece of string 4 to 5 feet long. You'll need the plumb bob to lay out your drawing in proper perspective.

Small Carpenter's Level. When you use a 6" to 8" long level in conjunction with the plumb

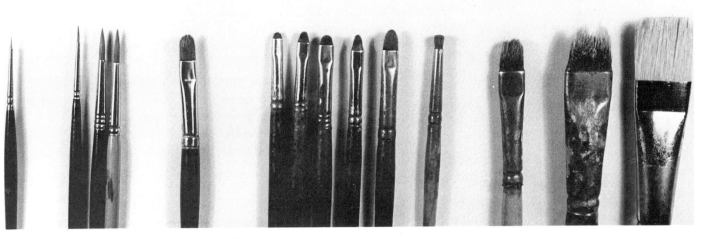

1. *Brushes (left to right): an 000 sable used for the smallest details; three round sables—a No. 1 and two No. 6, a filbert sable with rounded top used for painting larger areas than the pointed sable; five old, worn filberts used to soften edges and blend small glazed areas; an old round sable, cut down with a razor blade and then smoothed with fine sandpaper used for softening edges and "scumbling"; and three bristles—two old, worn ones used for scumbling large, coarse textures and a newer one for blocking in large areas.*

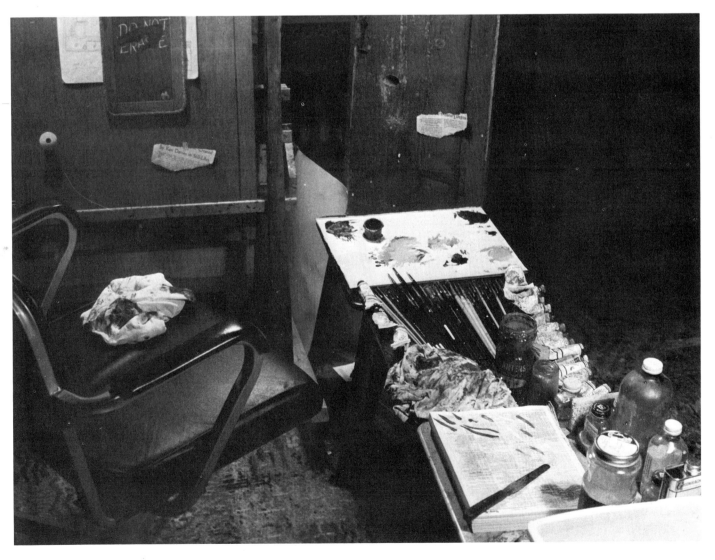

2. *The author's work area*

bob, you'll be able to line up vertical and horizontal checkpoints to sharpen the perspective of your drawings. You can buy the level at any hardware store.

Ruler. You're going to have to draw straight lines, and I believe that even the best-trained hand can have trouble accomplishing this without a ruler. I'd say that the most convenient length for a ruler is about 18".

Fixative. Buy a large economy-size can of spray fixative. It will keep charcoal pencil lines from smudging, which will be a definite benefit in both the drawing and painting exercises.

PAINTS AND BRUSHES

My own preferences in oil colors are listed below. Even though the group is limited, I feel it makes up an adequate palette. Please bear in mind, however, that this is only a *suggested* group of colors for those just breaking into the oil medium. As your painting experience grows, you'll surely want to add, or perhaps subtract, colors and experiment with new pigments on the market.

Each time a project or exercise requires a palette with a full range of colors, use all of the ones listed here:

Titanium white	Yellow ochre
Ivory black	Cadmium red light
Cobalt blue	Cadmium vermilion
Ultramarine blue	Cadmium red deep
Cerulean blue	Alizarin crimson
Viridian green	Burnt umber
Permanent green light	Burnt sienna
Sap green	Raw umber
Cadmium yellow light	Raw sienna

Sable Brushes. Personal preference applies to the choice of brushes as well as paints. (Figure 1.) Although sable brushes are very expensive (they will probably be one of your largest expenditures), they are essential in the type of oil painting with which this book deals. In spite of their delicate appearance, they're surprisingly durable. As they wear down, which of course they will, they can be trimmed to new shapes.

Sables come in round and flat shapes plus a variation of the two. For my course I recommend round, flat, and filbert types. The hairs of round sables are fitted into round metal ferrules and taper to a fine point. Flat sables are either short, in which case they are called "brights," or long. In either case they are flattened to a chisel edge. Filberts are a cross between the two. They are flat yet taper to rounded tips. As you become familiar with them, you'll discover that each has its own "personality" and its own kind of stroke. The different sizes of brushes are indicated by numbers. I recommend you start out by getting the following brushes:

Round: Nos. 3, 6, and 10

Flat: Nos. 4, 8, and 12

Filbert: Nos. 4, 8, and 12

Bristle Brushes. Bristle brushes produce textural effects that are quite different from the smooth strokes you can get with sables. Like sables, bristles come in flat, round, and filbert shapes. I suggest you start with the following:

Round: Nos. 2, 4, and 8

Flat: Nos. 4, 8, and 12

Filbert: Nos. 2, 4, and 8

How to Clean Brushes. Fill a large glass jar almost to the top with turpentine. Dip the brush in the turpentine, and wipe the excess paint off on the pages of the old telephone book. Wipe the brush with a paint rag to remove all remaining paint from the brush. Then dip the brush into the turpentine again and work the bristles up against the inside of the jar. When the brush is finally clean, wipe it again with a fresh rag. I find this method not only saves rags but prevents the turpentine from becoming dirty right away. Most painters finish the cleaning by washing the brush with ivory soap and lukewarm water.

OTHER PAINTING SUPPLIES AND EQUIPMENT

All the supplies that you'll need in the drawing and painting assignments should be placed on a table or taboret (a small portable table available at any art or office supply store) and kept close to your working area. It's a great convenience not to have to go hunting for some small item when you're in the middle of a difficult passage. (Figure 2.)

Mediums. Oil paint as it's squeezed straight from the tube has a lustrous appearance, but for most painters its consistency is too sticky to work with. Just a few drops of a medium, such as a mixture of linseed oil and damar varnish, added to the paint will give it a buttery texture and enable you to move it around easily on the canvas. Most painters feel that painting in oils without a medium is like roller skating without ball bearings in the wheels.

Good-quality turpentine is another extremely useful medium. Add just a small amount to the linseed oil/damar varnish mixture to thin your paint for making washes. Because turpentine is a solvent, you can also use it for cleaning brushes and removing paint from your skin and clothing. (Be sure to wash your hands after removing paint from them with turpentine.)

My own favorite medium is a mixture of ⅔ linseed oil and ⅓ damar varnish, but you're welcome to experiment with others whenever you feel ready.

Paint Rags. Don't shortchange yourself on rags. It's a pleasant luxury to have plenty of them around when you're in a hurry to clean your brushes and do a general mop-up after a particularly messy painting session. My favorite rag is an old cotton tee shirt.

Telephone Book. Rather than using just rags to clean my brushes I use the pages of an outdated telephone book. I wipe the dirty brush on the paper, tear out the soiled pages and throw them away.

Palette and Palette Knife. Your art supply store can sell you a white paper palette that's shaped like the traditional wooden one but with an updated feature that I find very convenient: when you're through painting for the day, you can simply rip off and throw away the top leaf of the paper palette. The surface underneath it, of course, will be clean and ready for the next painting session.

Another reason that I like paper palettes is that I prefer mixing my paints on a very white background. That way, I can see exactly what color I'm getting for painting on a white canvas or board.

A strong, flexible palette knife is essential for scraping off unwanted paint strokes and for mixing colors.

Metal Cups and Other Containers. Quantities of linseed oil and turpentine should be kept close at hand at all times. The twin metal cups sold in art supply stores are just the right depth for dipping brushes into, and they conveniently clip onto your palette. I like to use these little metal cups to hold linseed oil and damar varnish. Since I use much more turpentine than any other liquid, I keep a medium-sized jar filled with it by my side.

Varnishes. While your painting is still wet it has a lively, glossy finish, but as the painting dries, parts of it may become flat or dull in appearance, certainly a discouraging development. Retouch varnish sprayed or brushed onto the surface will revive the luster. But remember that the retouch varnish must be allowed to dry before you continue to paint over it.

Semi-matte varnish, a mixture of damar and matte varnishes, is applied only after the completed painting is thoroughly dry. It will give the painted surface a moderate luster rather than a slick shine. I prefer to apply it with a 2″ varnishing brush. The surface should be completely free from dust before varnish is applied.

Painting Surfaces. Because their surfaces are rigid I prefer canvas board and Masonite panel to stretched canvas. The tension of stretched canvas can vary, while canvas board and Masonite are predictably firm. An incident which involved my son sold me finally on rigid surfaces. At the age of two, he decided to practice with one of my golf clubs and swung a 3-iron into one of my first major paintings, *Lighthouse In the Alps*. The result was a sizable hole in the lower center of the painting. It has been repaired, but the experience left me with a staggering aversion to anything less sturdy than canvas board or Masonite.

Color Wheel. Purchase a basic color wheel at your art supply store. Unless you are totally familiar with the color wheel, you should have one for reference while mixing colors.

Mahlstick. Sharp focus still life painting is ex-

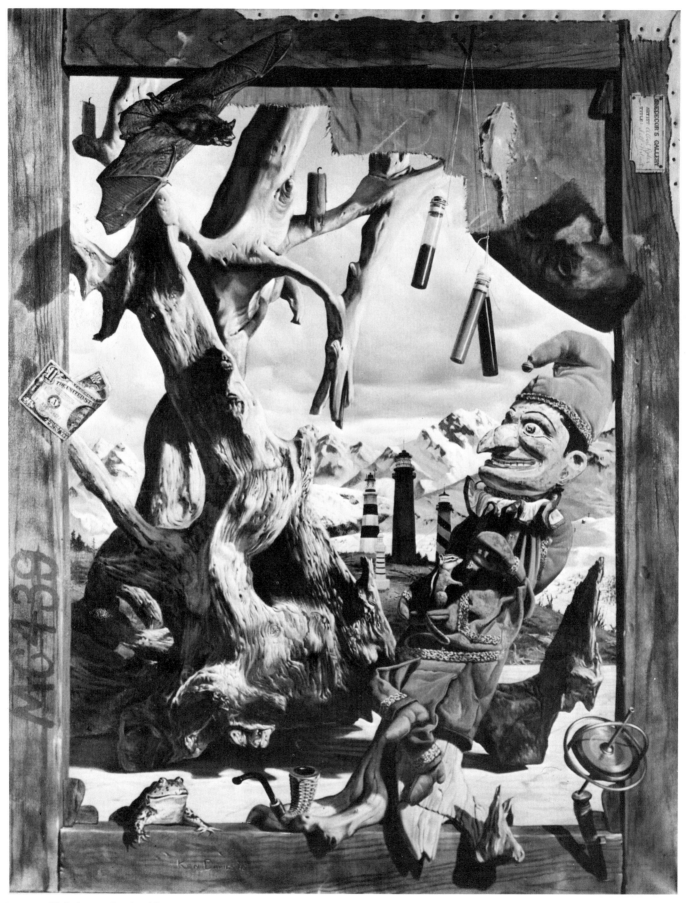

Lighthouse in the Alps

tremely precise and requires a steady hand. I use a mahlstick to give me the support needed to keep my wrist steady. If my wrist is steady I can keep my hand and brush in almost perfect control. You can make your own mahlstick by tapering an end of a 6-foot length of 1x2 lumber. To use it properly, stand one end on the floor and lean the other end across the painting, but not touching it, allowing it to rest against the easel. (Figure 3.)

LIGHTING

Lighting is an essential part of your work setup. It can alter the way your subject appears as well as the color of the pigments on your palette and work surface.

Natural Light. Because it varies tremendously, I prefer not to work under traditional north light. On sunny days, north light is blue. But even on cloudy or dull days when the light is neutral and therefore desirable, it changes intensity during the passing of the day. I use a neutral fluorescent bulb in my work area because its constant illumination is the most stable and reliable source, and I light my still life setups with a warm incandescent bulb.

Artificial Light. When you start to paint with oils, the color of the light you use will affect the tones you mix on your palette. An ordinary incandescent bulb is quite yellowish, while some of the fluorescent tubes cast a cold or even blue light on a subject. A good way to observe the effect of fluorescent versus incandescent light is by taking a walk through city streets at night. Look at the windows of office buildings and apartment houses and try to distinguish the windows that are lit with incandescent light from ones lit with fluorescent light. Notice the difference in their color. The difference in the warmth and coolness of the tones is quite spectacular.

If you paint under a yellow incandescent light, there will be a tendency to add too little yellow or warm color to the pigment. That's because the light tinges the color of the pigment with a degree of yellow. To eliminate this problem, use a neutral fluorescent bulb.

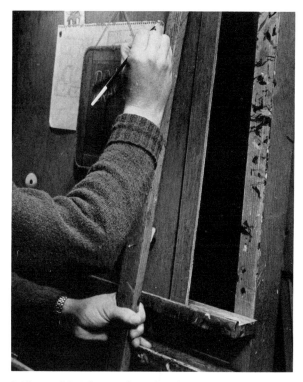

3. *The mahlstick is anchored with the fifth finger of the left hand against the easel while the right hand is steadied by resting on it.*

The spot in which the finished painting will be displayed has a direct relationship to the light under which it's painted. In art galleries, the lighting is generally on the warm side, whereas in commercial establishments cold fluorescent light is more often used. Although you can't really predict where your painting will be shown, I believe the use of a neutral fluorescent light will give you a good middle-of-the-road choice.

When I began to work commercially, I painted under yellow light. The paintings looked fine in the studio, but when I delivered them to a New York City advertising agency and displayed them under their cold fluorescent light, I was appalled by the change the color underwent.

In the projects and exercises that follow, I recommend using an incandescent bulb on the still life setup because it gives a more direct pinpointed source of light than a long fluorescent tube. These bulbs are inexpensive and certainly satisfactory for practice paintings.

A LESSON IN PERSPECTIVE

The subject of perspective deserves an entire book in itself, and there are, of course, many books devoted to this area. I urge every student of art to acquire one or two of them in order to become thoroughly familiar with this fascinating aspect of drawing and painting.

I won't go deeply into the study of perspective here, nor is it necessary if you limit yourself to still life painting, as you will see later, but I do want to talk about a few rules and facts that I feel are indispensable in their application to sharp focus still lifes. If you understand and memorize these facts, drawing and painting in correct perspective will become much simpler.

THE LINE IN PERSPECTIVE

The first consideration in a study of perspective is what happens to the simple line which is used to draw the objects in your setup.

Rule 1. *All receding parallel lines vanish at the same point.* Perhaps the simplest and most easily understood illustration of this rule is the classic one of the railroad tracks converging at a single point on the horizon.

Rule 2. *All receding horizontal lines have their vanishing points on the horizon line.* The horizon line, which will be referred to in the illustrations as H.L., represents your eye level. When you're in a sitting position, your eye level is naturally lower than when you're standing.

The key word here is *horizontal*, and by that I mean any receding line that is level with or parallel to the ground. Every straight line in your still life setup will be either horizontal, vertical, or inclining at an angle. Rule 2 applies only to receding horizontal lines. Figure 1A shows three rectangular blocks on a tabletop. Notice that the receding lines on all three blocks and the receding lines of the two sides of the table converge at the same vanishing point. Although the block at the far left extends above your eye level (or horizon line), the top edges still converge at the van-

ishing point. This is a simple illustration of *one-point perspective.*

Figure 1B shows the same setup in *plan view*, or looking straight down from above. The front and back edges of the table and the three boxes are all at right angles to each other. In other words, they are perpendicular to the line of sight. This fact alone determines the use of one-point perspective.

The plan view in Figure 2A shows the same three boxes. The boxes at far left and far right have been moved. Figure 2B is a perspective drawing of the three boxes. The boxes at the far left and far right are at different angles, and now each has two vanishing points. The perspective drawing required the use of *two-point perspective*. Use two-point perspective when an object is not at right angles to the viewer's line of sight. The center box in Figure 2B and the tabletop remain in one-point perspective.

Rule 3. *All inclined lines have their vanishing points either above or below the horizon line.* Figure 3 shows a drawing of a piece of folded paper with half resting horizontally on the table and half raised above it. The parallel sides of the raised half of the paper (*ac* and *bd*) are at an angle and vanish at a point above the horizon and directly above the vanishing point of the lower half (*ce* and *df*). The upper edge of the raised half (*ab*) vanishes at the same point on the horizon line as its corresponding edges resting on the table (*ef*). Being parallel to the ground *ab, ef,* and *cd* vanish at the same point.

For our purposes, all the vertical lines in your setup will remain vertical in your drawing. This statement doesn't apply in three-point perspective, but the still life and trompe l'oeil painter rarely finds it necessary to use three-point perspective. If you thoroughly understand these few simple rules and diagrams, no straight line in your still life setup will be a mystery to you. If you accurately plot your still life drawings with the horizontal and vertical check points using the plumb bob and carpenter's level (see Project 1), you

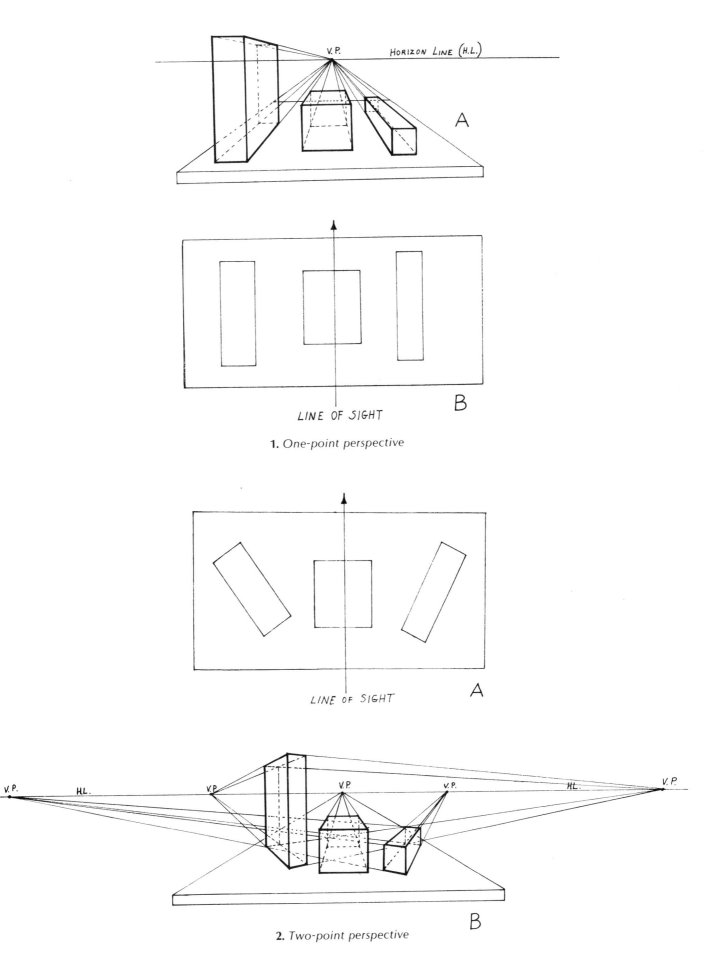

V.P.   HORIZON LINE (H.L.)

A

LINE OF SIGHT   B

1. *One-point perspective*

LINE OF SIGHT   A

V.P. H.L.   V.P.   V.P.   V.P.   H.L.   V.P.

B

2. *Two-point perspective*

17

don't actually need to know anything about perspective!

Of course, when you're ready to paint serious finished pictures for exhibition, you won't be restricted to copying your setup exactly as it is. You may want to enlarge or reduce an object or even change or exaggerate its shape. Your knowledge of perspective will then become a valuable, practical tool.

THE CIRCLE IN PERSPECTIVE

Another important subject in this extremely simplified discourse is the circle in perspective. A circle tilted into perspective becomes an ellipse. The closer a circle is tilted toward the horizon line the narrower it becomes. When it is tilted to coincide with the horizon line it's no longer an ellipse but a straight line (Figure 4). The narrower the ellipse, the easier it is to draw. You'll discover this when you start to draw ellipses in Project 1.

A geometric ellipse (Figure 5A) has a major axis (a–b) and a minor axis (c–d). The intersection of these two axes is the geometric center of the geometric ellipse. But the geometric center is *not* the center of the perspective circle. Even though the outline shape of a geometric ellipse is used for a perspective circle, the center of the two figures is not the same. A circle fits into a square, a geometric ellipse fits into a rectangle, and a perspective circle fits into a perspective square (Figure 5B and 5C). In the perspective circle (5C) the distance from the front to the center is greater than the distance from the center to the back. But notice that in the geometric ellipse (5A) the center is equidistant from the front to the back. Dot a is the center of the perspective circle, and dot b is the center of the geometric ellipse. Keep these facts in mind whenever you need to indicate the center of a circle in a drawing.

Here's one more important bit of information that will help you to draw the circle in perspective: When a circular object such as a cylinder or bottle is absolutely vertical, the major axis of its ellipse is always horizontal and the minor axis is always vertical. But if the object is tilted at any angle or is resting on its side, the situation changes.

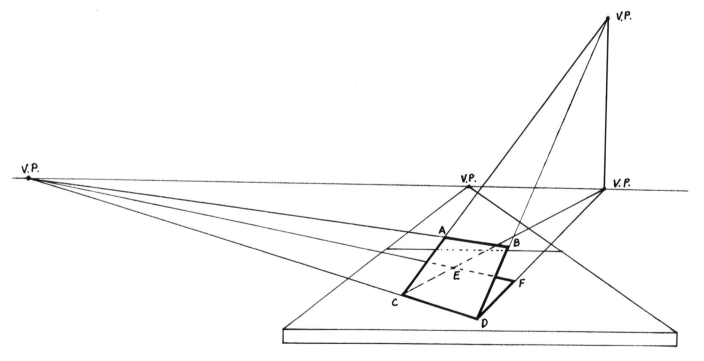

3. *Position of vanishing point of inclined plane shown directly above ground vanishing point.*

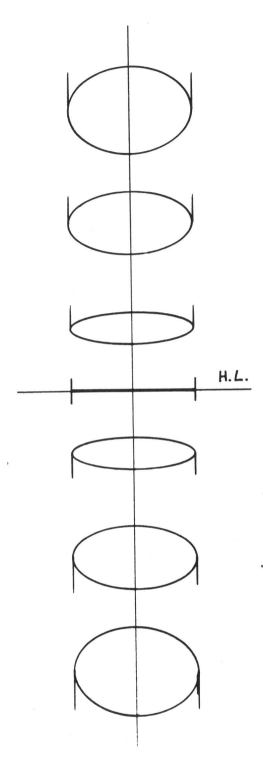

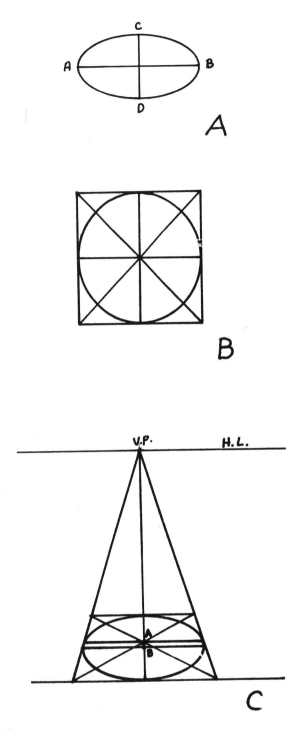

4. *Ellipses in perspective*

5. *Geometric ellipses*

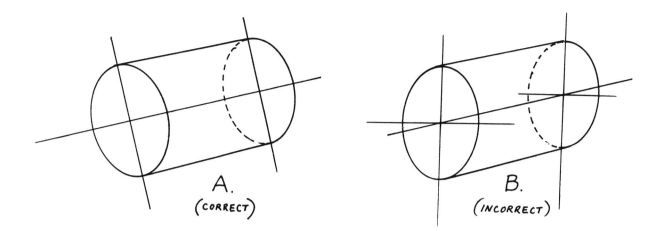

6. *Tilted circular objects*

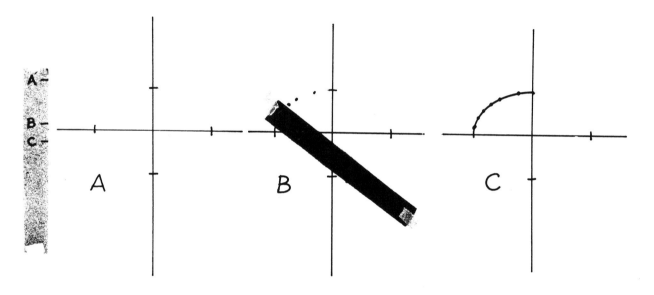

7. *Drawing an ellipse*

Rule. *The minor axis of the ellipse coincides with the center line of the object.* This rule is illustrated in Figure 6, which shows the common error made in drawing tilted circular objects.

MECHANICAL METHODS OF DRAWING ELLIPSES

It's possible to buy ellipse template guides and other gadgets to help you draw ellipses. One of the drawbacks of using a template ellipse guide is that the ellipse you want to draw may not be the size of the template. When you use a template you're limited to its size. The method I recommend allows you to draw any size ellipse. All you need is a pencil, a ruler, and a piece of paper.

First determine the length and width of the ellipse (major and minor axes). On the edge of a strip of paper, mark off half of the major axis and half of the minor axis (Figure 7A); *ac* is half the major and *ab* is half the minor. Line up point *b* on the major axis and point *c* on the minor axis. Move the paper strip counterclockwise making dots as you go (Figure 7B). Make as many dots as you need to draw one-quarter of the ellipse (Figure 7C). To complete the ellipse, repeat the procedure for the remaining three quarters, or if you prefer, simply trace the finished quarter and transfer it to the other three quarters.

We've barely scratched the surface of a most fascinating science. I've tried to touch on what I think are the major basic rules of perspective that will help in still life painting. But if your curiosity has been aroused, I once more strongly recommend that you investigate the subject more fully.

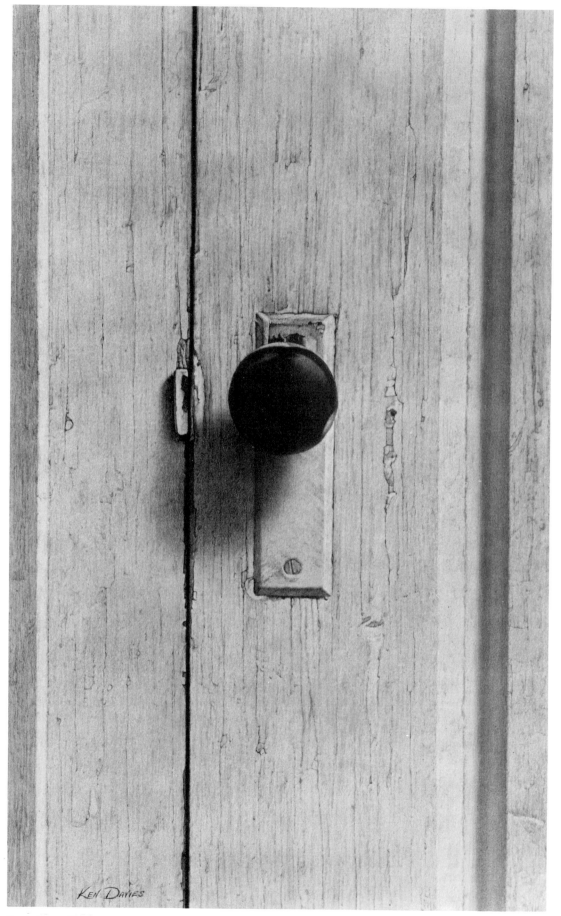

Back Door Knob

PART ONE **PROJECTS**

1 LINE DRAWING

Assignment 1 **Simple Shapes**

Assignment 2 **Complicated Shapes**

Assignment 3 **Crumpled Paper Bag**

Assignment 4 **Symmetrical Objects**

Assignment 5 **Ellipses**

2 BLACK AND WHITE VALUE DRAWING

Assignment 1 **Ball, Cone, Cylinder, and Block**

Assignment 2 **Still Life on White Charcoal Paper**

Assignment 3 **Still Life on Gray Charcoal Paper**

3 BLACK AND WHITE VALUE PAINTING

4 COLOR PAINTING

Assignment 1 **Value Scale**

Assignment 2 **Matching Chart**

These projects, and the exercises which follow in
Part Two, are designed to give you some practice
in seeing *shapes*, *values*, and *colors* and recording them accurately with oil paint.

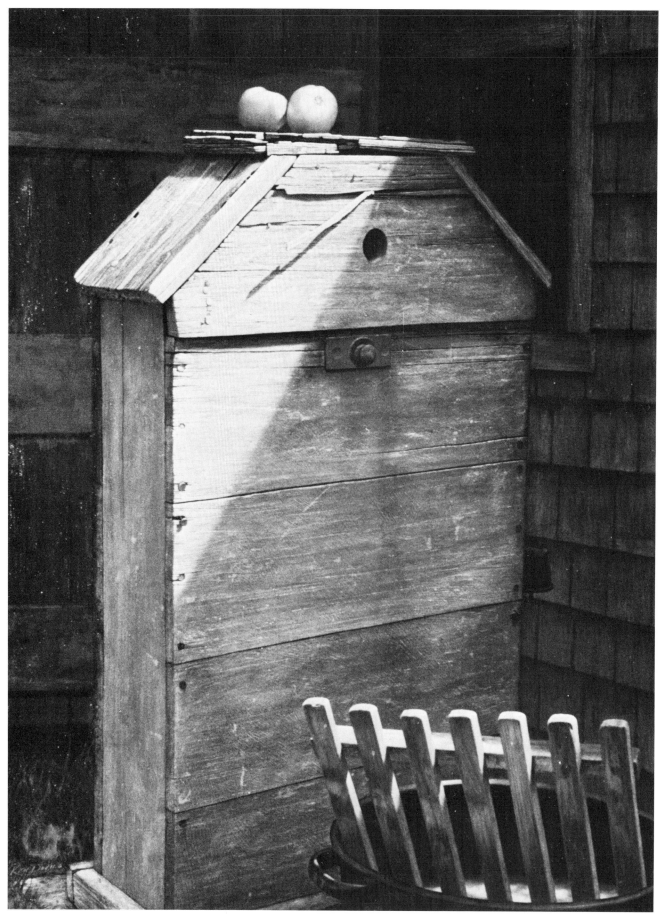

Ripe Fruit

PROJECT 1 **LINE DRAWING**

Beneath every good painting there should be an accurate line drawing. In painting still lifes, sharp illusions of reality will depend partially on that drawing. In sharp focus painting the line drawing can be defined as a rendering of the outline shapes of objects. The textures of the objects will be disregarded for the present.

There are five assignments in this first project which should enable you, with practice, to produce a still life drawing that is accurate in shape and perspective. Mechanical methods will be used, and learning to master them will give you satisfaction in the knowledge that your eye and hand together are capable of producing a correct drawing. Practice and repetition of the assignments will eventually obviate the further use of mechanical aids to drawing. I can't stress too much how important it is to keep making one drawing after the other, for a good line drawing is an important foundation to a good painting.

MATERIALS AND EQUIPMENT

Bond pad, 14" x 17"
Drafting pencil with HB and 2H leads
Eraser
Plumb bob
Carpenter's level
Ruler
Tracing pad, 14" x 17"
Masking tape

In each of the following assignments, place the still life objects on a flat surface, making certain the setup is slightly below eye level. If you prefer to stand at an easel, raise the setup so that you are viewing it from slightly above.

Assignment 1 **Simple Shapes**

Use a group of simple objects, such as a wooden block from a child's set, a rubber ball, a cardboard cereal or cracker box with the outer paper removed, a cone, and a cylinder (Figure 1). Make the cone by twisting a piece of white paper into shape and taping it in place. The cylinder can be made by covering an empty salt container with white paper. Since you'll be drawing only the outline shapes or edges, of these objects, their surfaces should be smooth. The textures of the objects and the shadows they cast will not be dealt with in this assignment.

Rough Sketch. View the setup and determine the proportions and relative sizes of the objects. Make a rough sketch of the setup on the bond pad, using a drafting pencil with an HB lead (Figure 2). Don't make your sketch too small; try to make the objects life-size. With the aid of the carpenter's level and the plumb bob, place dots locating the corners and tops of the objects in the rough sketch. The dots will make it simpler to correct the drawing.

Correcting Perspective. Check for correct perspective in the rough sketch using the carpenter's level and the plumb bob. Hold the carpenter's level at arm's length between you and the setup (Figure 3). Move the level until the small air bubble in the glass cylinder is centered. This will enable you to determine whether the top of the ball is lower than the top of the box, whether the top of the cylinder is higher or lower than the cone, and so on. In this way, check the *horizontal* position of each object in relation to the others. As you check these measurements, refine your rough drawing. It may be necessary to raise or lower the position of an object.

To illustrate the measurements made by the level and plumb bob, I have added horizontal and vertical lines to the rough sketch (Figure 4). It is not necessary to draw these lines on your rough sketch.

With the plumb bob held between you and the setup, check the vertical measures to find where one object overlaps the other (Figure 5). Using the pencil dots, correct the drawing.

Completing the Drawing. Using the dots as checkpoints, it should now be relatively simple to finish the outline drawing of the objects. The final drawing should show a neat outline of each object in its correct relationship to the others. Erase all remaining rough sketch lines (Figure 6).

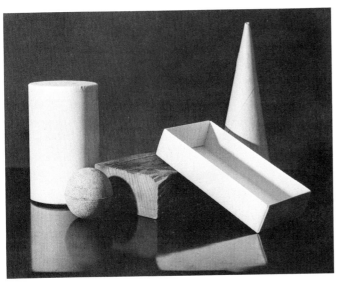

1. *Setup of simple shapes*

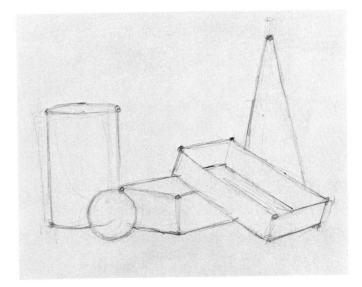

2. *Rough sketch*

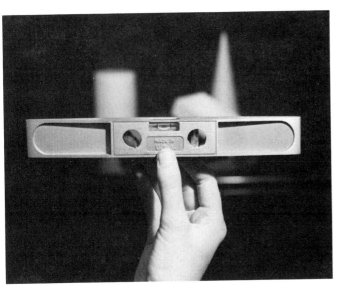

3. *Carpenter's level*

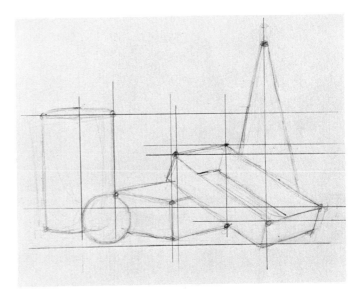

4. *Correcting perspective*

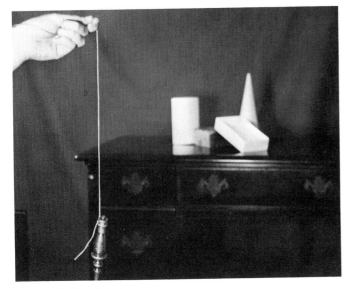

5. *Plumb bob*

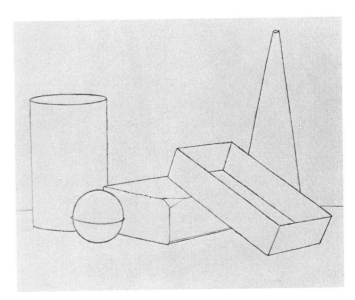

6. *Completed drawing*

Assignment 2   **Complicated Shapes**

Select a cup, an apple, a jug, a book, a saucer, and a cardboard box (with the cover left open). The objects should have no lettering or decoration on them.

Rough sketch. Repeat the drawing procedure as in Assignment 1, drawing with the HB pencil on the bond pad.

Correcting Perspective. Using carpenter's level and plumb bob, correct your drawing as you did in Assignment 1.

Completing the Drawing. Complete the outline of the still life setup; then erase all superfluous sketch lines (Figure 7).

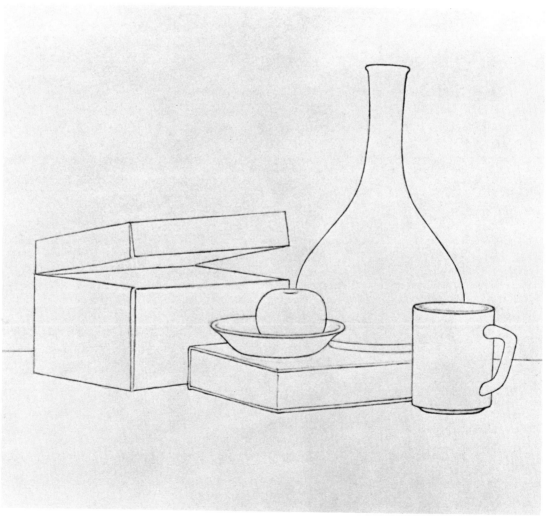

7. *Completed drawing*

Assignment 3 Crumpled Paper Bag

In this assignment, you'll draw one of the most complicated shapes of all—a crumpled paper bag. Use a plain brown paper bag, crumpled down to about half its original size.

Correcting Perspective. With the carpenter's level and plumb bob, check one wrinkle against the other. This is the real test of what you learned in the first two drawings but made more complicated by the shapes within the bag.

Completing the Drawing. The finished drawing should contain not only the outline of the bag itself but all of the interior wrinkles as well (Figure 8).

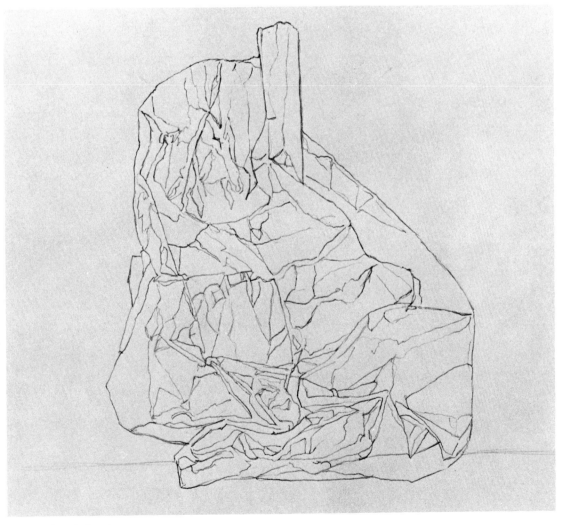

8. *Completed drawing*

Assignment 4 **Symmetrical Objects**

Choose a symmetrical object, that is, one in which both sides are identical—if it were cut down the middle, each half would be a mirror image of the other. A bottle or jar is suitable. Place the object on a table, just below your eye level.

Rough Sketch. Using the bond pad and the HB pencil, make a rough drawing of the object.

Refining the Drawing. On the rough drawing, find the center of the *top* of the object with your eye and place a pencil dot at that point. Find the center of the *bottom* of the object with your eye and place a pencil dot at that point. With the ruler, draw a line from the top dot to the bottom dot, extending the line slightly above and below the object. Correct one side of the drawing, and darken the outline. Place a piece of tracing paper over the outline of the corrected side and tape each top corner lightly to the drawing with bits of masking tape. With a very sharp 2H pencil, trace the center line that you've ruled in. Trace the corrected side of the object. Lift the tracing paper; turn it over, and place the drawn side face down on the uncorrected side of the rough sketch. The tracing of the corrected side is now on top of the uncorrected half of the drawing. When the center-line top and bottom dots are in perfect register, tape the tracing paper down again. Retrace the outline of the perfect side. It will transfer to the drawing paper. Remove the tracing paper and darken the outline (Figure 9).

Completing the Drawing. Erase the center line and all rough sketch lines.

Note. This is a mechanical method of drawing a symmetrical shape, but precision is necessary in sharp focus still life painting. The purist may claim that this is an artificial way of drawing, but I find that it's rare that the hand can be trained to draw precisely without the use of instruments. I don't like to sound dogmatic—after all, there may be the exceptional person who can draw with perfect accuracy—but the beginner will surely need mechanical aids. And, quite frankly, I still use them.

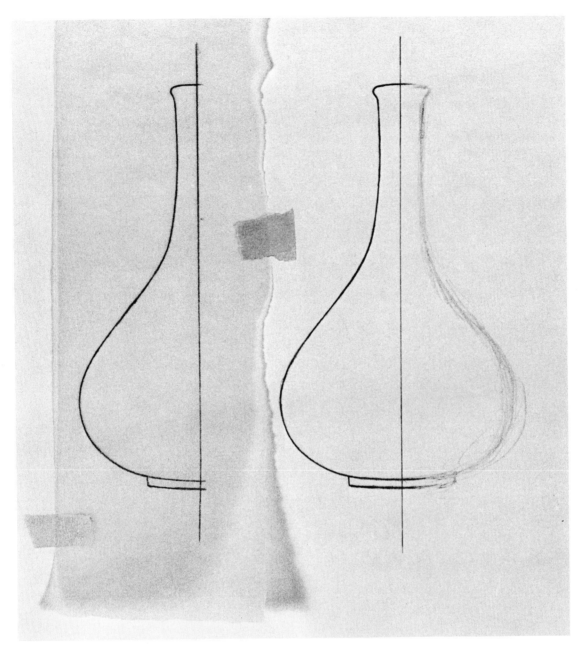

9. *Refining the rough sketch*

Assignment 5 **Ellipses**

Because ellipses are difficult to draw, this assignment is designed to give you lots of practice in drawing them. For your setup, you'll need a selection of round or cylindrical objects. You'll find that *any* circle in perspective becomes an ellipse (see A Lesson in Perspective). Place the objects on a table slightly below your eye level, tilting each of them to create ellipses at varying angles (Figure 10). Some ellipses are almost full circles while others are flattened.

Rough Sketch. Make a line drawing of the objects on the bond pad with the HB pencil.

Refining the Drawing. With the carpenter's level and plumb bob, correct and refine the drawing and erase all rough sketch lines (Figure 11). Eventually you should be able to eliminate the level and plumb bob entirely. As you develop skill through repetition of these assignments, you'll find that locating check points becomes automatic.

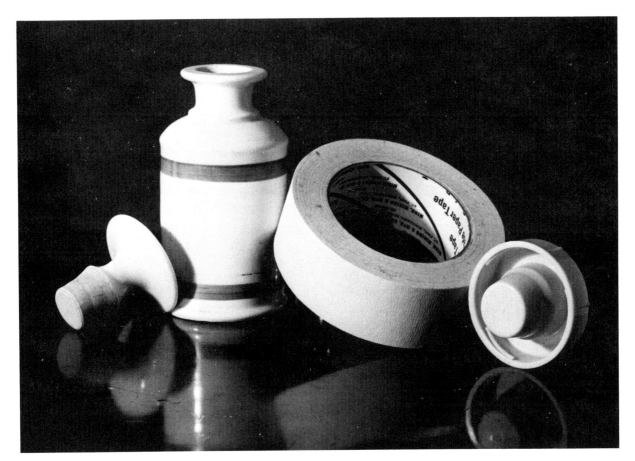

10. *Setup of ellipses*

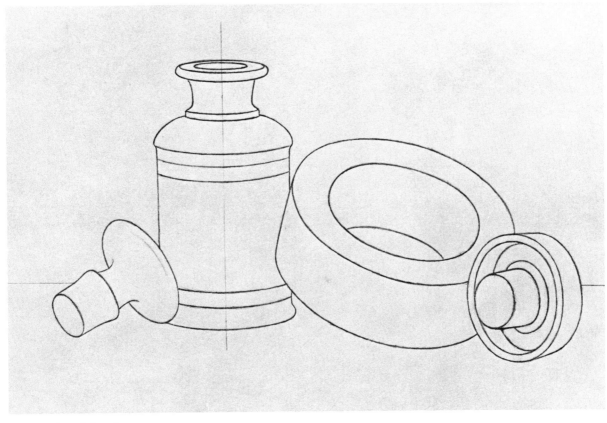

11. *Completed drawing*

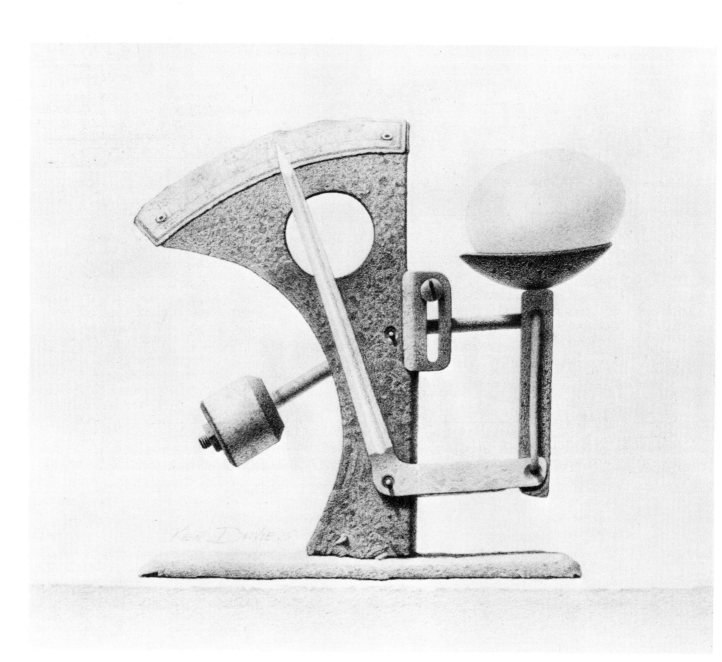

Egg Grader (study)

PROJECT 2
BLACK AND WHITE VALUE DRAWING

My students at Paier School got so tired of hearing me scream, "Darker, darker!" that they finally tacked signs up around the studio that read "Darker." After that incident, all I had to do was point mutely at the signs in order to get the idea across that they had the beginner's overwhelming tendency to make the dark areas of their drawings and paintings read too light. If you can become aware of what creates values, you won't be afraid of the darks!

WHAT IS VALUE?

Value refers to amounts of light and dark that you see. Simply speaking, a white piece of cloth is a *light value*, a black piece of cloth is a *dark value*, and a gray piece of cloth is a *middle value*. However, in addition, *the value of an object is primarily determined by its local color and the amount of light shining on it*. Local color refers to the color of an object. For example, the local color of an apple is usually red. Since this project deals with black and white value drawing and not with color, let's concentrate here only on the amount of light shining on the surface of an object.

When a light shines directly on a matte surface you'll see *dark, light,* and *middle* values depending on how much light is reaching the surface. If the object is curved, such as an egg, the values will be graduated without discernable boundaries along the curved surface. If the surface is flat and contains two or more planes, such as a block of wood or a paper box, the change in values will be sharply delineated (Figure 1).

In the study of light and shade, we can reduce the values into five basic types: (1) *direct light*, or light that hits a surface straight on to create a highlight; (2) *halftones*, or tones which are created when the surface planes turn away from the light source to receive less light; (3) *shadow*, or planes facing away from the light source which receive no direct light at all; (4) *reflected light*, or light coming from the direct source which has ricocheted off another surface into the shadow area (this light prevents shadows from being totally black); and (5) *cast shadows*, or the dark area caused when an object is placed between the light source and another surface (a good example is the darkness during a solar eclipse which is caused by the cast shadow of the moon passing between the sun and the earth).

LEARNING TO SEE VALUES

Let's return to the problem of getting darks in a drawing to read as dark as they really are. Although difficult, it's vital when *recording* values accurately that you *see* them correctly. The following hints may help you to overcome this fairly predictable problem.

Squint. Narrow your eyes and peer at your setup, then at your drawing. Setup, drawing; back and forth. Squinting makes the values appear sharper, and they are therefore easier to correct.

Cup Your Hand into a Tunnel. Peer through the tunnel at the setup, then at the drawing. Cross-check as you did while squinting.

Be Aware of the Values Surrounding an Object. The value of the object you're sketching can be deceiving depending upon the values around it. A gray square surrounded by white appears darker than a gray square surrounded by black, yet they are both the same value of gray (Figure 2). Train yourself to see these relationships.

Refer to the Value Scale. Compare the grays in your drawing and setup to the values on the *Value Scale* in the color section.

Don't Be Discouraged. The best way to overcome the problem of seeing darks and lights correctly is through experience. Keep making value drawings. Don't be discouraged by failure. Sometimes even fourth-year students find themselves wrestling with this problem.

MATERIALS AND EQUIPMENT

White charcoal paper, 19" x 25"
Gray charcoal paper, 19" x 25"
Charcoal pencils, 2B, 4B, 6B
White Conté pencil
Sandpaper block
Single-edged razor blade
Kneaded eraser
Carpenter's level
Plumb bob
Shadow box
Clip-on light with incandescent bulb
Drafting table lamp with neutral fluorescent tube
Fixative

In each of the three assignments that follow, be sure that the setup is slightly below eye level as you work. Use the clip-on light to illuminate each setup. Use the drafting table lamp to light your work surface. Pad your work surface with several sheets of paper so that the irregularities of the tabletop do not show up on your drawing.

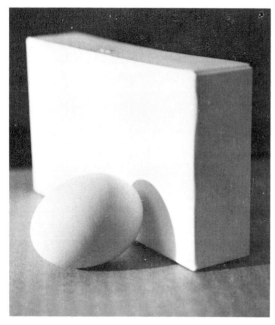

1. *Value variation on objects with different shapes*

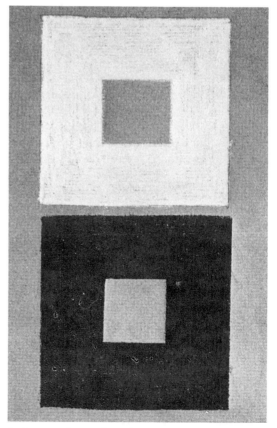

2. *Surrounding value change causing visual shift*

Assignment 1   **Ball, Cone, Cylinder, and Block**

Place the ball, cone, cylinder, and block side by side on a table. Don't let them overlap each other. Light and shadow can be controlled by changing the angle of the shade on the clip-on light (Figure 3).

Line Drawing. Use the carpenter's level and plumb bob to aid you in making a line drawing of the setup in correct perspective. However, if you've practiced the Line Drawing Assignment in Project 1, you may not feel that you need tools any longer to draw in perspective. Sketch the outlines of the objects and the shapes of the shadows. When the line drawing is complete, check it for correct perspective.

Shading Process. It will be possible for you to shade the ball, cone, cylinder, and block with confidence if you first reproduce the Shading Chart (Figure 4). Do this slowly and carefully, then proceed to shade your line drawing in the same manner.

Holding the 2B charcoal pencil lightly, move the pencil in a gentle, circular motion, in back-and-forth movements, or with a cross-hatching effect. Use the 2B pencil for producing light values, the 4B pencil for middle values, and the 6B pencil for dark values. Prevent your pencil leads from becoming stubby by sharpening them to elongated points with a razor blade. Rub the points frequently on the sandpaper block. Build up the shadows until you arrive at the correct values. The slower you build up the shadows, the smoother your rendering will be (Figure 5).

At this stage, don't use your fingers to smudge the shadows. Beginners can make a drawing look too overworked in this way. Avoid using paper stumps (see Glossary) as well. They are often fine for blending, but, improperly used, they can ruin a clean drawing. For the time being, learn to shade the hard way. That is, by using many fine pencil strokes (Figure 6).

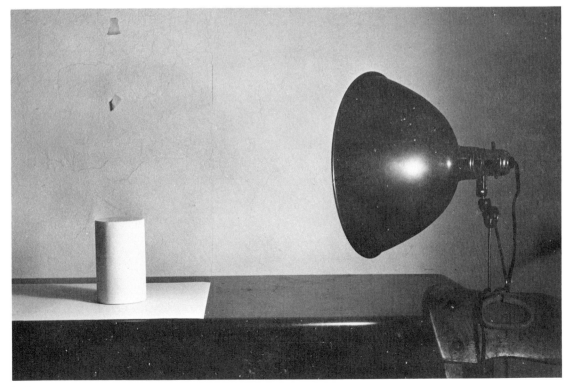

3. *Setup*

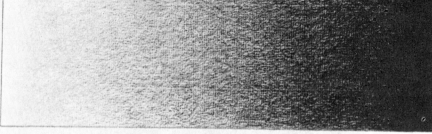

4. *Shading chart*

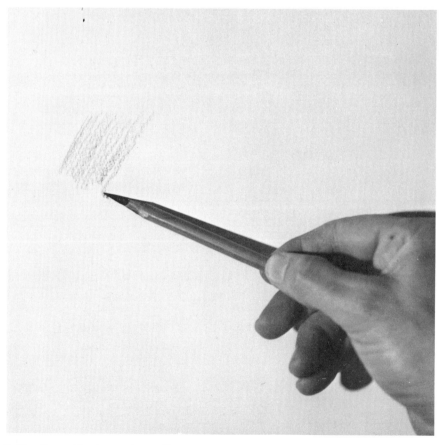

5. *Shading with charcoal pencil*

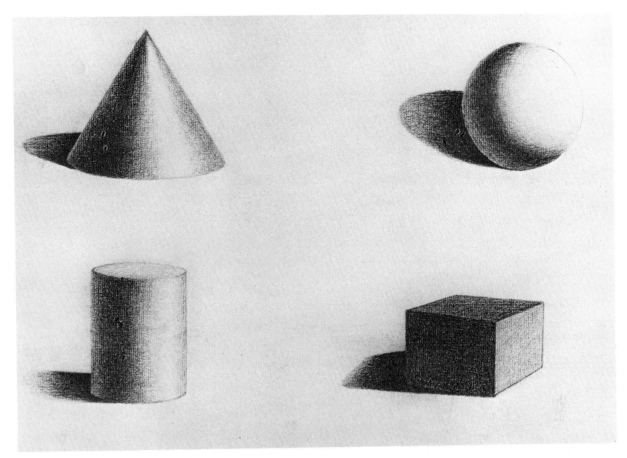

6. *Shaded forms*

Assignment 2   **Still Life on White Charcoal Paper**

In a shadow box, arrange the objects to your own taste. Light the setup with the clip-on light. The shadow box must shut out most of the light within the room. Control the light on the setup in the shadow box with the clip-on lamp to create one main source of light.

Line Drawing. Make a line drawing on a half-sheet of white charcoal paper with the 2B charcoal pencil. Correct the perspective with the carpenter's level and plumb bob, if necessary.

Shading Process. Repeat the shading procedure as in Assignment 1. As you continue to shade the drawing, remember to work from the background to the foreground objects. Keep checking the related values for correctness. Spray the completed drawing with fixative to prevent smudging (Figure 7).

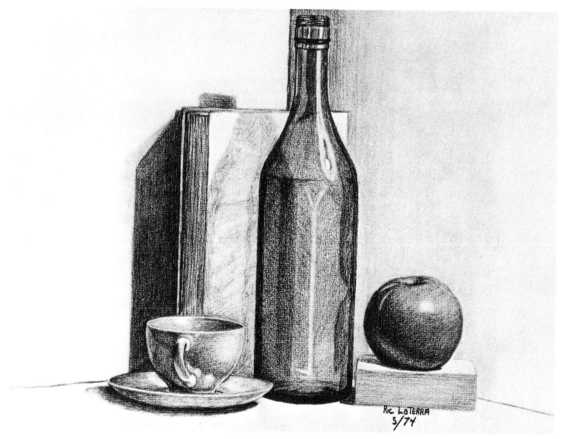

7. *Completed drawing*

Assignment 3   Still Life on Gray Charcoal Paper

Set up a still life using the same objects as in Assignment 2. Rearrange them to form a different composition in the shadow box. Light them with the clip-on light.

Line Drawing. On a half-sheet of gray charcoal paper, make a line drawing of the setup with charcoal pencils. Check for correct perspective.

Shading Process. The only notable difference between shading on white paper and shading on gray paper is that the gray paper acts as a value and the white Conté pencil is used for highlights. The gray paper is approximately a middle-gray value. Each area in the setup equal to the value of the gray paper should be left untouched. Each area in the setup that is darker than the value of the gray paper should be shaded with charcoal pencils. Any area that is lighter than the gray paper should be highlighted with white Conté pencil (Figure 8). Let me caution you not to blend the white and black pencil strokes together. If you do, you'll get a muddy or dirty tone quality that's inconsistent with the clarity of values you are trying to achieve in your drawing.

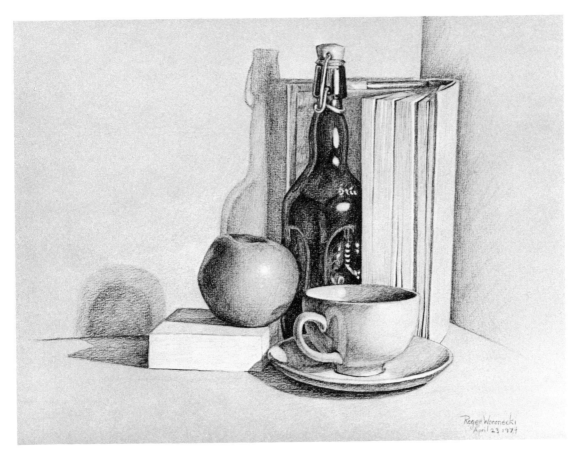

8. *Completed drawing*

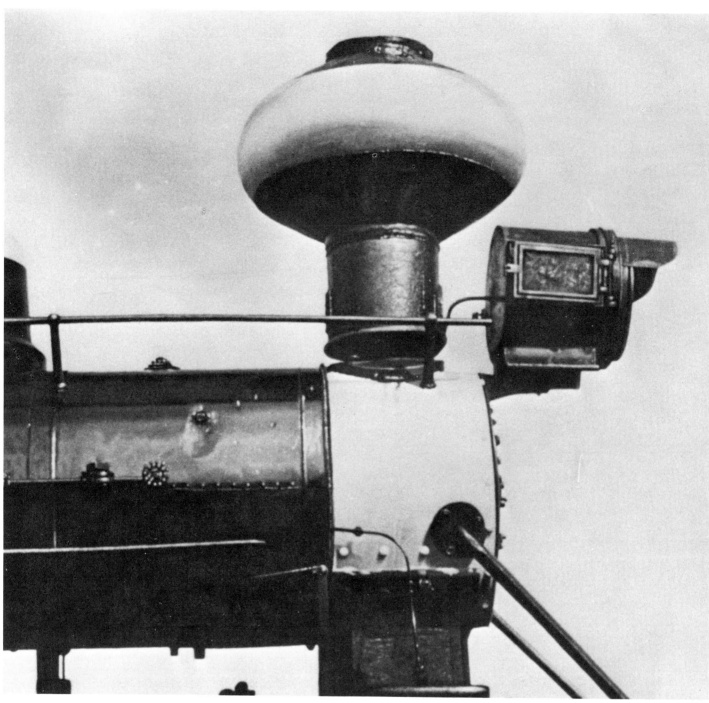

Edaville Railroad

PROJECT 3
BLACK AND WHITE VALUE PAINTING

With a good understanding of the nature of values, it's relatively easy to make the transition from charcoal pencils to oil paints. Only black and white oil colors will be used in this assignment. As you continue to increase your perception of values you'll also start to familiarize yourself with oil paints. If you've never used them before, now is the time to get used to handling them without the added complication of mixing colors.

MATERIALS AND EQUIPMENT

Drawing supplies (same as in Projects 1 and 2)
Fixative
Canvas boards (two or more), 11" x 14"
Ivory black oil paint
Titanium white oil paint
Linseed oil
Small metal cup
Turpentine
Palette knife
Palette
A mahlstick, used for painting details or whenever you want finer control of the brush
Paint rags and a large phone book for cleaning brushes
Use the same five objects as in Assignment 1 of Project 2: a ball, cone, cylinder, block, and box. Arrange them in the shadow box. Light the setup with the clip-on light.

Time limit: four hours for each painting.

Line Drawing. Make a line drawing on an 11" x 14" canvas board with the 2B charcoal pencil. Draw the outlines of each object and the shapes of the shadows (Figure 1).

Correcting Perspective. Correct the perspective of your drawing, using the carpenter's level and plumb bob.

Fixing the Drawing. Spray the finished drawing with fixative to set the charcoal lines and prevent smudging.

Preparing the Paints. On your palette, squeeze out some black paint about the size of a quarter. Squeeze out an equal quantity of white paint. Pour a small amount of linseed oil into a metal cup. When mixing oil paints, you usually add a medium to make the paint spreadable yet not so thin that it is transparent. I suggest you use linseed oil for the time being; however, there are many other types of artist's mediums in the stores and the painter should eventually experiment with all of them.

Mixing the Paints. View the setup and estimate the values. Then mix the black and white paints on your palette in varying proportions until you've obtained the right gray for each corresponding value in the setup.

Direct Painting. Always start by painting the background, then move into the foreground. This procedure makes it easier to determine the value of a foreground object as it's seen against its actual background. Keep mixing and applying the grays to the proper areas. Choose a brush suitable to the size of the area in which you're working; for example, a broad area should not be covered with a very small brush (Figure 2).

Blending. When one value merges with another you'll need to blend the area. To do this, determine each and every square inch of value in the area. Then mix each of the corresponding grays, and apply them correcting the values as you go (Figure 3).

If the values on an object change gradually, special brush techniques can be used for blending. Use a dabbing and/or stroking motion with your brush along the edge to be blended. If the values are sharply defined, the edges should be left hard and unblended. Don't be too concerned with perfect blending at this point. You'll find that it will become easier as you discover your own methods through experience. Right now consider it more important to achieve the accurate values in each area (Figure 4).

Painting Practice. On an 11" x 14" canvas board, make another black and white oil painting using more complicated objects in your setup—jugs, bottles, cups, books. This will further test your skill in determining values and using oil paints. Don't stop with just two black and white oil paintings; keep on arranging new setups with even more complicated objects.

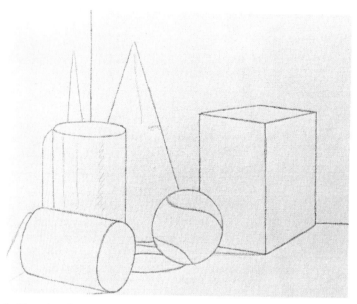

1. *Line drawing*

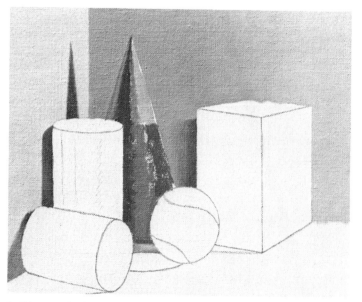

2. *Direct painting*

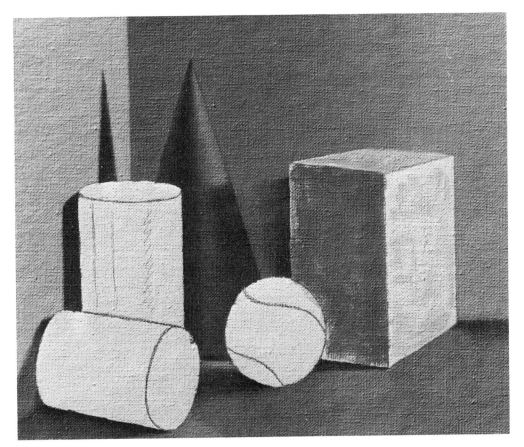

3. *Blending*

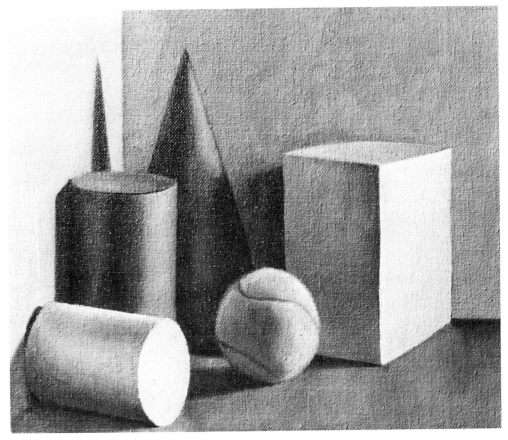

4. *Completed painting*

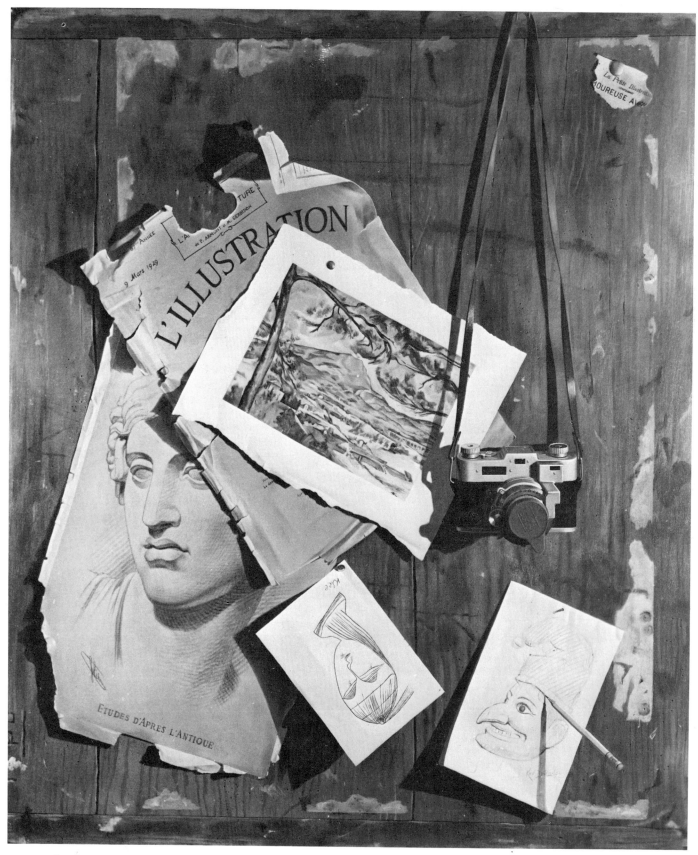

Academic Procession

COLOR PLATES FOR THE EXERCISES

The final steps of the exercises presented in *Part Two: Exercises* (pages 67–128) are reproduced on the pages that follow.

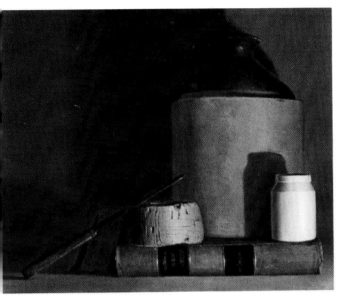

Exercise 1 *Color Still Life*

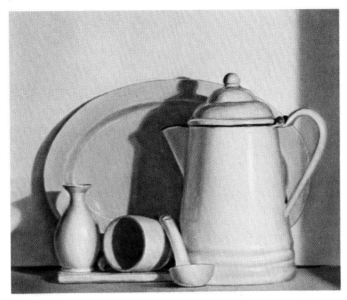

Exercise 2 *All-White Painting*

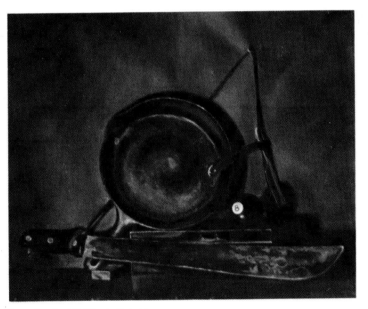

Exercise 3 *All-Black Painting*

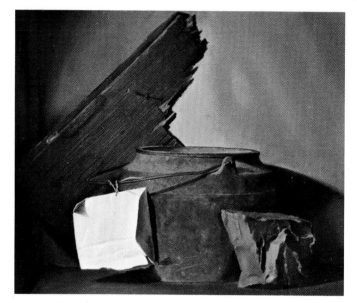

Exercise 4 *Rough Textures*

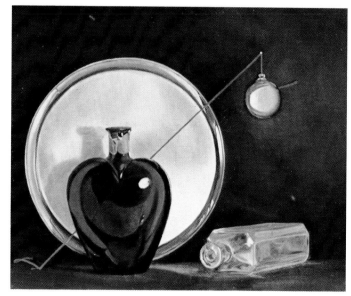

Exercise 5 *Smooth Textures*

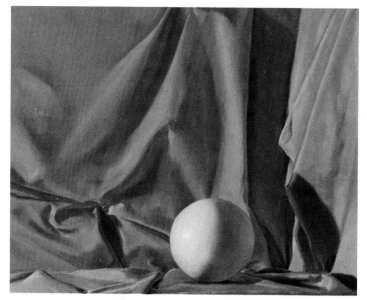

Exercise 6 *Reflected Light*

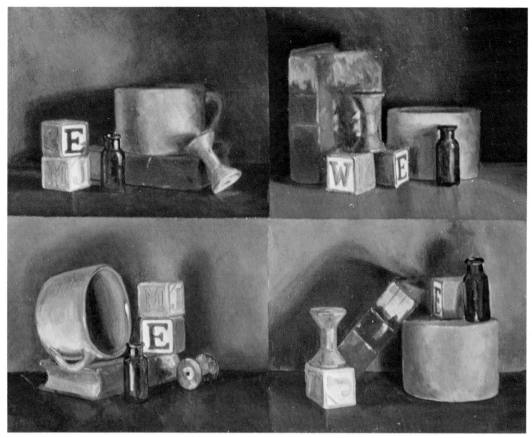

Exercise 7 *Speed Painting*

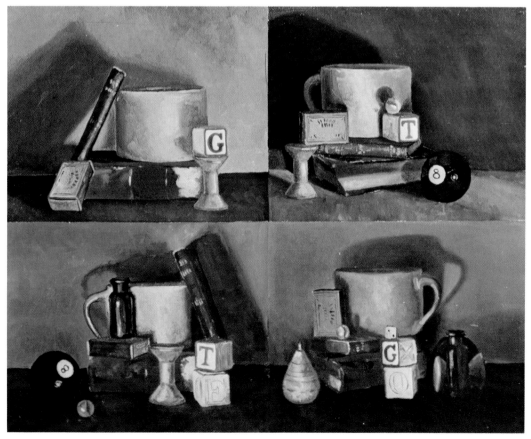

Exercise 8 *Speed Painting*

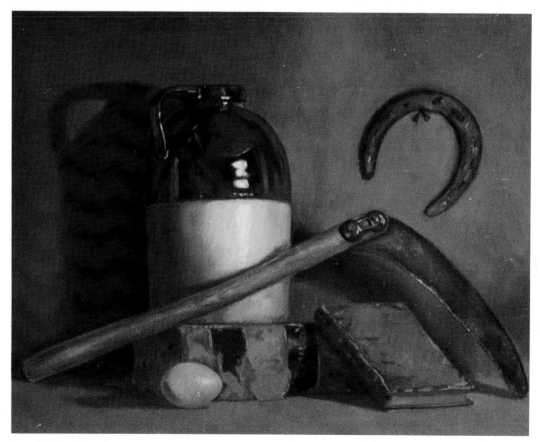

Exercise 9 *Monochrome Wet-into-Wet*

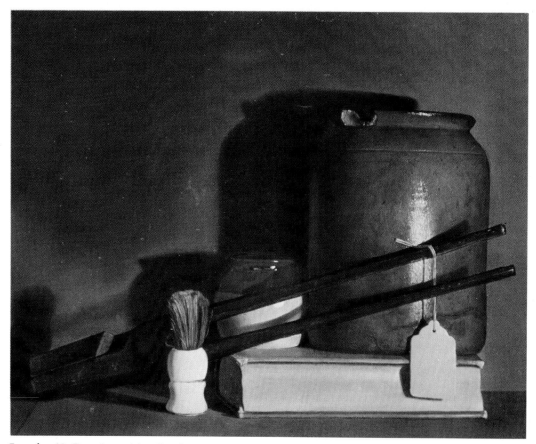

Exercise 10 *Drawing with a Brush*

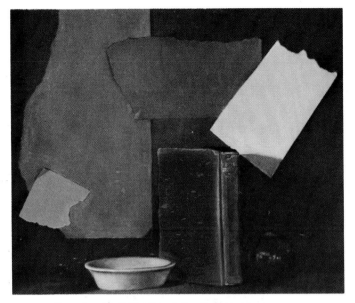

Exercise 11 *Still Life under Red Light*

Exercise 12 *Still Life under Green Light*

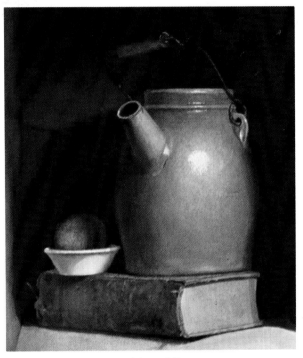

Exercise 13 *Glazing and Scumbling*

COLOR PLATES FOR THE DEMONSTRATIONS

The wash-in and block-in stages of the demonstrations presented in *Part Three: Demonstrations* (pages 145–186) are reproduced on the pages that follow.

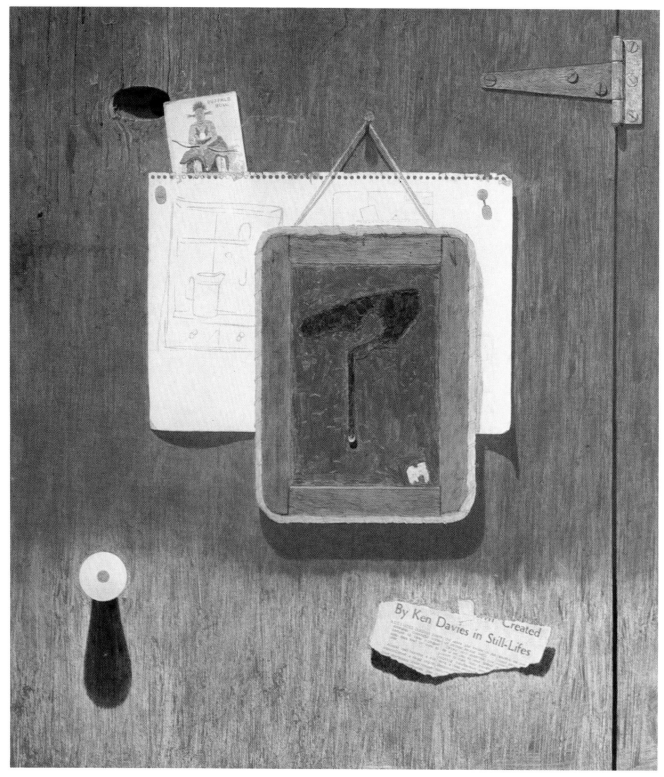

Demonstration 1 *From the Sketchbook. Wash-in*

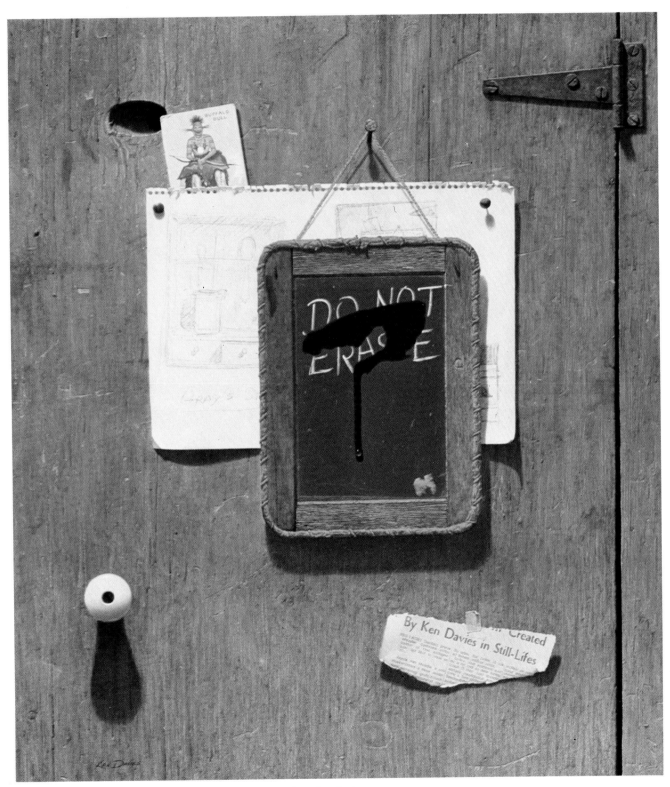

Demonstration 1 *From the Sketchbook. Completed painting*

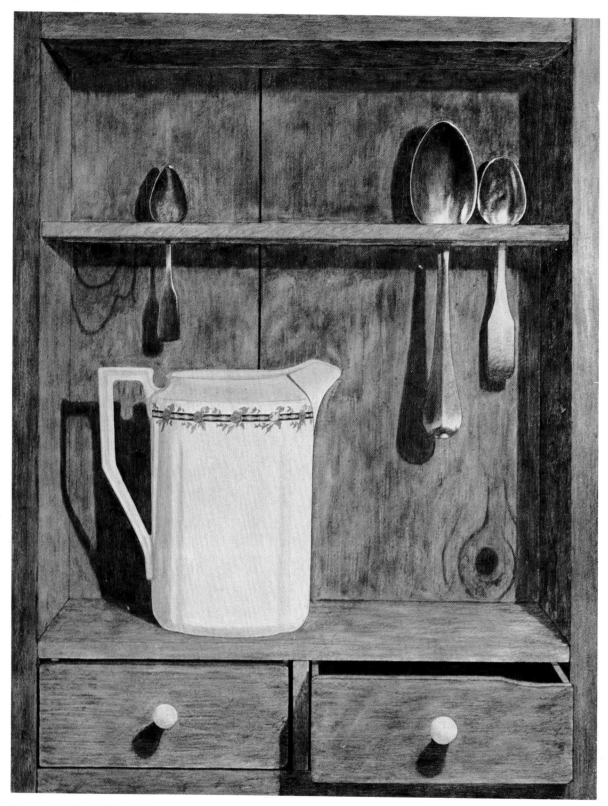

Demonstration 2 *Gray's Spoons. Wash-in*

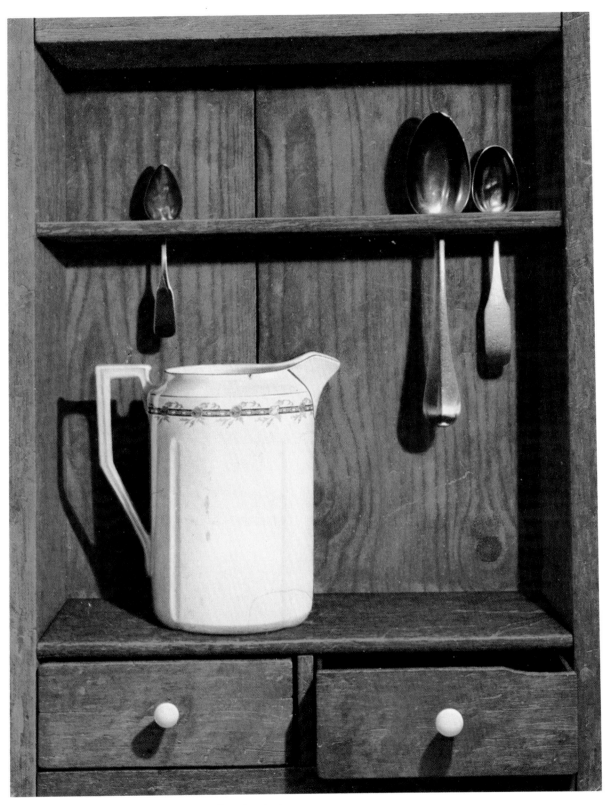

Demonstration 2 *Gray's Spoons. Completed painting*

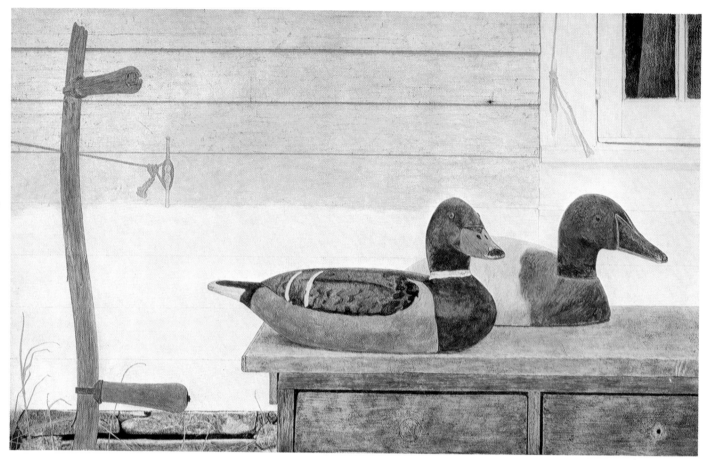

Demonstration 3 *A Gisler Mallard. Wash-in*

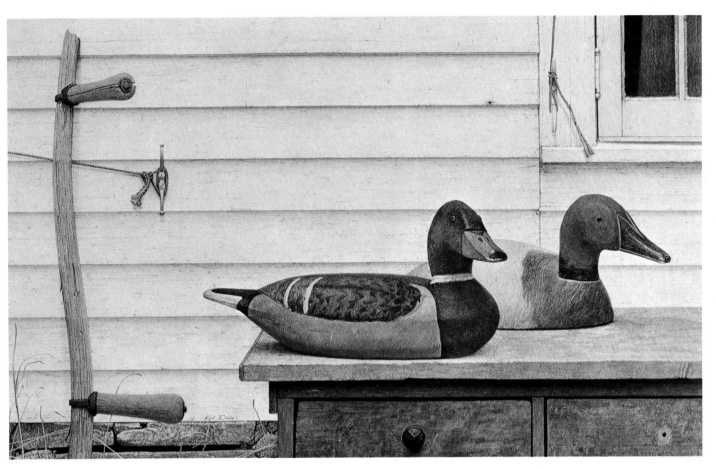

Demonstration 3 *A Gisler Mallard. Completed painting*

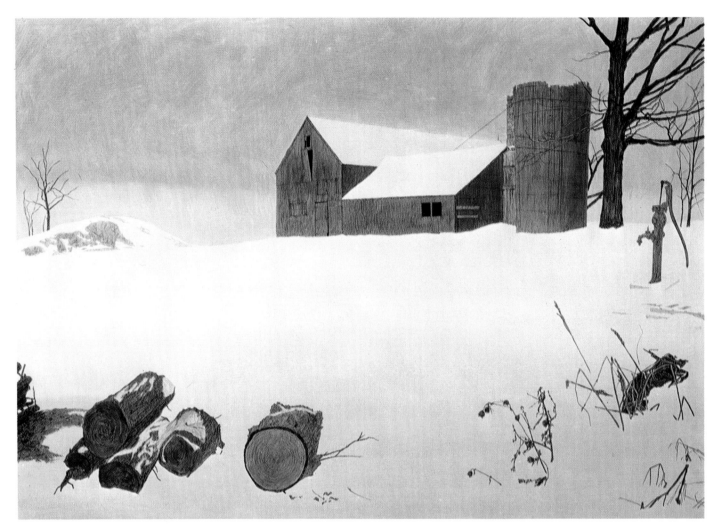

Demonstration 4 *On 139 Near 80. Wash-in*

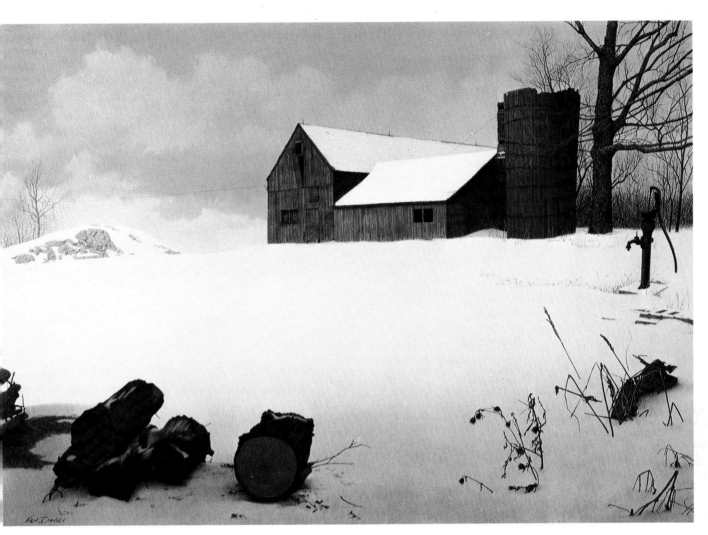

Demonstration 4 *On 139 Near 80. Completed painting*

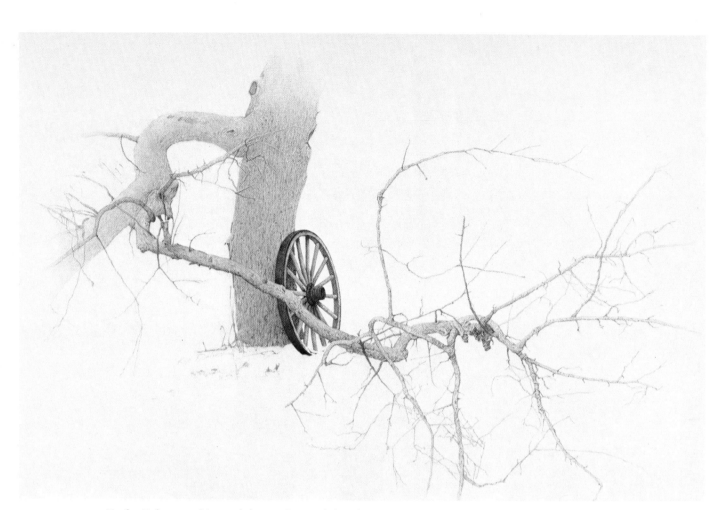

By the Driveway. *Many of the studies and sketches such as this one are a marvelous change-of-pace from the time-consuming finished paintings on Masonite panel. I paint them on double-weight illustration board using a 95% transparent oil wash (mixed with linseed oil and damar varnish) with a bare minimum of opaque color, generally only in the highlight areas. These paintings are often mistaken for watercolors.*

Assignment 1   **Value Scale**

Painting this chart will give the beginning oil painter the experience of mixing and then matching each of the six basic colors on the color wheel at each value on the Value Scale reproduced on page 49.

MATERIALS AND EQUIPMENT

Two canvas boards, 16″ x 20″
Palette spread with full range of colors (see list in the chapter on Materials and Equipment)
Painting supplies
50 different colored paint chip samples from the paint store
Brushes
Pencil
Ruler

Preparing the Grid. Using a pencil and ruler, divide the canvas board into seven vertical columns and nine horizontal columns.

Painting the Grays. The first vertical column on the left is the black and white Value Scale, which ranges in nine steps from just off-white to just off-black. The exact middle of the Value Scale can be found in the fifth rectangle from the top. To reproduce this column, mix the grays by using ivory black and titanium white. Match all the grays and paint them in their corresponding rectangles.

Painting the Colors. Paint the remaining columns in reds, yellows, oranges, greens, blues, and violets to reproduce each of the six basic colors of the color wheel at each of the nine values found in the first column of the Value Scale.

When you've finished, squint at the values across any given line from left to right. You should find that the colors change while the values remain the same.

Assignment 2   **Matching Chart**

Examine the Matching Chart reproduced on page 50. The mounted color chips, which were obtained from a paint store, are initialed in ink. Just above each color chip is a rectangle in which the color of the chip was exactly matched and painted in oil colors.

How to Mix Black. In the Value Scale we've used ivory black primarily to darken the cooler colors. From this point on, eliminate ivory black from your palette. Why? Because very often the warm colors become muddy when darkened with ivory black. This is especially true for inexperienced oil painters.

It's possible to produce your own black by mixing *burnt umber* and *ultramarine blue*, and the resulting black is almost identical to the ivory black from the tube.

Mixing Grays. Handsome grays can be mixed quite successfully from various combinations of colors without using ivory black. Experiment with these on your palette:
(1) different combinations of *blues* and *browns* plus *white*;
(2) different combinations of *violets* and *yellows* plus *white*;
(3) different combinations of *reds* and *greens* plus *white*.
(Notice that what I'm saying is that complementary colors neutralize each other.)

You can get infinite variety and subtlety in gray tones by mixing them with colors rather than just black and white. This brings us to the small outcast rectangle on the left of the Value Scale. When mixing that gray use *no black paint*. That gray should be identical to the fifth rectangle in the first vertical column of the Value Scale. That small rectangle is final proof that you need never use black paint to mix gray.

Preparing the Grid. On the canvas board, measure ten vertical and ten horizontal rows as shown on the Matching Chart. In every other vertical row paste the color chips.

Mixing and Painting the Colors. Using the colors on your palette, mix the color of each paint chip and apply it to the space adjacent to it. Refer to the mixing instructions presented earlier in this project when necessary.

Painting Hints. Remember that complements neutralize each other; white paint cools, lightens, and grays a color. Matching the color chips correctly will mean much trial and error; some of the color chips will be much simpler to match than others. For example, those with tones closest to the tube colors will be easier to achieve. The more subtle tones will require more complicated mixing. Don't waste time struggling with a particular color if you can't get it to match the color chip. Give it your best try, then leave it alone. Go on to the next color and return to the problem color later. It's best to mix the easy colors first and to build your skill and ability gradually.

When you have finally surmounted the frustrations of completing the Matching Chart, you should be quite expert at matching almost any color you can see.

PART TWO **EXERCISES**

It isn't my intention that you paint completed works during these exercises. I hope instead that, like practicing the scales on the piano, you practice the development of hand-eye coordination toward the time you'll be producing a serious, finished painting.

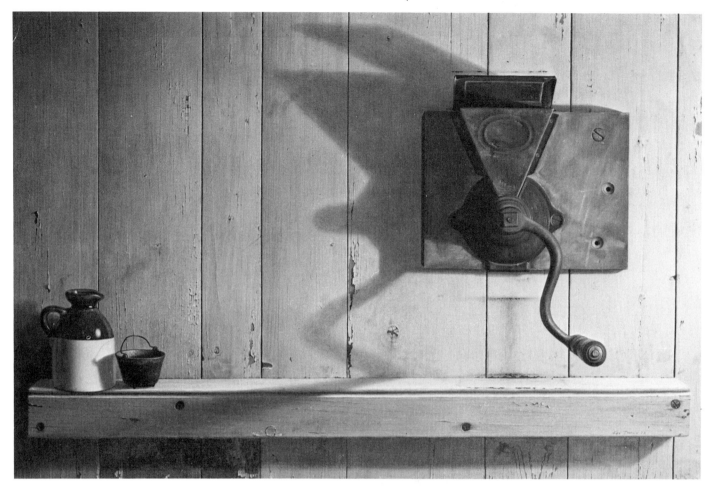

Antiques

EXERCISE 1 COLOR STILL LIFE

If you've accomplished the projects in the first part of this book, you already have a basis to paint a still life in oil colors. Skills that are faithfully developed are an important foundation of good painting, and if you're ready to develop your skills even further—to combine your knowledge of values with the use of colors—this is the moment you've been working for.

MATERIALS AND EQUIPMENT (Assignments 1 and 2)

Drawing supplies
Palette spread with full range of colors
Brushes
Canvas board, 16" x 20"
Turpentine
Linseed oil
Shadow box (made from a large cardboard box)
Extra piece of cardboard to overhang top of shadow box and block out studio lighting
Clip-on light with incandescent bulb
Construction paper of any color
Masking tape
Retouch varnish
Varnishing brush, 2"
Choose any six objects, each a different color. Line the shadow box with colored construction paper. Light the setup with the clip-on light (Figure 1). Notice that the clip-on light is placed at an angle that maximizes the forms of the objects.

Time limit: eight hours.

Line Drawing. Using the drafting pencil on the canvas board, make a line drawing including the outline form of the objects and the cast shadows (Figure 2). Spray the drawing with fixative to prevent smudging.

Wash-in. Thin the paint with a mixture of ⅔ linseed oil and ⅓ turpentine. Wash the value and color of the background and each object into the foreground (Figure 3). The paint should be transparent, allowing the lines of the drawing to show through. Cover the canvas with paint as quickly as possible in order to get a rough impression of the finished painting. The immediacy of the wash-in is a good icebreaker between you and the empty, white canvas.

Drying Period. Allow the painting to dry at least overnight. Reds and yellows may take longer to dry than some of the blues and greens. Be patient; wait until the surface is thoroughly dry before you continue.

Block-in. Starting with the background and working forward, block in each area by mixing the value and color of each object, its shadows and light areas (Figure 4). Use opaque paint. If you must thin it, use only linseed oil in very sparing amounts. The paint must be workable yet not transparent.

Blending. Blend the edges that need softening by dabbing or stroking them with a filbert sable brush. Any brush or implement that will do the job is fine—you can even use your finger. Keep the hard edges very sharp, just as you see them in your setup.

Drying Period. Allow the painting to dry thoroughly before proceeding with the next step.

Details and Highlights. On the dry painting add the final details and highlights.

Varnish. Again allow the painting to dry thoroughly. Clean all lint from the surface with masking tape. With a 2″ varnishing brush, coat the finished painting with retouch varnish to bring out color in dead or sunk-in (matte) areas. A final varnish coat can be brushed on later if you think the painting is good enough to exhibit. (This step will be discussed more fully in the demonstrations in Part Three.)

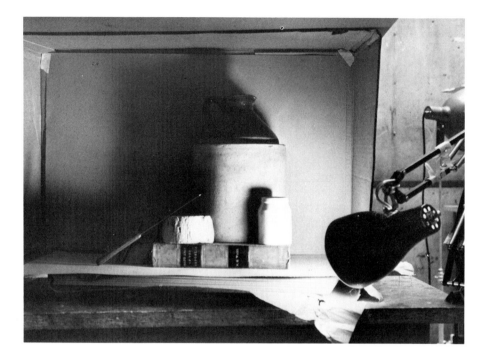

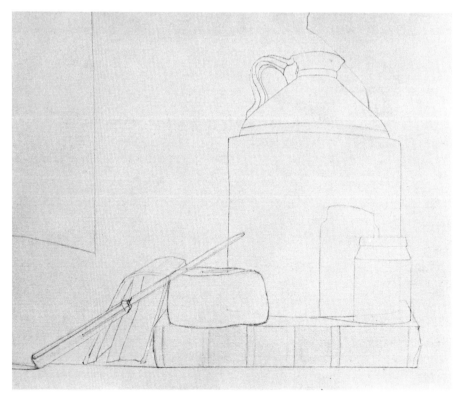

2. *Line drawing*

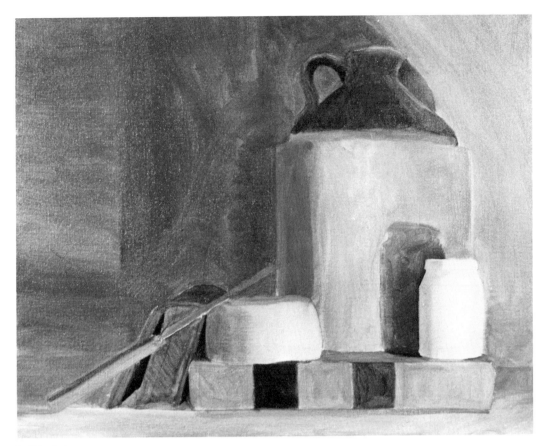

3. *Wash-in*

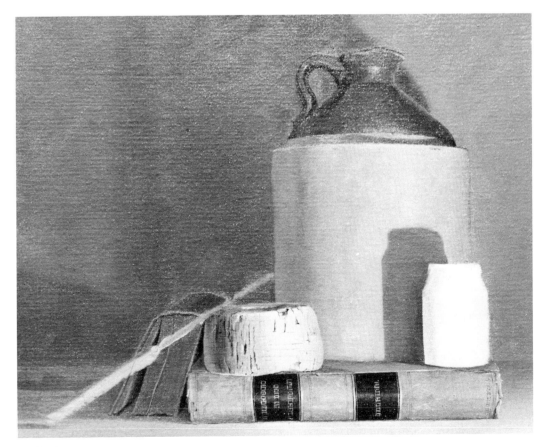

4. *Block-in*

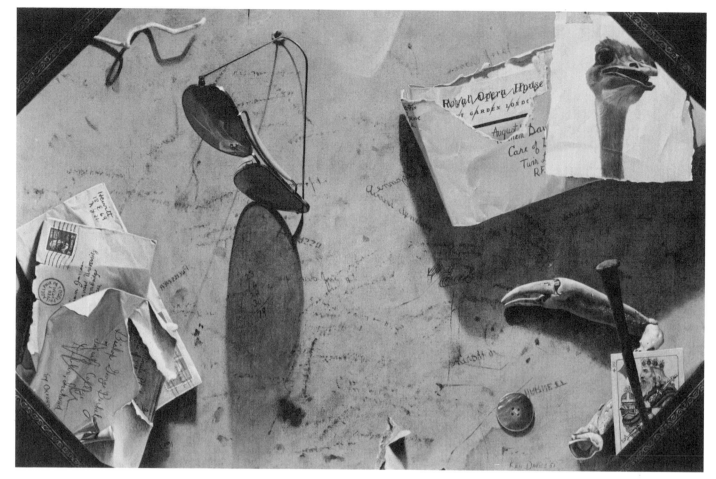

The Blotter

EXERCISE 2   ALL-WHITE PAINTING

All-white objects against a white background present a surprising variety of values and tones. If you look at a group of white objects, you'll see that each is a slightly different color. As you study and illustrate white objects and surfaces you'll find that you use no white paint straight from the tube. Even the brightest highlights, which may seem a very pure white, will have a slight trace of yellow from the incandescent bulb of the clip-on light.

Pay special attention to the values of the shadows cast by the white objects, as there is a tendency to paint them too light. After you've carefully determined the *values* of the shadows, study their *colors*. Many of the values and colors will present problems; their variations may be extremely subtle and hard to differentiate. Approach values and colors boldly!

MATERIALS AND EQUIPMENT

Drawing supplies
Palette with full range of colors
Brushes
Canvas board, 16" x 20"
Turpentine
Linseed oil
Shadow box with extra flap to block out room lighting
Clip-on light with incandescent bulb
White construction paper
Retouch varnish
Varnishing brush, 2"

Line the shadow box with heavy white paper. Place in it any six white objects. Arrange them in a still life and light them with the clip-on light (Figure 1).

Time limit: eight hours.

Line Drawing. On the canvas board, make a line drawing of the setup. Spray it with fixative to prevent smudging.

Wash-in. Wash in the background and the local color of each white object. Mix the grays in various combinations of complementary colors, using no black. Notice that the incandescent light bulb casts a warm, slightly yellow light on the subject (Figure 2). Allow the painting to dry thoroughly.

Block-in. Carefully determine the values and colors of the shadows and highlights; with more opaque paint, block in the background and then the foreground objects (Figure 3). Notice that the values of the shadows are very dark even though all the objects are white. Blend the edges and allow the painting to dry.

Highlights. Using no white paint straight from the tube, paint the highlights. Allow the painting to dry thoroughly. Apply retouch varnish to the dry surface.

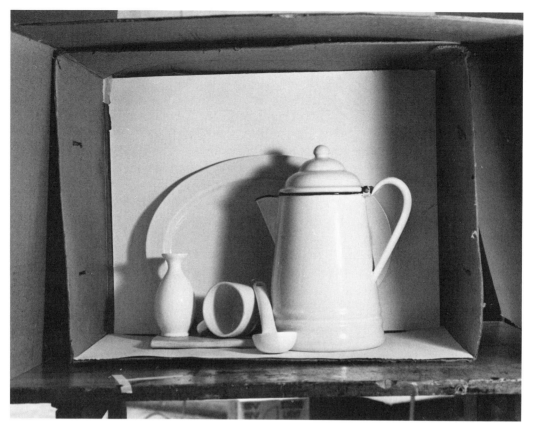

1. *Setup in shadow box*

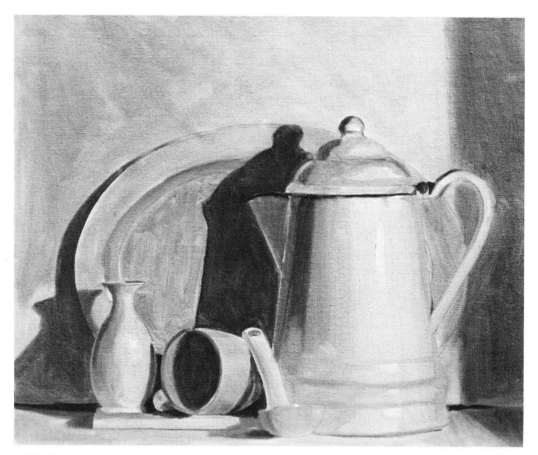

2. *Wash-in*

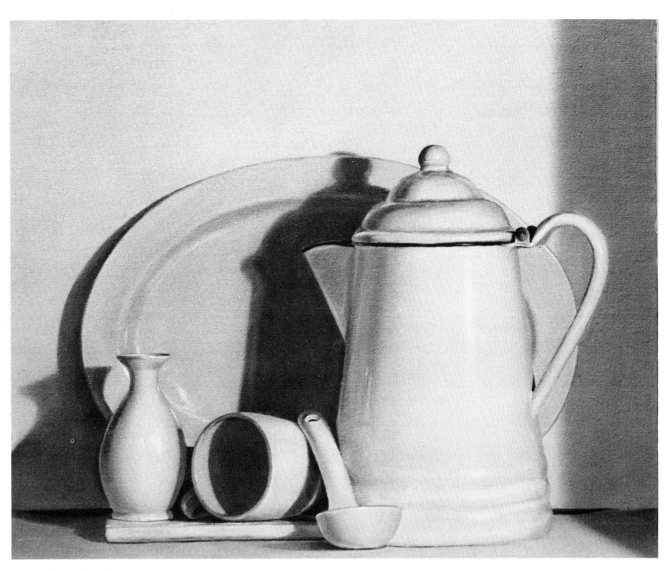

3. *Completed painting*

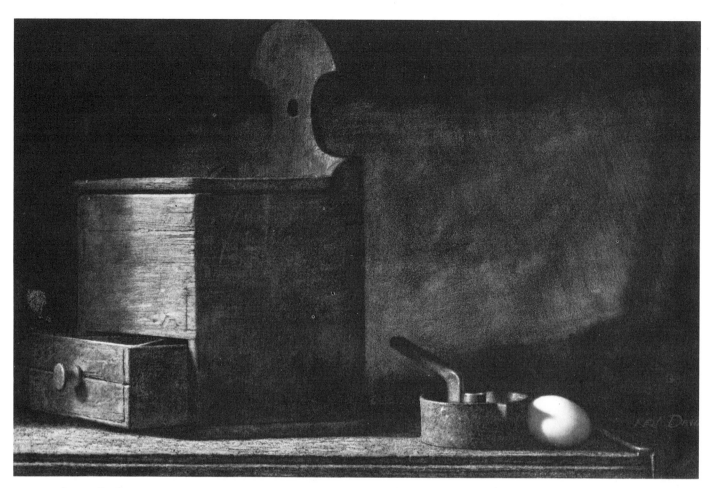

Pantry Shelf

EXERCISE 3 ALL-BLACK PAINTING

Black is pure only in the total absence of light. Unless you're in a completely unlighted space such as a photographic darkroom, from the moment black paint is squeezed from the tube it's no longer black. When light of any type or intensity reaches black, technically it becomes gray. Bearing this in mind, study the value and color of black by painting six black objects under an incandescent light with a minimum of black paint.

I suggest that you reduce your use of black paint for two reasons: (1) it's slow-drying; (2) it tends to produce a dirty mixture that looks as though you mixed coal dust with the paint. In place of ivory black, use a mixture of burnt umber and ultramarine blue; it's faster-drying and richer in tone. My tube of black paint was purchased 20 years ago, and there's still plenty left. The only time I use black from the tube is to paint the very darkest of darks, such as a small hole in a piece of wood or an extremely dark shadow cast on a black object.

This is a challenging experiment that will enhance your understanding of the variations in blacks.

MATERIALS AND EQUIPMENT

Drawing supplies
Palette with full range of colors
Brushes
Canvas board, 16" x 20"
Turpentine
Linseed oil
Shadow box
Clip-on light with incandescent bulb
Black construction paper
Retouch varnish
Varnishing brush, 2"

Line the shadow box with black construction paper. Place in it any six black objects. Arrange them in a still life and light them with the clip-on light (Figure 1). Although not completely black, the eight ball is used because its shiny surface reflects the other parts of the setup. You can experiment by moving the clip-on light around to find the most descriptive combination of lights and shadows in the setup before starting to work.

Time limit: eight hours.

PAINTING HINTS

When painting the setup, pay strict attention to the light areas; there's a tendency to paint them too dark. (The opposite is true with an all-white setup; dark areas are usually painted too light.)

The warm incandescant light cast on the black objects will give them a warm tint. If you choose to add yellow ochre or any other yellow or ivory tone to the black paint, a greenish mixture will result. To neutralize the greenish mixture, add cadmium red light. This is a very practical application of your knowledge of the color wheel; *green* plus its complement, *red*, is grayed or neutralized.

When dark colors dry, they have a tendency to become matte or dull. This can totally change the value of a color. To remedy this, spray or paint retouch varnish on any area that has gone "dead." The retouch varnish will revive the color to its original value. This is an important step to repeat, since you'll need to keep relating one value to another during the painting procedure. One incorrect area left undetected can set you on the wrong course. Pay careful attention to any area that is drying; add retouch varnish to bring the values up. You can continue to paint directly over the retouch varnish, which dries very quickly.

Line Drawing. On the canvas board, make a line drawing of the setup (Figure 2). Spray it with fixative.

Wash-in. Wash in the background and objects (Figure 3). Continue to use a mixture of paint thinned with ⅔ linseed oil and ⅓ turpentine. Allow the painting to dry thoroughly.

Block-in. With opaque paint, thinned only with linseed oil, block in every value and color (Figure 4). Blend the edges and allow the painting to dry.

Highlights. Add the details and highlights, then allow to dry. Apply retouch varnish to the clean, dry surface.

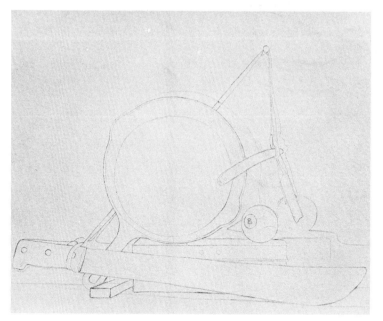

1. *Setup*

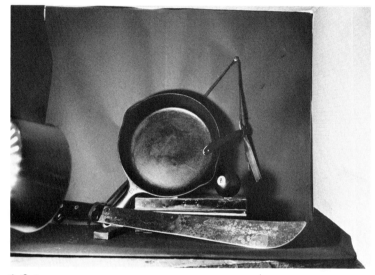

2. *Line drawing*

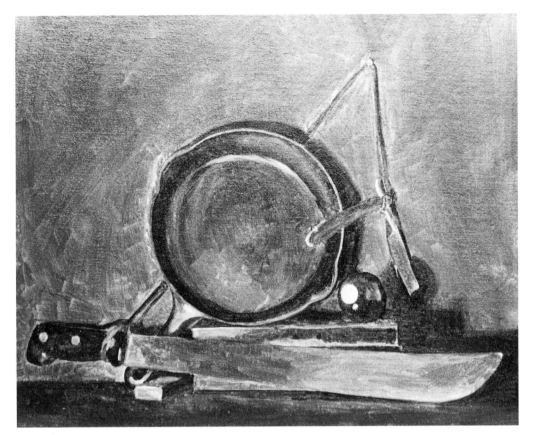

3. *Wash-in*

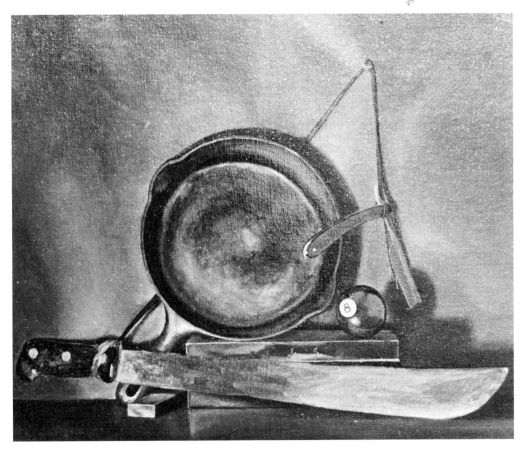

4. *Block-in*

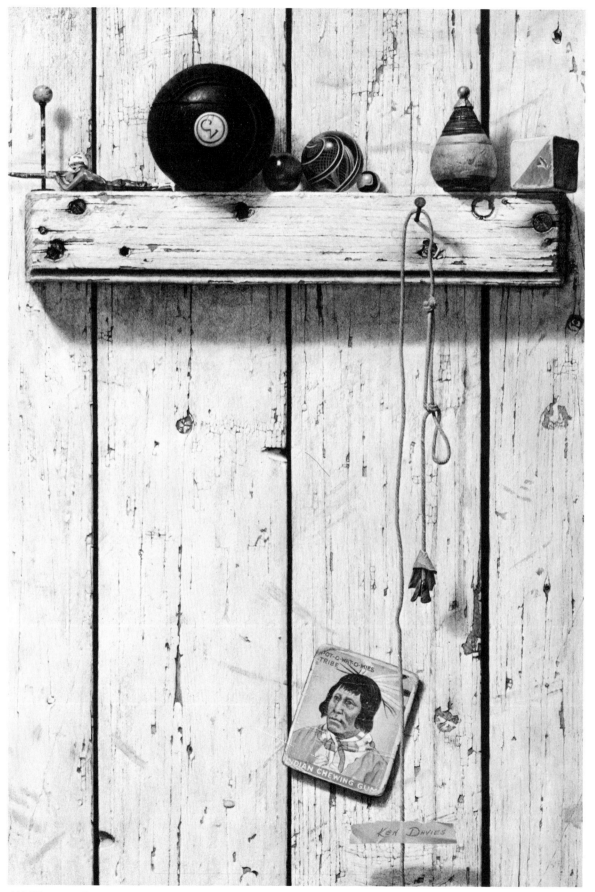

116 Chestnut Street

EXERCISE 4 **ROUGH TEXTURES**

Observing and learning to paint the many different textures that exist in natural and man-made objects can present a problem. How can we paint them as they truly are? It would be impossible to answer that question if we tried to cover *all* the textures that exist, so let's concentrate on only four: wood, iron, paper, and stone. They are the textures I paint most often in still life.

As you might imagine, wood, iron, paper, and stone categorically offer textures within texture. For example, wood can be either highly polished or rough and unfinished. The grain on some wood surfaces is so defined that it is actually three-dimensional. The surface of cast iron, similarly, can be either smooth or pitted and rusty.

Each of these four textures presents its own painting problem. After tackling them, it would be helpful for you to experiment with as many other textures as you can find. Leather, rough fabrics such as burlap or natural linen, or surfaces found in foliage may be interesting to you.

TEXTURES IN LIGHT AND SHADOW

When painting textured objects, you're actually painting a still life within a still life. Pinpoint an area of a rough-textured object and you can see that it's a tiny landscape of hills and valleys which are either maximized or minimized by the light cast on its surface.

An oblique angle of light cast on the object will give a pronounced texture, whereas a direct angle of light will minimize it.

In lighted areas, texture is more emphasized; in shadow areas, it is less pronounced.

Texture is most dramatically apparent in halftone areas where light glances off the object at an oblique angle.

TEXTURES IN REFLECTED LIGHT

Little or no texture is perceived in reflected light. You can observe this in nature, for example, in the light cast by the moon. Moonlight, you may recall, is reflected light. In moonlight there is little definition of the earth's texture. The same is true of the reflected light in your still life setup. Find the areas of reflected light and observe how little texture is apparent. Now compare the textures in the reflected light areas to those in the direct light areas. Notice that texture is minimized under reflected light and maximized under direct light.

Critical virtues for achieving realistic results in sharp focus still life painting are patience and fidelity. Careless, hurried work almost invariably results in sloppy, amateurish paintings. Close attention to each textured area and faithful rendering separate the professional from the amateur.

MATERIALS AND EQUIPMENT

Drawing supplies
Palette with full range of colors
Brushes
Canvas board, 16″ x 20″
Turpentine
Linseed oil
Shadow box
Clip-on light with incandescent bulb
Retouch varnish
Varnishing brush, 2″

Set up a still life arrangement, using wood, iron, paper, and stone objects. Attempt to find rough-grained wood and pitted iron. The shadow box can be either lined or unlined. Experiment with the angle of the light on the setup in order to heighten textures. You can bring out the textures of the objects by placing the clip-on light at an oblique angle to create deep shadows (Figure 1). The nail that secures the piece of wood to the back wall of the shadow box will be painted as part of the still life. The upper left corner of the piece of paper has been bent forward to create an interesting shadow; the right side of the paper is folded forward to create a large shadow area on the side of the cast-iron pot. The rock is carefully arranged so its lighted side shows up against the shadow side of the pot.

Time limit: eight hours

Line Drawing. On the canvas board, make a line drawing of the setup (Figure 2). Spray with fixative.

Wash-in. Wash in the background and local color of each object (Figure 3). At this stage none of the textures has yet been suggested. Allow to dry thoroughly.

Block-in. Block in the values and colors of the background and objects. Now you can begin to suggest the textures of the objects. Start to paint the wood grain and the stone by working directly into the wet paint with a small sable brush. Suggest the pitted areas of the cast-iron object by stippling or dabbing at the wet surface with a round bristle brush. If there are wrinkles or folds in the paper object, paint in only the major areas. Don't attempt to render complete details while the painting is wet. Complete all the major textural shapes in this block-in stage and leave the details and highlights for later. Allow the painting to dry thoroughly.

Completing the Painting. Use a small sable brush to carefully paint the details. Each line of the wood grain must be painted individually and literally. The same is true for the stone and iron objects. The success of the reality you achieve will be in direct proportion to the amount of time devoted to painting these textural details (Figure 4). After allowing the painting to dry thoroughly, apply retouch varnish.

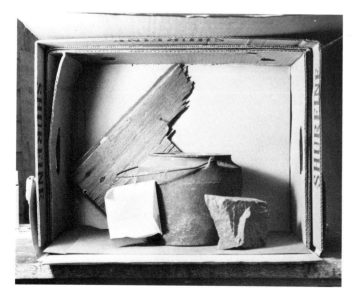

1. *Setup*

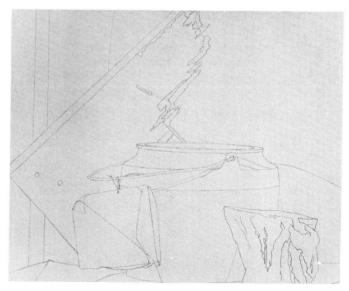

2. *Line drawing*

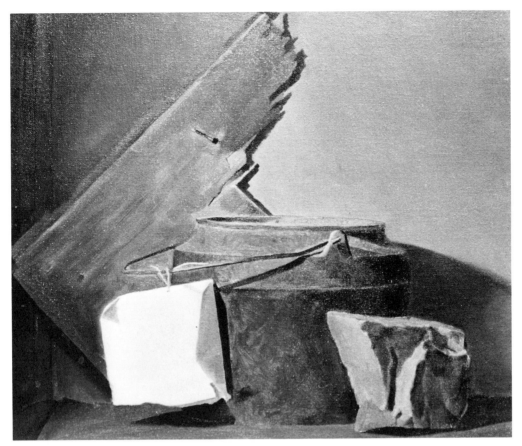

3. *Wash-in*

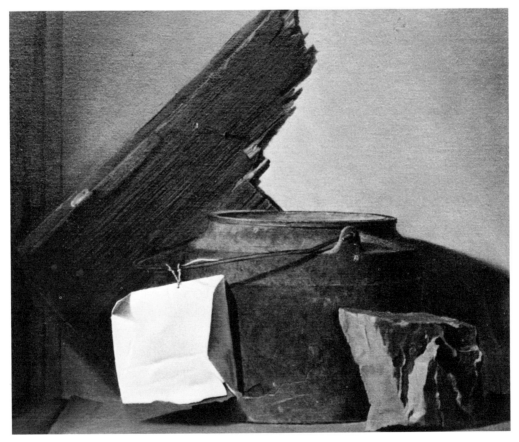

4. *Completed painting*

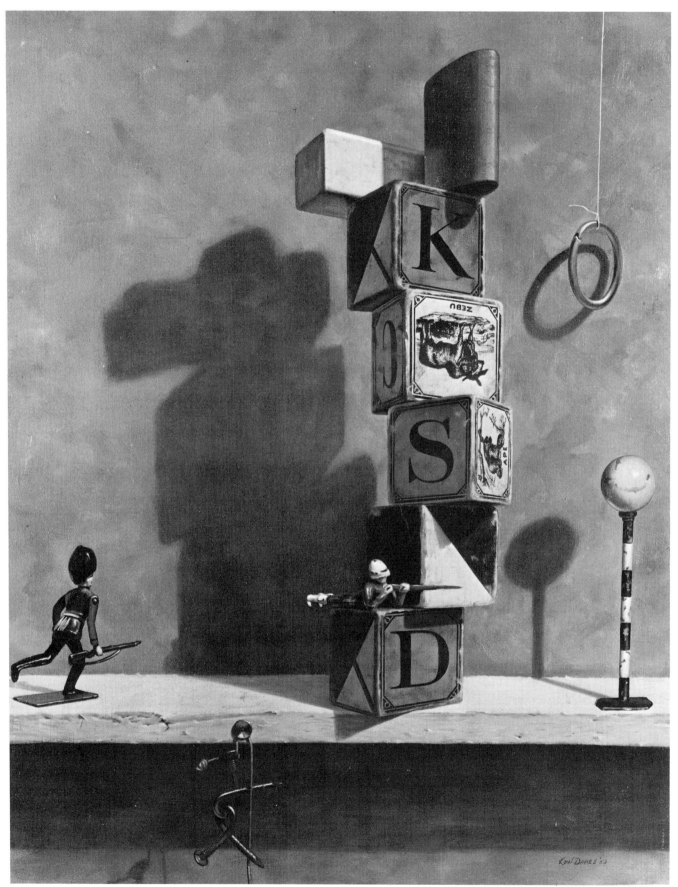

Kid's Things

EXERCISE 5 **SMOOTH TEXTURES**

Most beginning painters (and many experienced painters, too) are baffled when faced with the transparency of glass and the highlights and reflections of metallic objects. They are apt to ask themselves: "How do I transform all this gloppy oil paint into a smooth, shiny surface?" It's one of the easiest things for a painter to do—and I'll prove it!

The first thing for you to do is convince yourself that the problem is all in your mind. Now, turn off that electric sign in your head that says "glass" or "metal," and start thinking "shape, value, color." Look at the reflection of the light on the glass vase in your setup: the reflection has its own *shape* contained within the outline of the vase, it has its own *value* in relation to all the other values you see, and it has its own *color*. All you have to do is draw the shape and match its color and value.

MATERIALS AND EQUIPMENT

Drawing supplies
Palette spread with full range of colors
Brushes
Canvas board, 16" x 20"
Turpentine
Linseed oil
Shadow box
Clip-on light
Retouch varnish and brush

In this exercise, I recommend that you use one object from four different categories to give yourself the chance to solve most of the problems that will arise in painting glass and metal surfaces. The objects should vary in size. They should be absolutely smooth rather than cut, carved, or embossed. The four objects should include a clear glass object, a colored glass object, a silver-colored object, and a gold-colored object. You will also need a shadow box lined with colored or neutral fabric or paper and a clip-on light with an incandescent bulb.

Time limit: eight hours.

Setup. Place the four objects in the shadow box in a still life arrangement. Light the setup with the clip-on light, maximizing shadows and highlights.

Line Drawing. Make an outline drawing of the still life setup (Figure 1). Draw the outlines of the major shapes of the reflections and highlights *within* each object. These inside shapes make the painted objects look realistically like glass and metal. Smooth objects naturally reflect shapes of other objects close to them, much like a mirror, and if those reflections are neglected, the essence of the surface is lost. Spray the drawing with fixative to prevent smudging as you start to paint.

Wash-in. Wash in the background and local color of each object and of the shapes of the reflections and highlights within them (Figure 2). Even now the effect of shiny glass and metal is evident. Allow the painting to dry thoroughly.

Block-in. Carefully determine the value and color of each outlined shape. Match the color of each shape (as you did on the Color Matching Chart, Project 4) and block the color into the proper area of the drawing (Figure 3).

Completing the Painting. Determine the relative softness or hardness and blend each edge. Then add the highlights. You'll obtain the most realistic effect by paying careful attention to details.

Now, for the first time, you're allowed to think "glass" or "metal." And, if the above procedure has been followed faithfully, I guarantee that your opaque, soft-textured oil paint will now look like transparent glass and shiny metal.

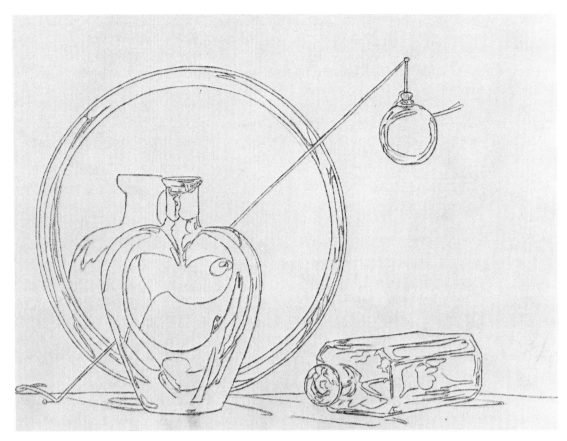

1. *Line drawing*

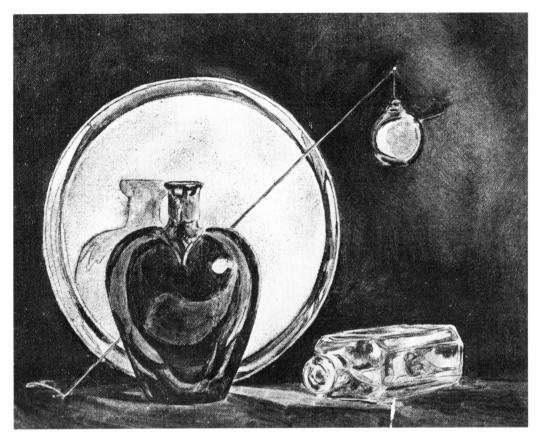

2. *Wash-in*

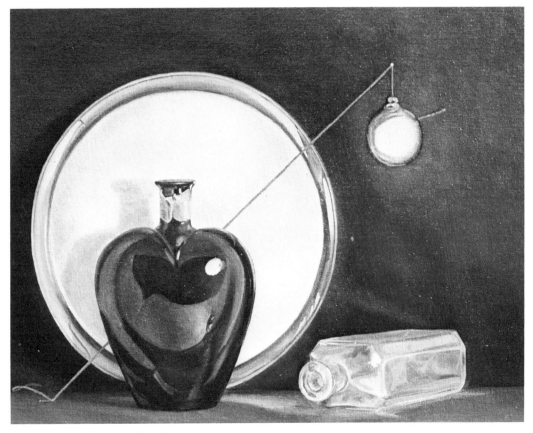

3. *Painting almost completed*

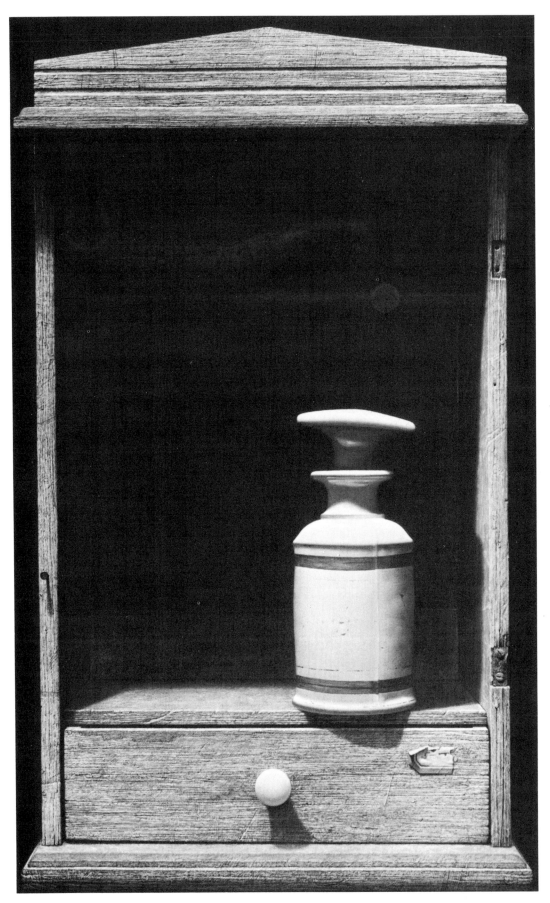

From Circuit Avenue

EXERCISE 6 **REFLECTED LIGHT**

Reflected light originates from a main light source, deflects off a surface, and bounces into a shadow area. Usually, reflected light is of a darker value than direct light. Its color is partially determined by the reflecting surface.

In this exercise we want to observe and study the intensity, color, and value of reflected light. A dramatic example that I use is to hold a bright green or blue piece of paper close to my face. Standing in front of a mirror, I aim a strong light at the right side of my face while holding the paper to the left side. I allow the light beam to illuminate the paper at the same time that it illuminates my face. The shadow side of my face shows the bright color of the reflected light.

Snow also provides good examples of reflected light. The shadows on snow reflect the light of the sky; shadows are blue if the sky is blue, gray if the sky is gray.

MATERIALS AND EQUIPMENT

Drawing supplies
Palette with full range of colors
Brushes
Canvas board, 16" x 20"
Turpentine
Linseed oil
Shadow box
Clip-on light
One piece each of red, yellow, and blue fabric
A smooth white ball
Retouch varnish and brush

Line the back wall, floor, and side of the shadow box with red, yellow, and blue fabric, respectively, draping the fabric in folds. Place the white ball in the center of the shadow box. Light the setup with the clip-on light, aimed from the left at approximately a 20° angle, and observe what has happened (Figure 1). The white ball reflects the color of the fabric. The reflected light comes into play on the folds of the draped fabric and influences the colors of various parts of the ball. Reflected light is often not as light in value as it appears. In order to determine accurate values, compare the value of the light side of the ball with the value of the shadow side.

Time limit: eight hours.

Line Drawing. Make a line drawing of the setup on the canvas board (Figure 2). Spray with fixative.

Wash-in. Wash in the background value and color and the white ball (Figure 3). Allow to dry.

Block-in. Block in the lights and shadows of the draped folds and the white ball. Allow to dry.

Completing the Painting. Paint the highlights. Allow to dry. Then apply retouch varnish.

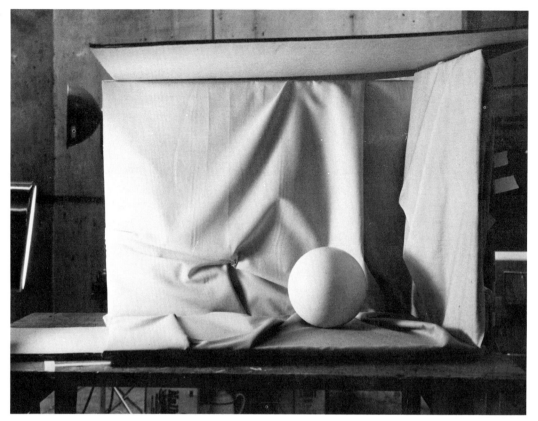

1. *Setup*

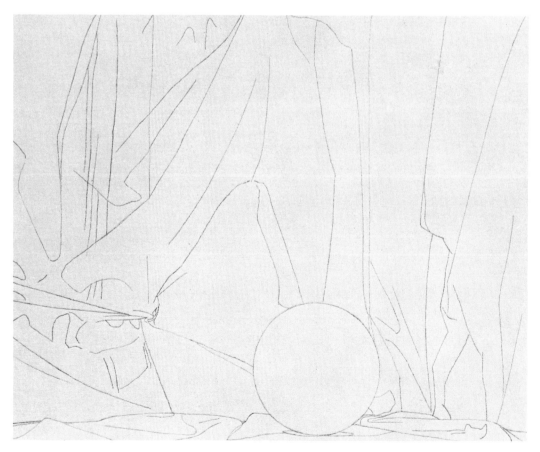

2. *Line drawing*

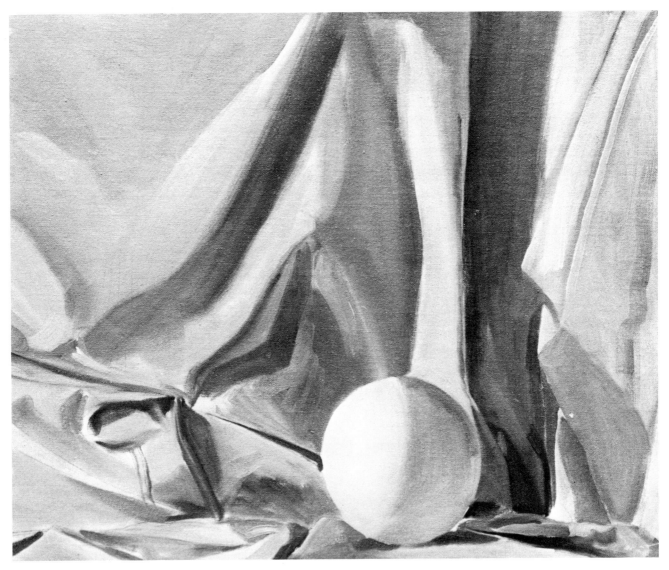

3. *Wash-in*

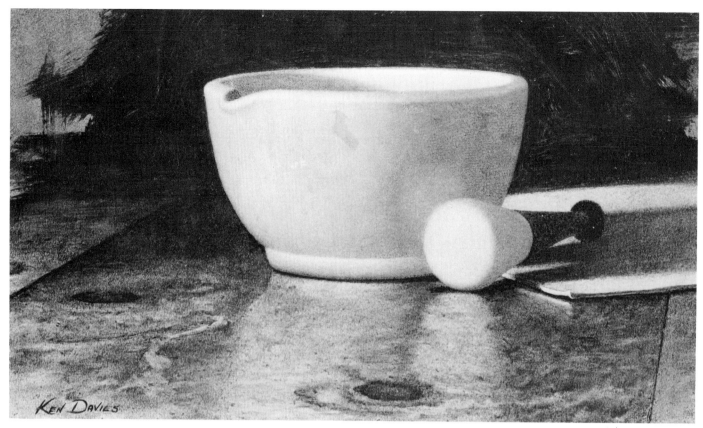

Study for Light and Props

EXERCISE 7 **SPEED PAINTING**

Hesitation in judging shapes, values, and colors, and trial-and-error color mixing are generally frustrating to the inexperienced painter. Decision-making of this sort during the painting procedure can be accelerated by: (1) imposing shorter time limits; (2) reducing the size of the painting area; and (3) using the direct painting method.

Your canvas board will be divided into quarters for this challenging experiment. In each quarter, you'll complete a mini-still life painting in a three-hour time limit. Small objects should be used for the setup, for example, spools of thread, tiny bottles, or children's blocks. Use the same objects in all four paintings, but for the sake of variety rearrange them in each setup. Use the direct painting method: determine the value and color of an area, mix the corresponding color, put it down, and leave it alone. There won't be time to change it. The wash-in, block-in, and drying periods are eliminated to speed up the procedure.

At first you may not be able to complete a painting in three hours, but at least attempt to complete all but the sharp details. Certainly all raw canvas should be covered.

If you're truly conscientious and can resist cheating on the time limit I've prescribed, you'll find that just the attempt at these four little paintings will considerably develop your ability to judge shapes, values, and colors more quickly and accurately.

MATERIALS AND EQUIPMENT

Drawing supplies
Palette with full range of colors
Brushes
Canvas board, 16" x 20"
Turpentine
Linseed oil
Shadow box
Clip-on light
Six small objects

Place the six small objects in an unlined shadow box. Light the setup with the clip-on light and incandescent bulb.

Time limit: three hours for each painting.

Rough Sketch. With a pencil and ruler, divide the canvas board into quarters. In the first quarter, make a quick, rough pencil sketch of the setup (Figure 1). Spray it with fixative.

Direct Painting. Apply the paint directly to the background areas (Figure 2).

Completing the Painting. In three hours complete as much as possible of the setup. You should try to cover all raw canvas, complete all objects, and suggest highlights (Figure 3).

Rough Sketch of the Second Quarter. Rearrange the same six objects in the shadow box and sketch the setup (Figure 4).

Direct Painting. Paint the second quarter as you did the first, being careful to accurately portray shapes and values (Figure 5). Complete this painting in three hours also.

Painting the Other Quarters. Rearrange the setup, sketch, and directly paint the remaining two quarters of the canvas as you did the first two (Figure 6).

Note: If you were able to complete the fourth painting, don't feel too sure of success until you've completed Exercise 8.

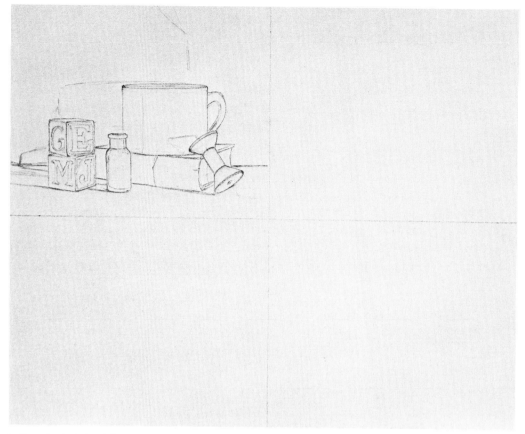

1. *Rough sketch of first quarter*

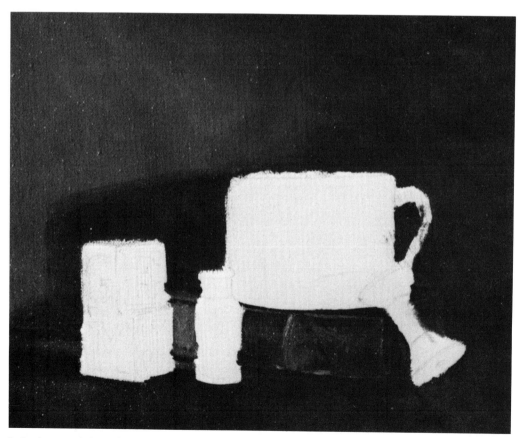

2. *Background directly painted*

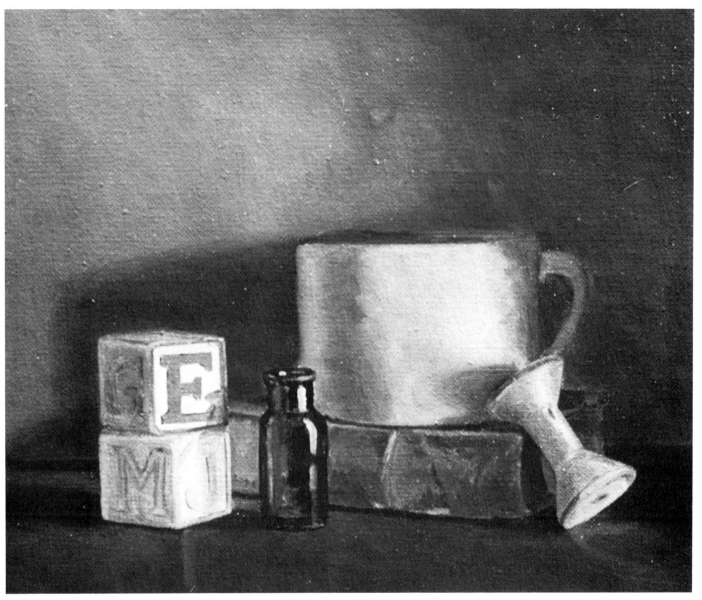

3. *Completed first quarter*

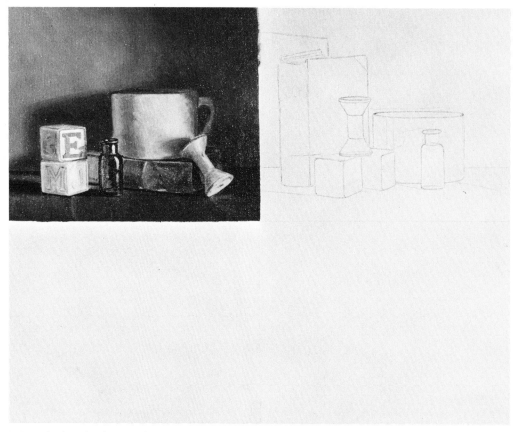

4. *Rough sketch of second quarter*

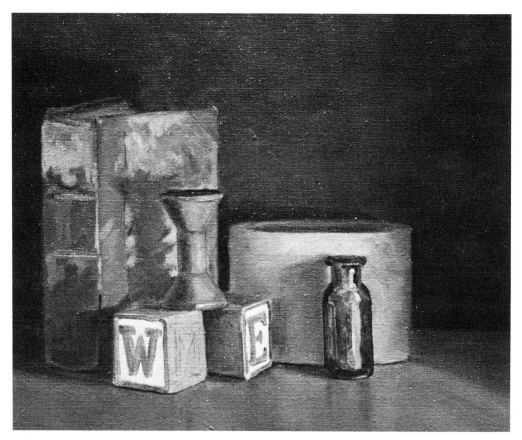

5. *Completed second quarter*

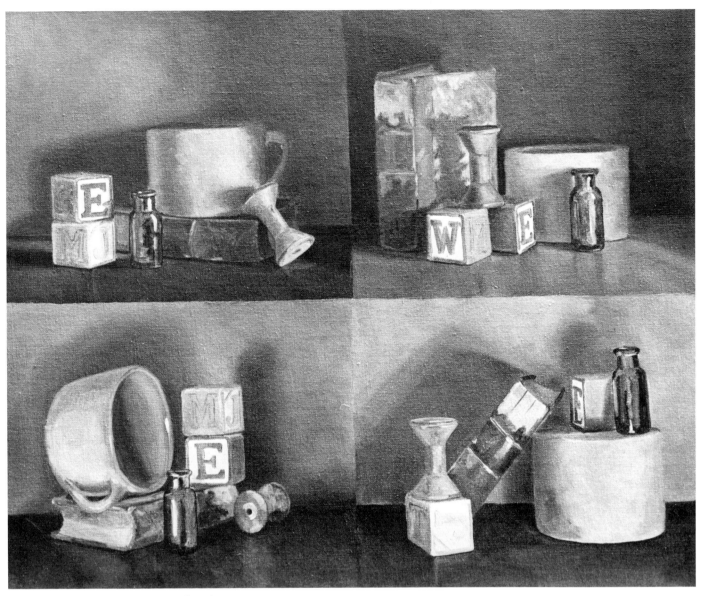

6. *All four quarters completed*

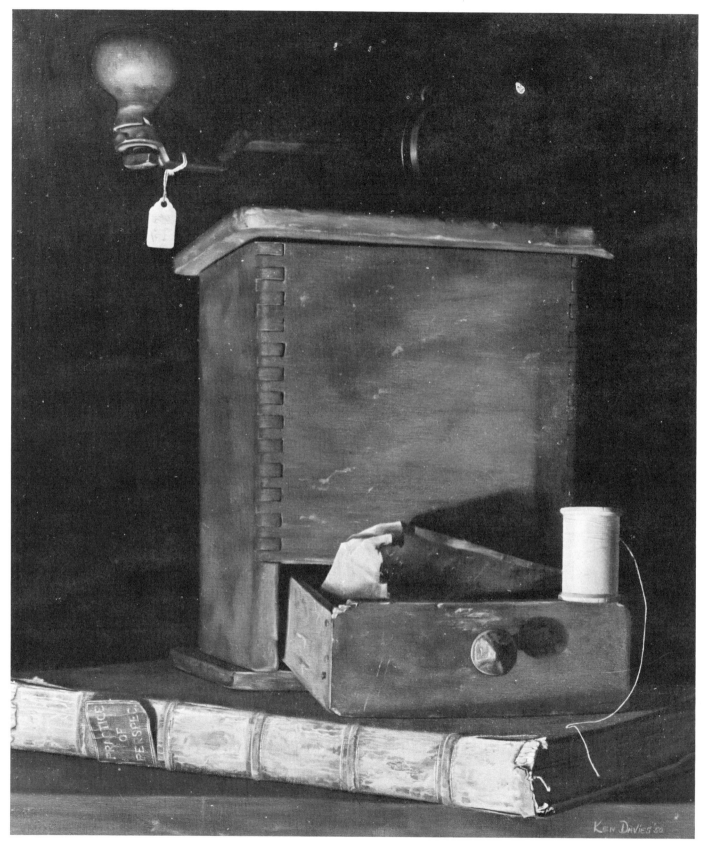

Coffee Grinder

EXERCISE 8   SPEED PAINTING

Insure the speed with which you make painting decisions about value, color, and shape by completing four more speed paintings. Again your canvas will be divided into quarters. In the first setup use six small objects; in the second use eight; in the third use ten; and in the fourth use 12 objects. As you see, the addition of two more objects to each speed painting increases the pressure on the painter, who must make his color and value choices at a much faster rate each time. The time limit for each painting is three hours.

Contrary to what you may think, this exercise is not designed merely to drive the student mad, but to train nimble eye-hand coordination. Good luck.

MATERIALS AND EQUIPMENT

Drawing supplies
Palette with full range of colors
Brushes
Canvas board, 16" x 20"
Turpentine
Linseed oil
Shadow box
Clip-on light
Twelve small still life objects

For each speed painting arrange the small objects in an unlined shadow box. Light the setup with the clip-on light and incandescent bulb. Divide the canvas into quarters with a pencil and ruler.

Time limit: three hours for each painting.

Painting the First Quarter. In the first quarter, arrange six objects in the shadow box, light the setup, make a quick rough sketch, and complete the painting in three hours as you did in Exercise 7.

Rough Sketch of the Second Quarter. Rearrange the setup, this time using eight objects. Make a rough sketch of this setup in the second quarter (Figure 1).

Direct Painting. Paint in the background areas and begin to paint the details of the foreground shapes, blending the soft edges (Figure 2).

Completing the Painting. Complete the painting in three hours, adding highlights if possible (Figure 3).

Painting the Other Quarters. In the remaining quarters, complete speed paintings using 10 and then 12 objects. Follow the procedure outlined above (Figures 4, 5, and 6).

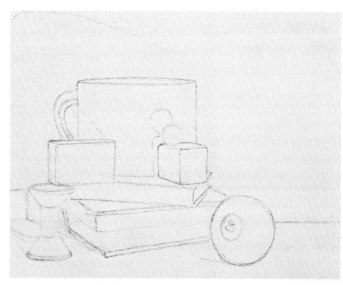

1. *Rough sketch of second quarter*

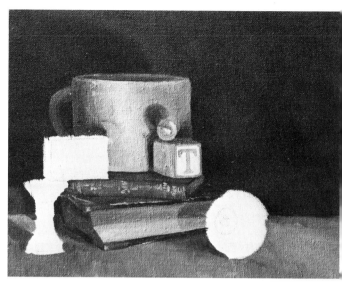

2. *Direct painting*

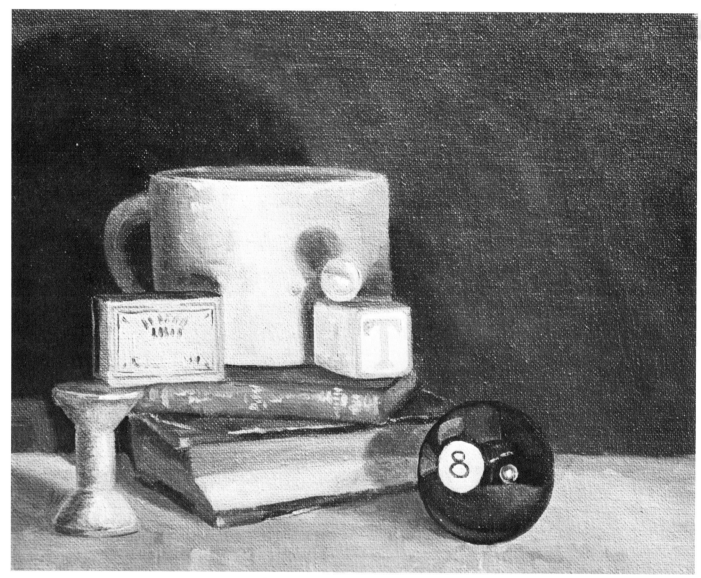

3. *Completed painting*

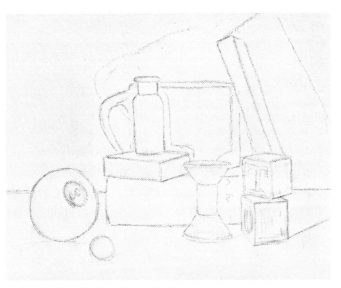

4. *Rough sketch of third quarter*

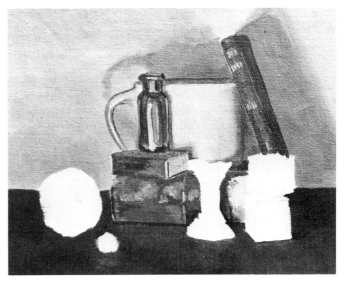

5. *Direct painting*

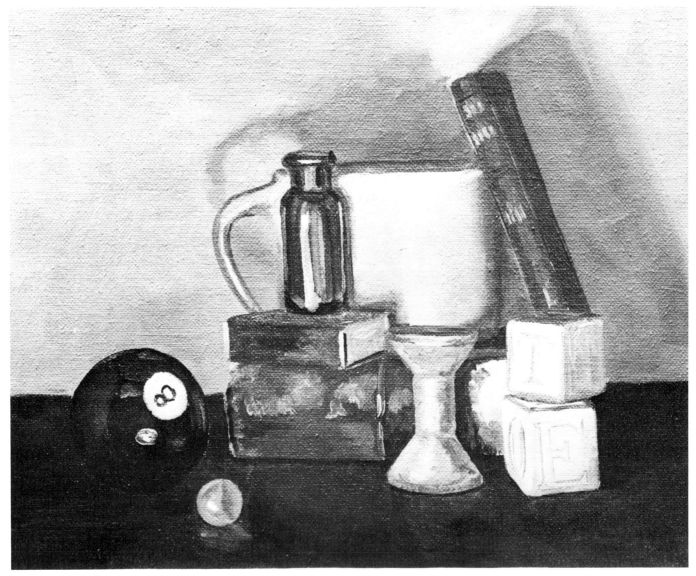

6. *Completed painting*

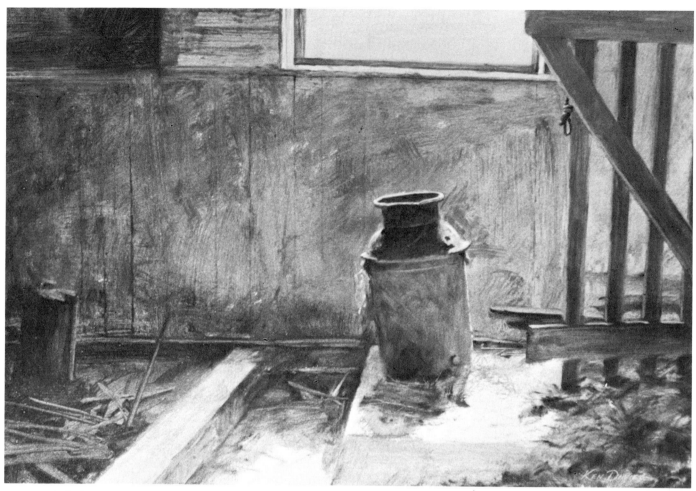

Milk Can

EXERCISE 9   MONOCHROME WET-INTO-WET

In previous exercises the wash-in and block-in stages were separated by long drying periods. Each time you applied a new color to the dry surface, you could anticipate the need to blend some edges and soften others.

By eliminating the drying periods between the wash-in and the block-in, softer edges can be achieved. The wash-in will still be wet while you work more opaque paint over it (block in). This is called working "wet-into-wet." Many still life painters prefer this method when they want to avoid hard edges.

Working wet-into-wet is a looser form of painting, and I think you'll find it an exciting change of pace. To lessen the complication of working with too many colors at the outset of this new method, use objects of the same general color in your setup.

MATERIALS AND EQUIPMENT

Drawing supplies
Palette with full range of colors
Brushes
Canvas board, 16" x 20"
Turpentine
Linseed oil
Shadow box
Clip-on light
Retouch varnish and brush

For the monochrome wet-into-wet painting, choose any six objects of the same general color. Be certain that the background color in the shadow box is in the same color range. The earthenware jug, brown egg, rusty horseshoe, old scythe, and book are all warm earth tones (Figure 1). Here the natural corrugated board of the shadow box works as a background. However, if you choose, for example, a blue monochromatic scheme, line the shadow box with a shade of blue.

Time limit: eight hours.

Setup. Place the six objects in the shadow box. Light the setup with the clip-on light (Figure 1).

Line Drawing. Make a line drawing of the setup on canvas board. Spray it with fixative.

Color Wash. Determine the approximate middle color value of the setup. Mix that color thinned with turpentine; the pigment must be transparent. Then brush the thinned color over the entire canvas. The drawing should be visible through the paint (Figure 2).

Block-in. While the wash is still wet, start painting with opaque tones. Block in the background, then the foreground. Block the objects in the setup directly into the wet paint, trying to get as close to the correct values and colors as you can while the paint is wet (Figure 3). Allow the painting to dry thoroughly.

Sharpening the Painting. Start to sharpen some areas of the painting, while leaving other areas in soft focus. A beautiful effect can be created, for instance, by sharpening the focus of the center of interest while all other areas remain soft, or you may want to sharpen just one object and leave the other parts of the setup unfinished.

When you're satisfied with the soft- and hard-edged effects, allow the painting to dry. Then brush on retouch varnish.

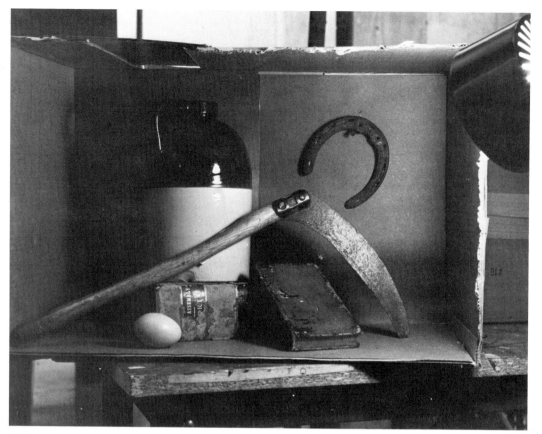

1. *Setup*

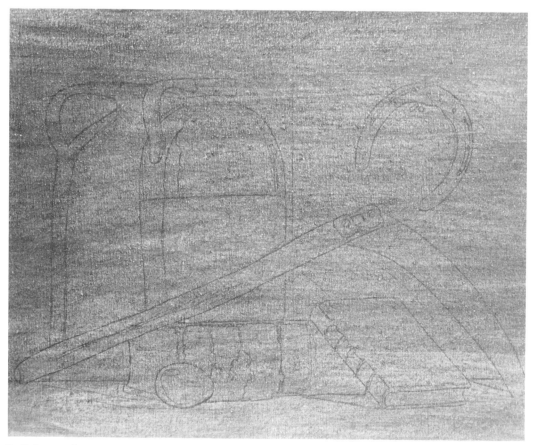

2. *Color wash*

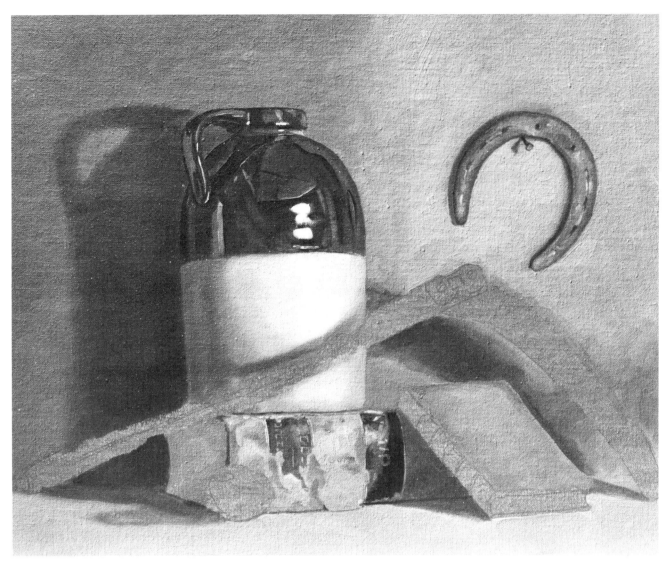

3. *Block-in partially completed*

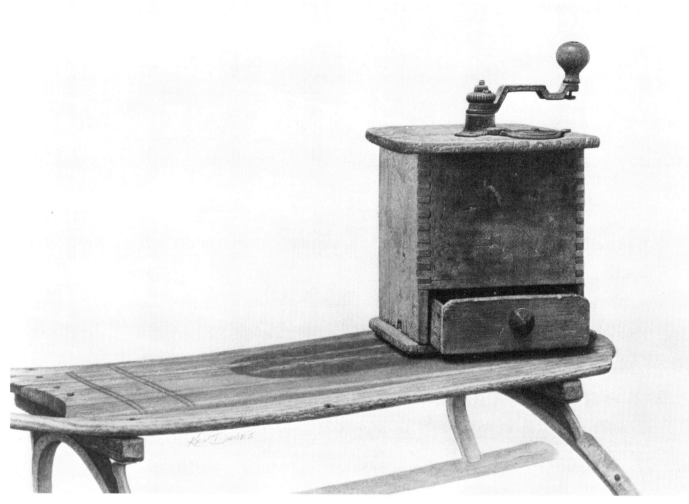

Williamsburg Coffee Grinder

EXERCISE 10 **DRAWING WITH A BRUSH**

If you're interested in a looser style, making your initial drawing of the setup with a brush on the canvas board can help you move in that direction. Drawing with a brush will give you more room for expression. However, in terms of perspective, your drawing should be almost as precise as when you were drawing with a pencil, although perhaps not as detailed. In this case, the drawing can and should be corrected during each painting stage rather than perfected at the start.

Test your skill in this exercise by drawing on the canvas board with a brush. It will give you the experience necessary for a softer-focus style of painting.

MATERIALS AND EQUIPMENT

Palette with full range of colors
Turpentine
Linseed oil
Brushes, including a No. 6 round sable
Canvas board, 16" x 20"
Turpentine
Linseed oil
Shadow box
Clip-on light
Retouch varnish and brush

Choose any five objects. In the beginning it is best to choose objects with uncomplicated silhouettes and little or no decoration. Arrange them in the shadow box. Light the setup with the clip-on light (Figure 1).

Time limit: eight hours.

Brush Drawing. Make a drawing of the setup on the canvas board, using the No. 6 round sable brush. Use paint of the color predominant in the setup thinned with turpentine. Although the drawing should be made in correct perspective, it isn't necessary to refine it in this stage (Figure 2). The thinned paint will dry quickly.

Wash-in. Thin your paint with turpentine and linseed oil and wash in the background, the local color of each object, and the shadows. Correct and refine the drawing at this stage (Figure 3). Allow the painting to dry thoroughly.

Block-in. Block in the background color and the color of each object in the setup with opaque paint (Figure 4).

Completing the Painting. Refine the drawing again by adding all details and highlights. Allow the painting to dry, then paint with retouch varnish.

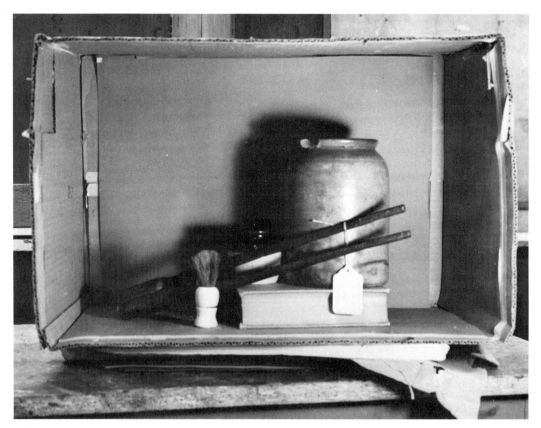

1. *Setup*

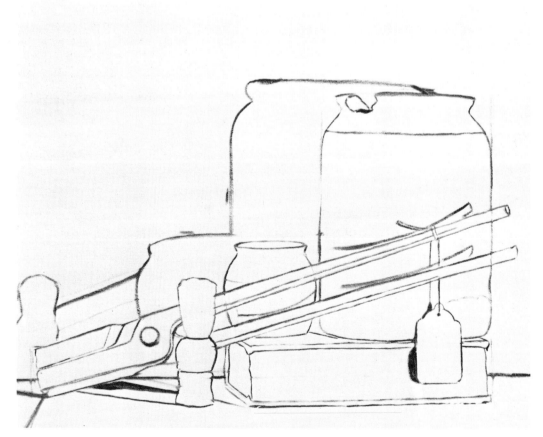

2. *Brush drawing*

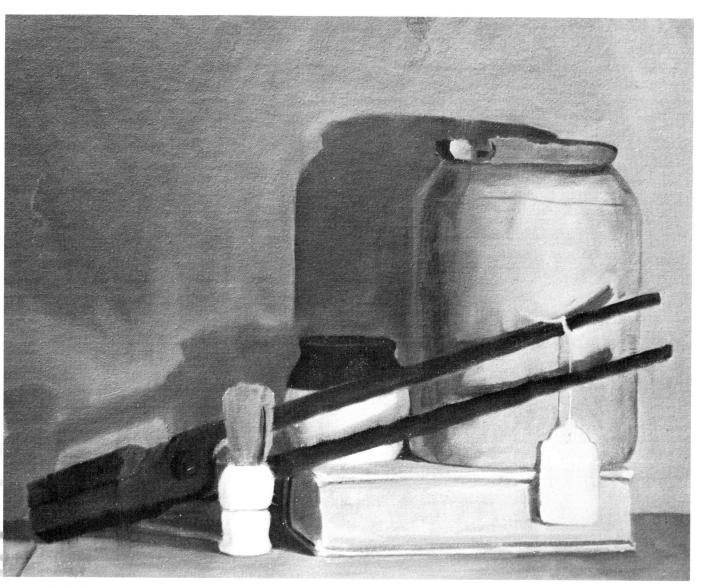

3. *Wash-in*

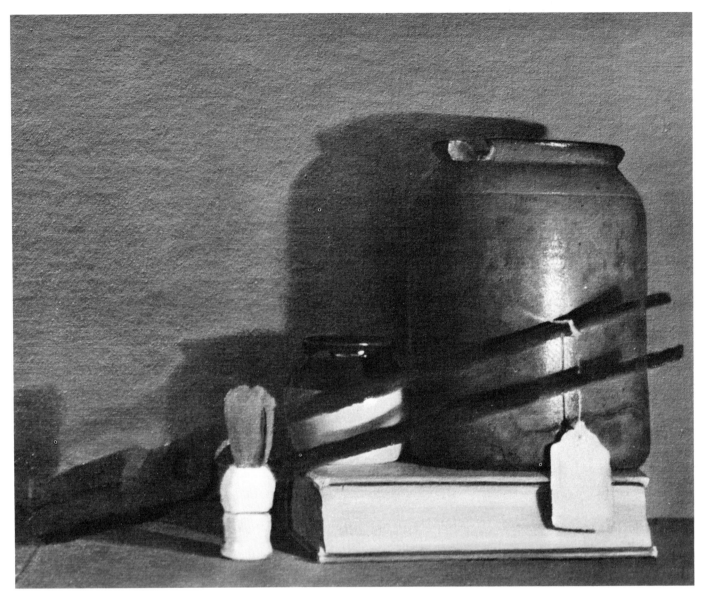

4. *Block-in*

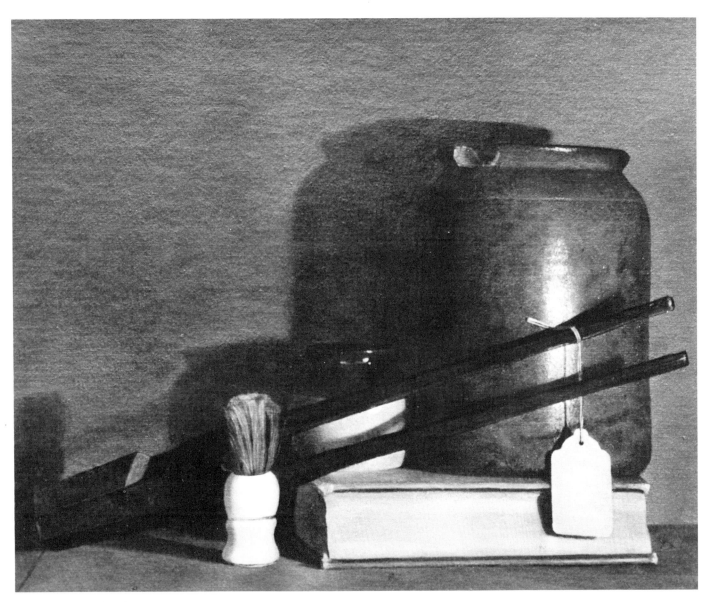

5. *Completed painting*

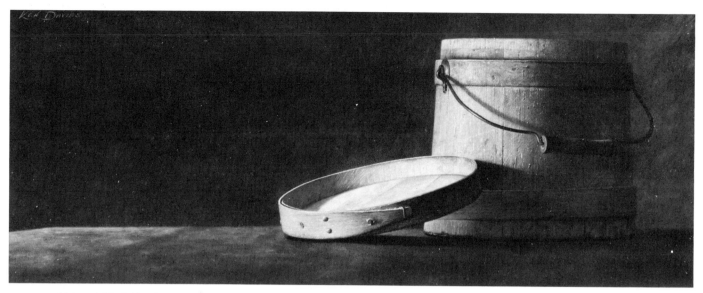

Old and Well Used

EXERCISE 11 **STILL LIFE UNDER RED LIGHT**

The color of light is fascinating to study. Let's approach this exercise by observing the effect of a colored light source on the local color of objects. Up to this point, we've been using an ordinary incandescent bulb to light the subject. The incandescent bulb, as you will have observed, gives a slightly yellowish tint to the objects, and this is how they are often normally seen. Now replace the incandescent bulb with a red one. You'll see that dramatic color changes occur as the red light shines on an area. Think of your setup as a stage set where performers will appear; you've just cast a red spotlight on the set. Under the red spotlight, whites appear a glowing red, whereas green objects turn gray and red objects glow with more insensity. Place blue, green, and yellow objects under the red spotlight and observe the color changes that occur.

It's said that human color perception is diminishing. If this is true, perhaps the remedy for the artist is to try harder to see color and to understand its nature. The study of the color of light and the color of paint is complicated and compelling. This exercise gives you the opportunity to make your own discoveries about our perception of color, a subject over which scientists have been at odds for centuries.

MATERIALS AND EQUIPMENT

Drawing supplies
Palette with full range of colors
Turpentine
Linseed oil
Brushes
Canvas board, 16" x 20"
Shadow box
Clip-on light and red bulb
Retouch varnish and brush

Choose five or six objects of any color and arrange them in the shadow box (Figure 1). Observe the setup under incandescent light. Now change the bulb to red. Notice the dramatic difference.

Time limit: eight hours.

Line Drawing. Make a line drawing of the setup on the canvas board. Be sure to include the outlines of all the shadows and details (Figure 2). Spray the drawing with fixative.

Wash-in. Wash in the background and local color of each object (Figure 3). Allow the painting to dry.

Block-in. Block in the entire setup (Figure 4). Allow to dry. Add highlights and details, then paint with retouch varnish.

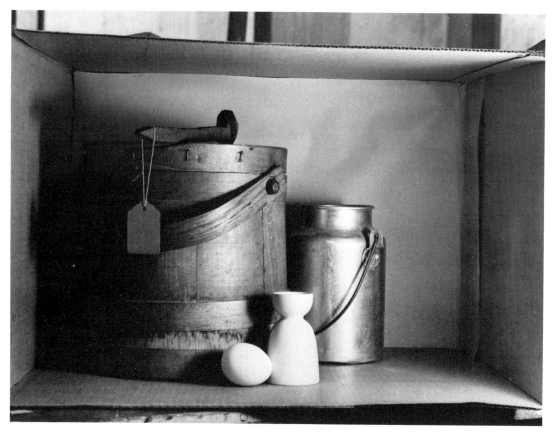

1. *Setup*

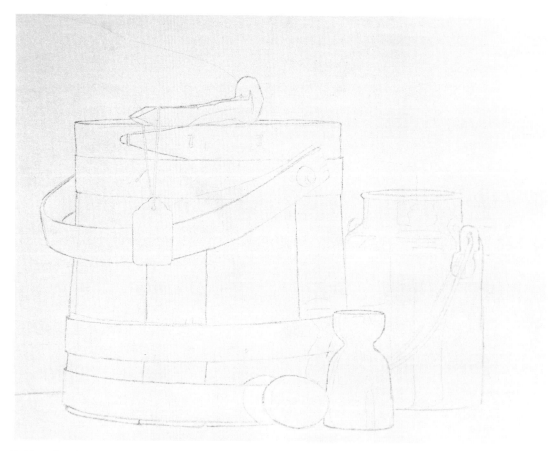

2. *Line drawing*

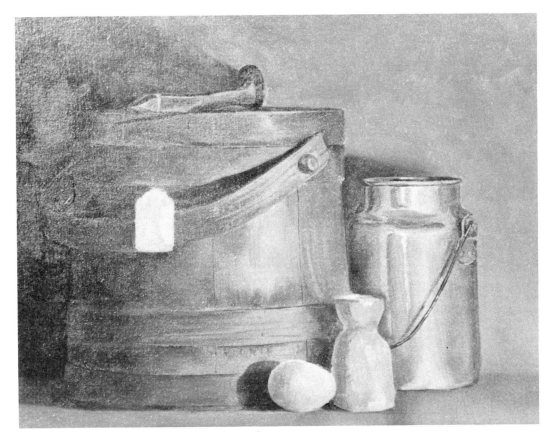

3. *Wash-in*

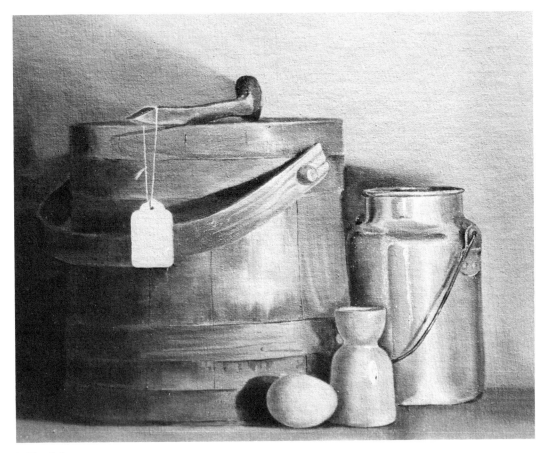

4. *Block-in*

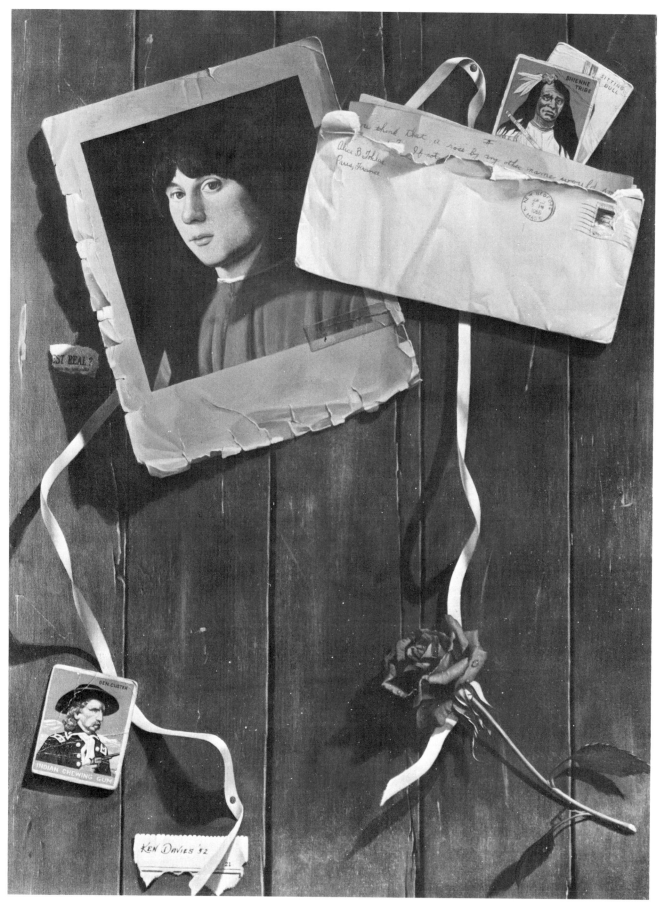

Is a Rose a Rose?

EXERCISE 12 **STILL LIFE UNDER GREEN LIGHT**

I hope that by completing Exercise 11 your color perception has been heightened. Now we will study the effect of a green light bulb. This time your setup will be composed of every color on the basic color wheel with the addition of a white and a black object. This isn't as complicated as it may seem. The exercise simply carries you one step further in the study of color and light. By now you know that you can change the color of an object by changing the color of the light shining on it. Or that you can increase the intensity of a color if the light source and the object are the same color.

Playing with color and light will help you to investigate the physics of light. You may find that the most intense colors you can create with light are *so* intense that they are impossible to reproduce with pigment. Don't expect a perfect match in such a case. Do try all sorts of combinations of your own by shining different colored lights on objects of varied colors. You'll be amazed at some of the results.

At some time in the future, you may want to use this newly gained knowledge to control the colors of your setup by lighting part of it with natural and part with colored light.

Color information of different kinds is also practical for professional illustrators, for example in an assignment to paint a stage set lit by colored spotlights, or in an interior of a room with light coming through a stained-glass window. Color study is particularly valuable to the artist, because often a painting or illustration must be invented in the studio.

MATERIALS AND EQUIPMENT

Drawing supplies
Palette with full range of colors
Turpentine
Linseed oil
Brushes
Canvas board, 16" x 20"
Eight colored objects, one each of: red, blue, yellow, green, violet, orange, black, and
    white
Shadow box
Clip-on light with green bulb
Colored construction papers (four of the above objects can be torn pieces of construc-
    tion paper)
Retouch varnish and brush

Tack four different colors of construction paper to the back wall of the shadow box. Place the black object, the white object, and the two remaining colored objects in the shadow box. Light the setup with the clip-on light containing a green bulb (Figure 1).

Time limit: eight hours.

Line Drawing. Make a line drawing of the setup on the canvas board (Figure 2). Spray the drawing with fixative.

Wash-in. Wash in the background and local color of each object (Figure 3). Allow to dry.

Block-in. Block in the background and local color of the objects, correcting the color as you go. Begin some of the details (Figure 4). Allow to dry.

Completing the Painting. Add details and highlights. Allow to dry thoroughly. Then you can add minute details, such as the torn binding of the book and the highlights on the billiard ball (Figure 5). Allow to dry and then paint on retouch varnish.

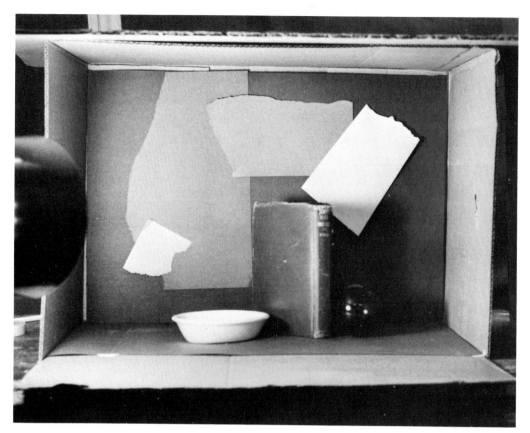

1. *Setup*

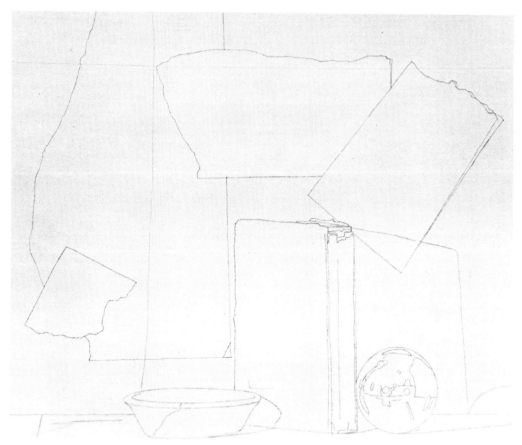

2. *Line drawing*

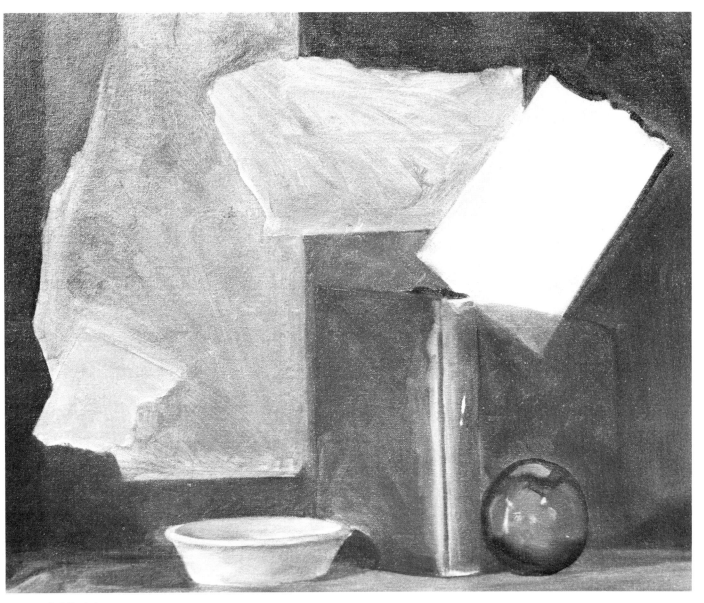

3. *Wash-in*

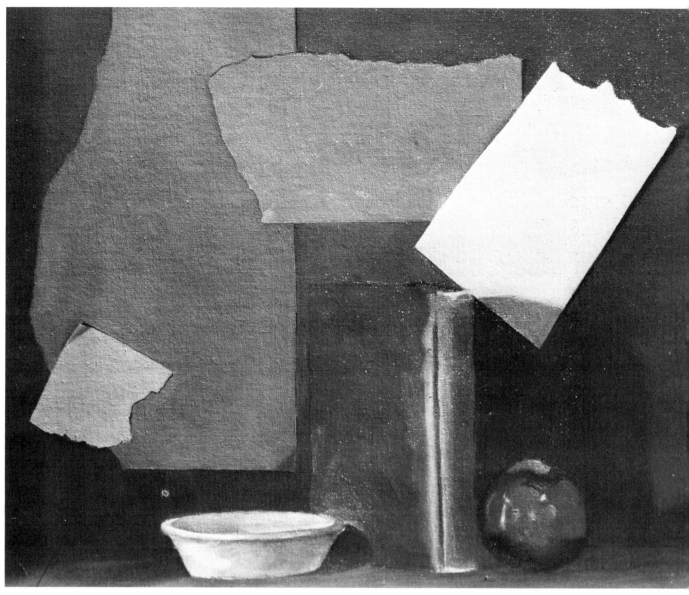

4. *Block-in*

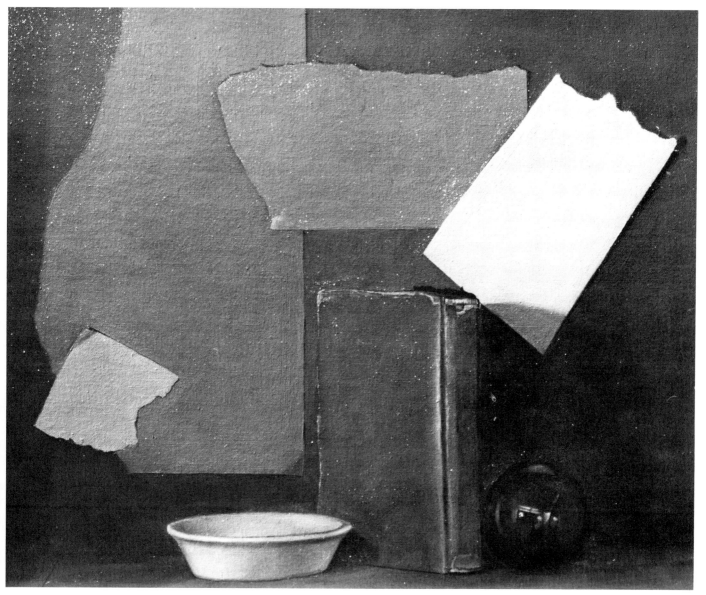

5. *Completed painting*

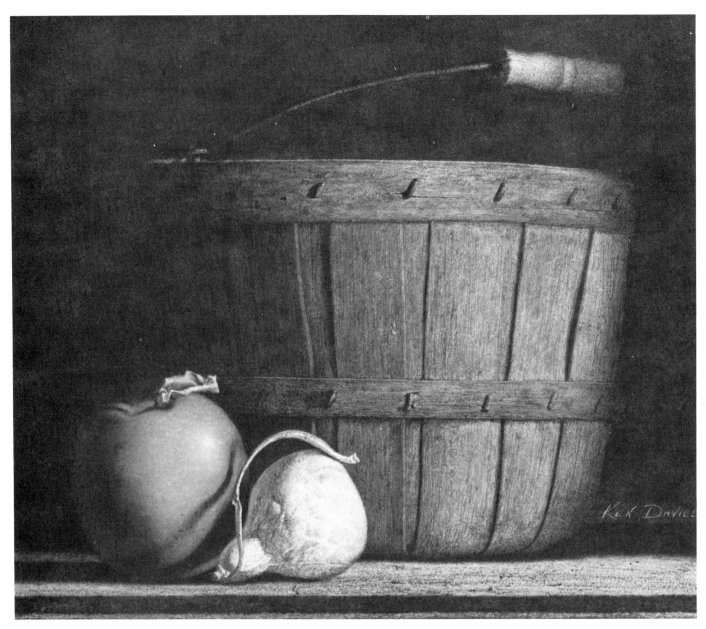

Red and White

EXERCISE 13 GLAZING AND SCUMBLING

The first two parts of this book are designed to give you the practical steps necessary to learning the techniques of direct painting. In direct painting, you're concentrating on achieving the right values and colors just as they are, from the very start to the finish of a painting. The paintings you produce from these projects and exercises are not intended to be exhibition quality but merely a series of practice pieces used to learn new skills and sharpen old ones.

This exercise marks a transition to a new plane of endeavor for the painter, one in which important exhibit-worthy paintings may be produced. Here we'll investigate two painting methods that have not been discussed up to now, glazing and scumbling. Glazing is a method by which one layer of paint is applied over another. The undercoat must be thoroughly dry before the glaze is brushed over it. A glaze is usually thinned paint of a dark value painted over a lighter value. The layer beneath the glaze shows through to give a luminous quality. It's the transparency of the glaze that makes the difference between the directly painted shadow and the glazed shadow.

The advantage of glazing in sharp focus realistic painting is most evident when applied to shadows and the details that fall within them. Glazed shadows appear more realistic than directly painted ones. They're convincing enough to give the feeling that one can reach deep into them. The details are minimized in glazed areas and seem mysterious.

The scumble, or scumbling technique, is a method of applying an opaque light-colored paint mixture on a dry layer of dark paint, just the opposite of glazing. In scumbling, fairly thick paint is either dry-brushed or applied in normal fashion to the surface. Scumbling gives the surface of the painting a sense of immediacy. Textures are maximized, giving the impression that the surface is real enough to touch.

The general rule I make is that *shadows are glazed down* and *light areas are scumbled*.

MATERIALS AND EQUIPMENT

Drawing supplies
Palette with full range of colors
Brushes
Canvas board, 16" x 20"
Turpentine
Linseed oil
Shadow box
Clip-on light
Still life objects
Masking tape
Retouch varnish and brush

Set up a still life in the shadow box using relatively simple objects. Light the setup with the clip-on light and incandescent bulb.

Time limit: eight hours.

Line Drawing. Make a line drawing of the setup on the canvas board. Spray it with fixative.

Wash-in. With transparent paint (thinned with a mixture of ⅔ linseed oil and ⅓ turpentine), wash in the background and local color of each object.

Block-in. In preparation for glazing, the block-in procedure is slightly different from before. Paint the shadows lighter than they appear in the setup. They will later be glazed down to the correct value.

Paint the light areas slightly darker than they appear in the setup. They will later be scumbled with light paint and brought up to the correct value.

Paint the details in the light areas. If some of the details in light areas continue into shadow areas, paint them a darker value in the shadow area yet slightly lighter than they actually are. At this stage allow the painting to dry thoroughly.

Glazing. All dust must be removed before glazing, otherwise the glazed area will appear gritty rather than smooth. Use masking tape to carefully lift all loose lint or dust from the surface.

Glaze all shadow areas as follows: Mix a transparent dark wash. With a filbert or flat brush, wash the color over the shadow areas. When you're glazing a surface that must appear round, find the area where the shadows blend into light areas. At those points feather out the paint with quick movements of the brush (Figure 5).

The transparent paint used for the wash must be neither too thin nor too opaque. Experience will eventually tell you how to reach the right consistency. When in doubt, make the wash on the thin side rather than too opaque. When a thin glaze has dried another darker layer can be added, but if a glaze that is too opaque is used it is much more difficult to correct.

Daubing. After the glaze is applied, it will look streaky and the details will be partially obliterated. To correct this, shape part of an old tee shirt into a dauber (Figure 6). Lift all loose lint and dust from the dauber with masking tape. Pat and blot the wet glaze until it is smooth and blended. The value of the glaze will now be considerably lighter (Figure 7).

Scumbling. Scumble the highlights and light areas with opaque paint of light value and add minute details. When dry, coat with retouch varnish. Glazing and scumbling will be illustrated further in the demonstrations in Part Three.

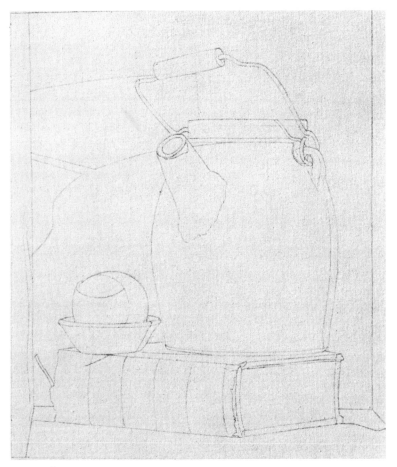

1. *Setup*

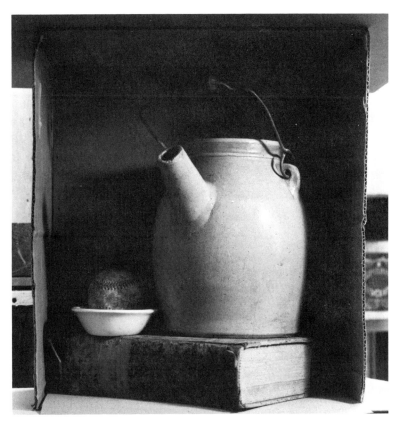

2. *Line drawing*

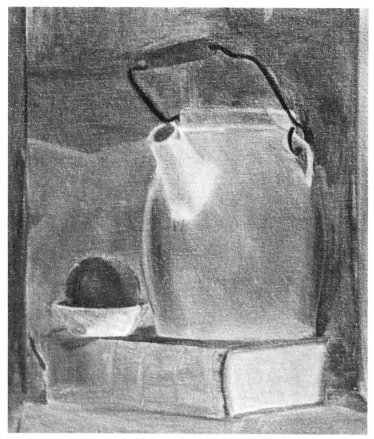

3. *Wash-in*

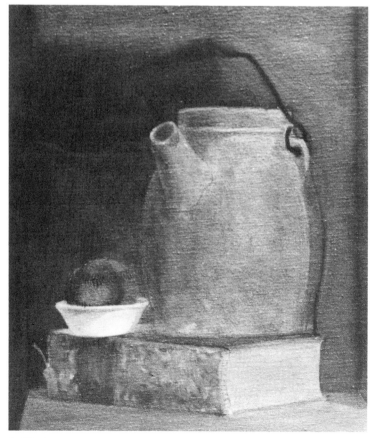

4. *Glazing*

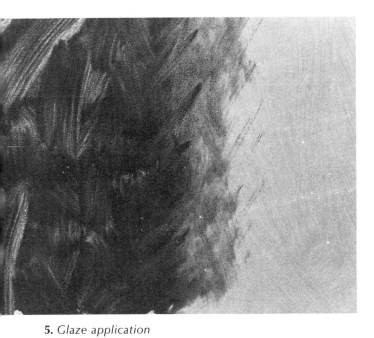

5. *Glaze application*

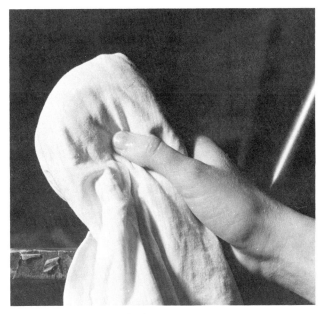

6. *Tee shirt used as a dauber*

7. *Glazed area after daubing*

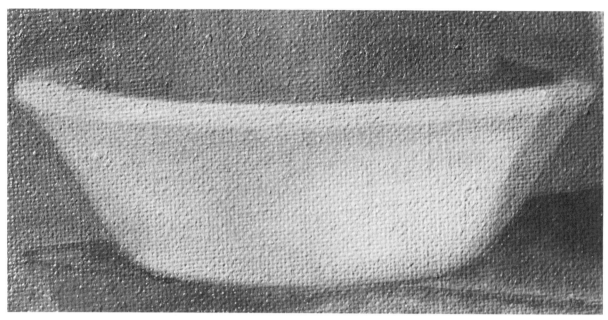

8. *Detail of block-in area before glazing*

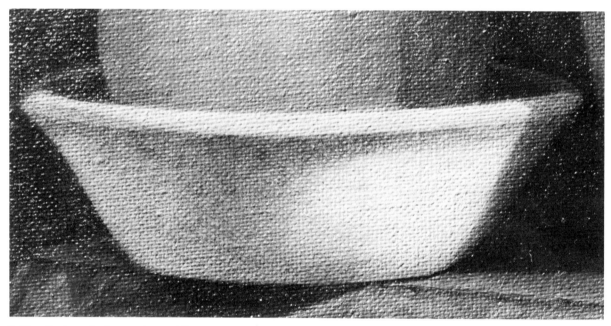

9. *Detail after glazing and scumbling*

A Commemorative *(Opposite page). In 1972 I was commissioned by the United States Postal Service to design the Pharmacy Stamp. Later I thought it would be amusing to paint a trompe l'oeil that would include the stamp. The mailbox which provides the setting was given to me by a student. The composition fell together quite easily, but painting the small postage stamp life size in oils was one of the most grueling jobs I've ever faced: for the first time in my career I had to use a magnifying glass while painting.*

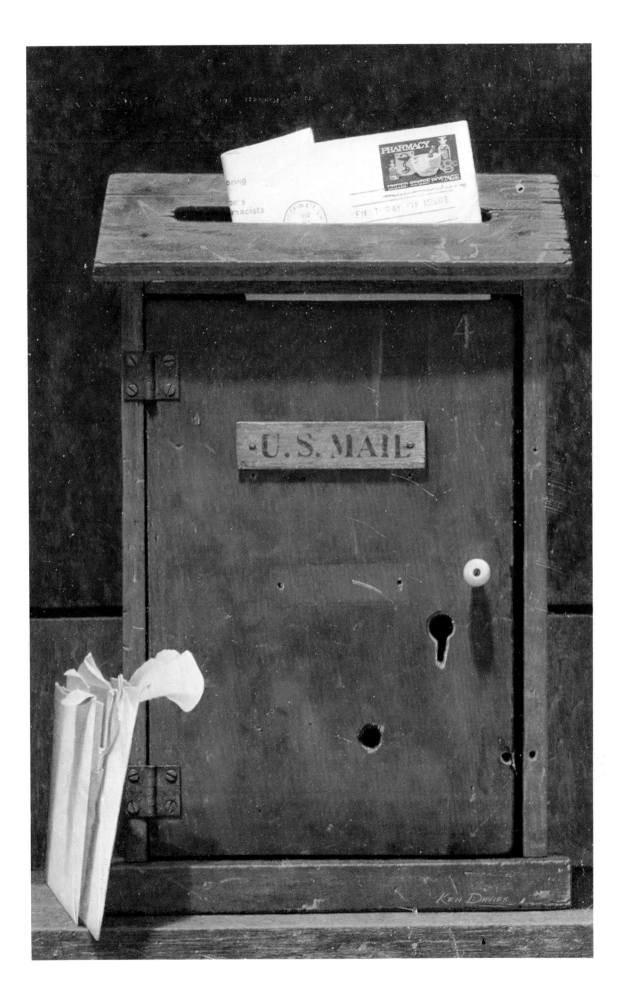

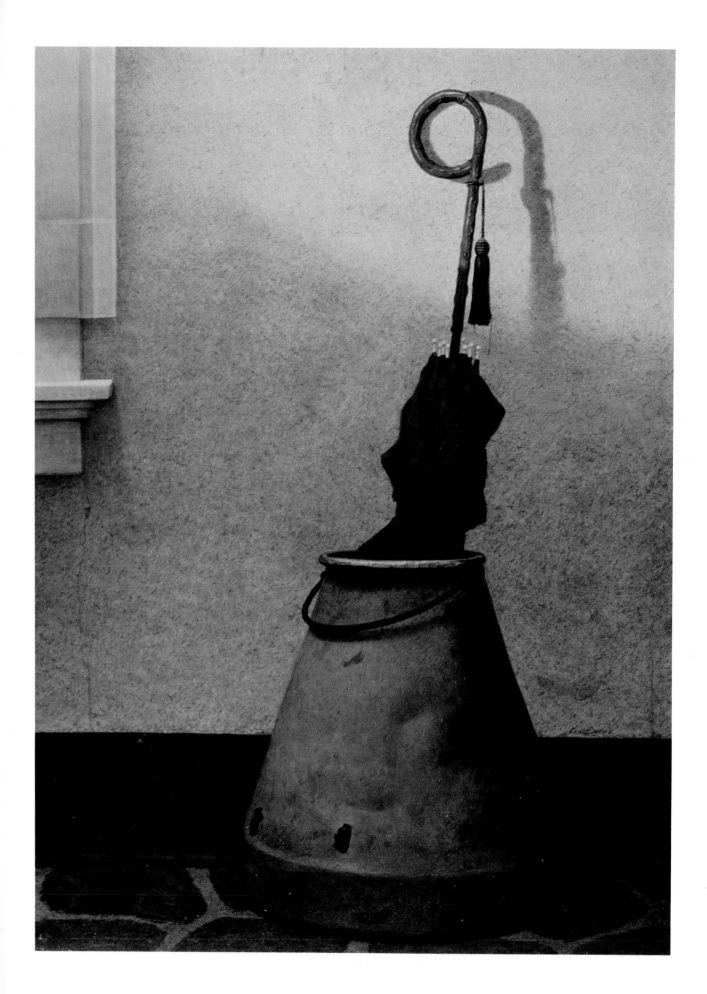

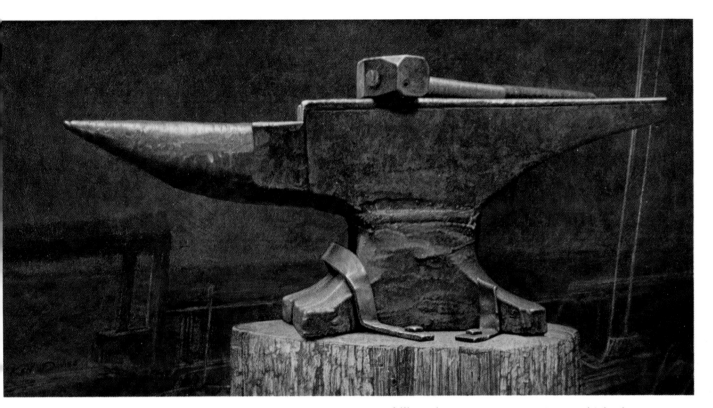

Umbrella Stand *(Left). One of my favorite pastimes is browsing through antique shops. To me they are a wonderfully rich source of paintable objects, and the excitement of discovering a subject for a new painting adds spice to the experience. The old milk can and umbrella were found on such an excursion. I had no specific plans for either of them until I arrived home and put the umbrella into the milk can for safekeeping. A few days later I glanced at the accidental arrangement and decided that the pair would be the subject for my next painting.*

Durability *(Above). Here's a situation in which a loose, suggestive background works well with a highly finished foreground object. The anvil is one of my favorite props because of its angular contour.*

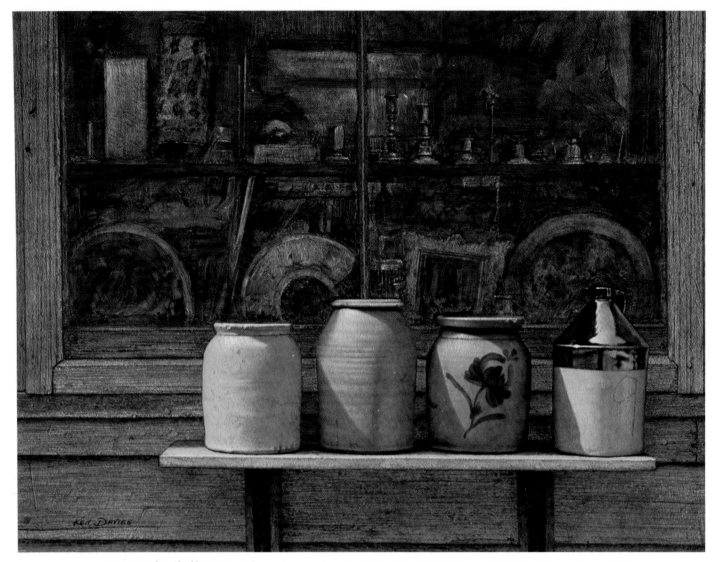

Four on the Shelf. *Driving through a rural part of New York State I caught sight of these four old jugs, arranged just as they are in the painting outside an antique shop. The background is painted in a much looser style than I ordinarily use (described in Exercise 9, Monochrome Wet-Into-Wet). In this painting I was particularly gratified at having achieved a contrast between the highly finished rendering of the foreground and the more loosely handled objects in the window.*

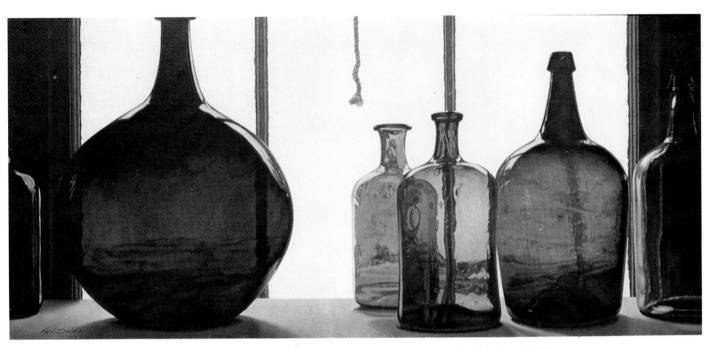

Transparencies. *In this, one of my most colorful paintings, I utilized clear glass bottles of different tones. This painting is a particularly good example of the techniques presented in Exercise 5, Smooth Textures.*

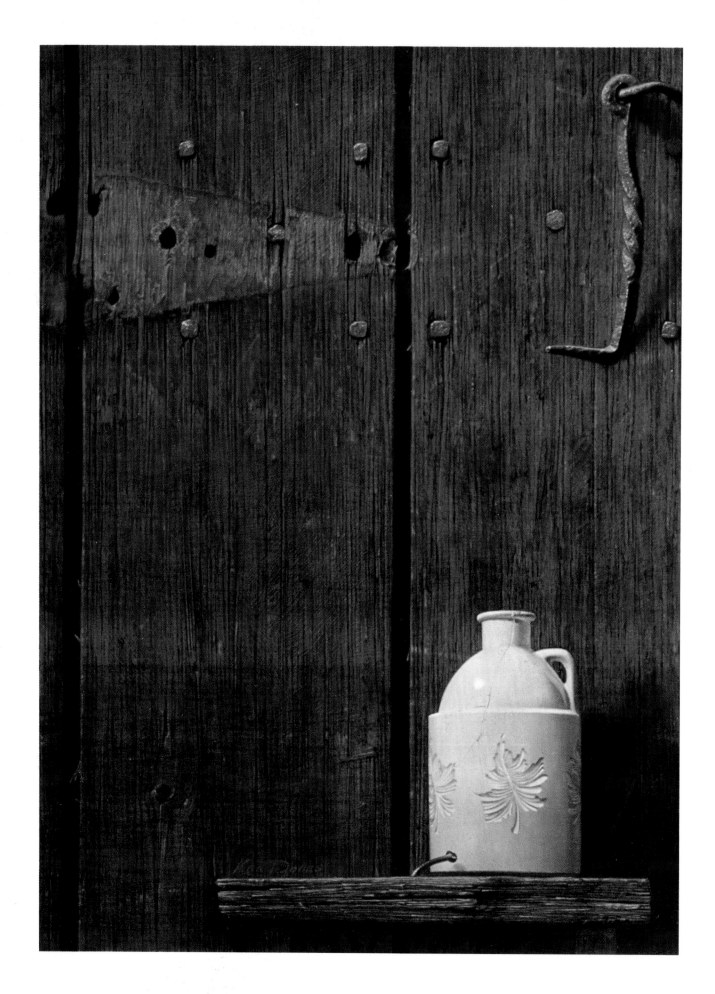

134

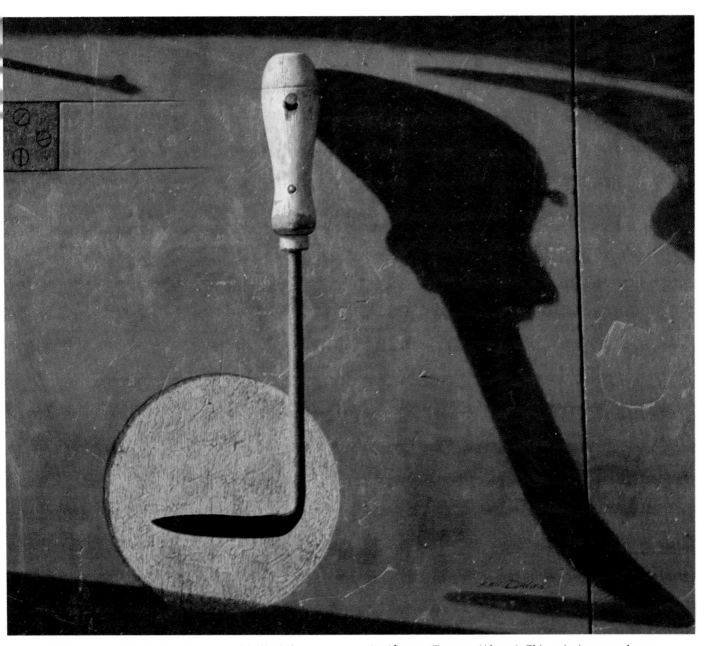

White Jug (Left). During the second half of their second year, students in the painting class at the Paier School are expected to produce what is referred to as their "major painting," the culmination of all they have learned by working through the course presented in this book. Each year I look forward to seeing the props brought in as subjects for these paintings. Occasionally I'll see ones that appeal to me for my own work and I'll negotiate with the student to either buy or borrow them. The white jug and wooden board were part of a student's setup which I borrowed for this stark, simple still life.

An Abstract Trompe (Above). This painting reveals my interest in combining ultra-realism with abstract design. The composition evolved from an old garden tool which I hung from a nail jutting through an old board. I left the board on my porch where I would be sure to see it again. As I hoped, the perfect moment occurred. It was late in the afternoon with the sun very low in the sky, and the shadow cast by the iron form onto the board fascinated me. The blue circle did not exist; I added it to enhance the abstract design.

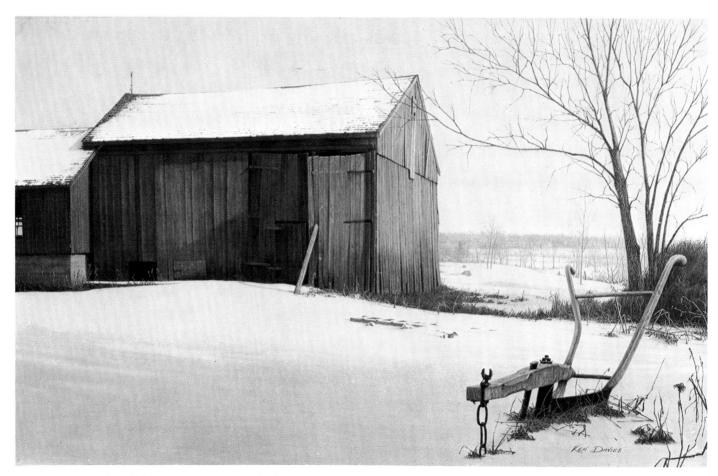

Last Winter. *I'm a true barn "buff," therefore painting old barns is a novelty that I find most enjoyable. The title of this painting suggests the fate of the barn: soon after the painting was completed the building was torn down, and now the foundation is all that remains.*

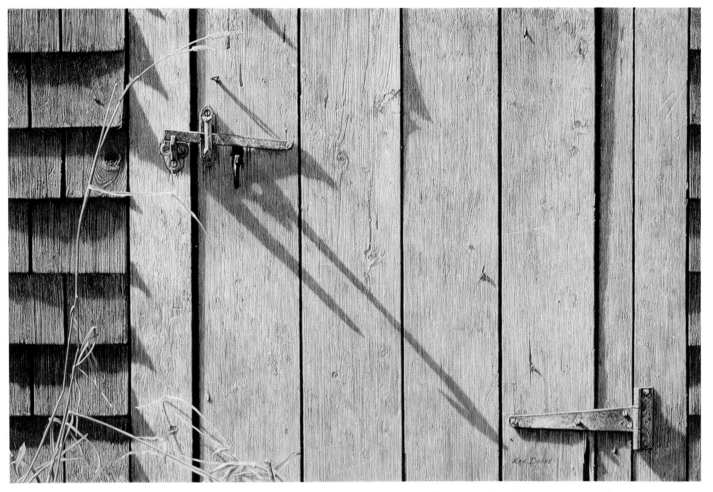

Chilmark Tool Shed. *The time I enjoy the most on Martha's Vineyard is off-season when the summer crowds have returned to the mainland. Then I can roam about unhampered by people and take in the treasures, natural and man-made, of the island. One crisp October afternoon, I happened on this scene in the yard of an old, uninhabited house in Chilmark. The perfect angle of the autumn sun on the hinge and the faded, worn wood latch was an ideal ready-made setup. I painted it exactly as I found it. And as late as the summer of 1974 it still remained, a bit faded from exposure but otherwise exactly as I recorded it.*

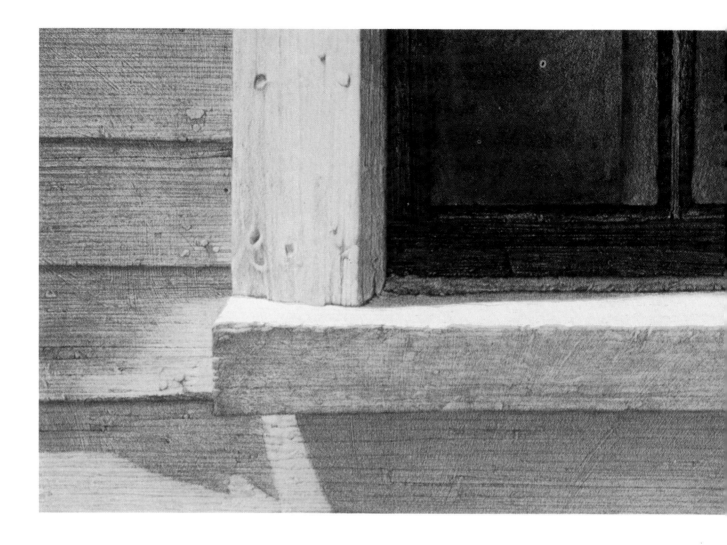

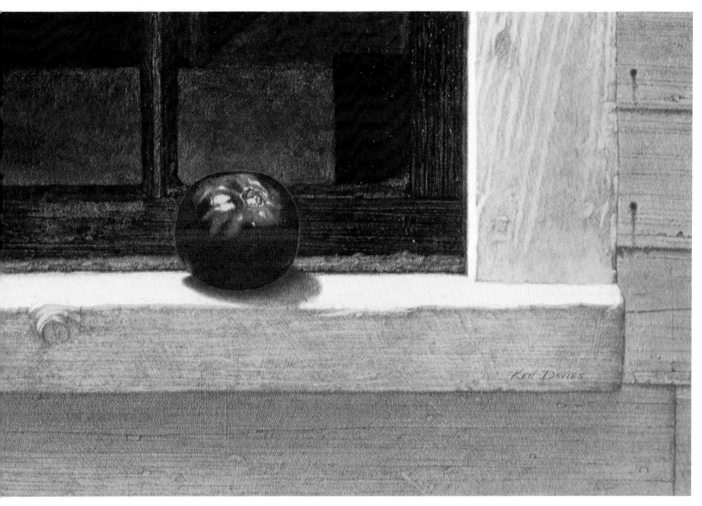

A Spot of Red. *I'm always happy when I'm able to combine realism with abstract composition, as in this painting. The subject, a tomato ripening on the windowsill of a house in New Hampshire, represents a memory of a visit to the summer home of a friend.*

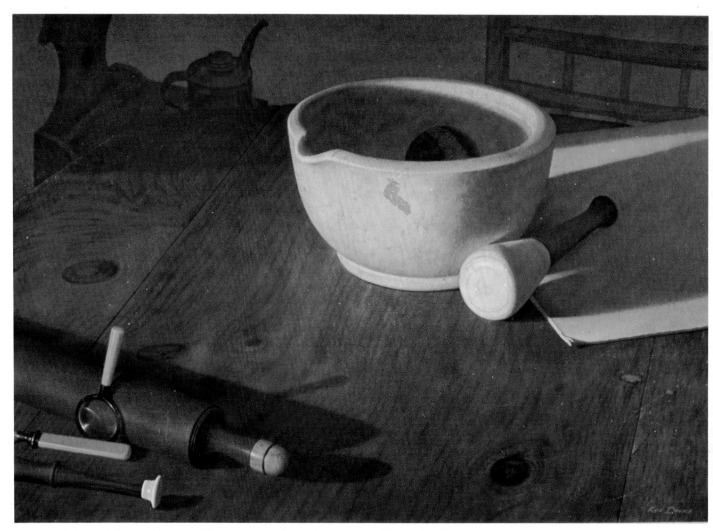

Light and Props (Above). The mortar and pestle are what I consider perfect subject matter, and I've used them again and again. I keep them on my living room mantle where I can glance at them every day for renewed inspiration.

White Eggs Plus (Right). When hung under proper lighting I can say that this is one of the most effective paintings I've done. I noticed the old bucket in a shop on Martha's Vineyard, and it was one of those occasions when an object created an instant impetus to paint—I visualized white eggs in the bucket the moment I saw it. I'm constantly foraging in antique shops for subject matter for still lifes, and usually when I find something I think I can use, I store it in my studio for months, or even years, while awaiting the proper moment to paint it.

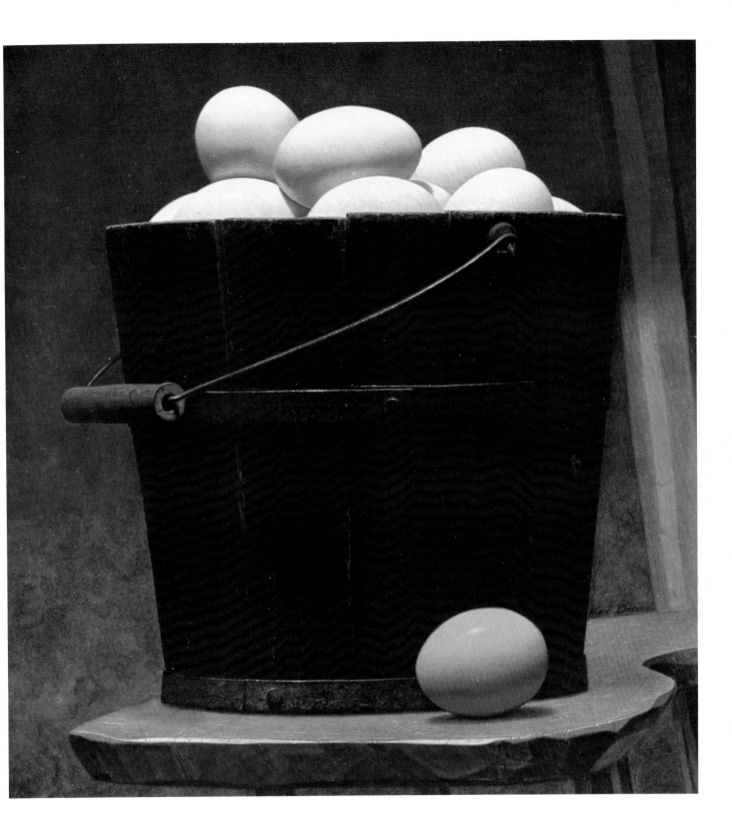

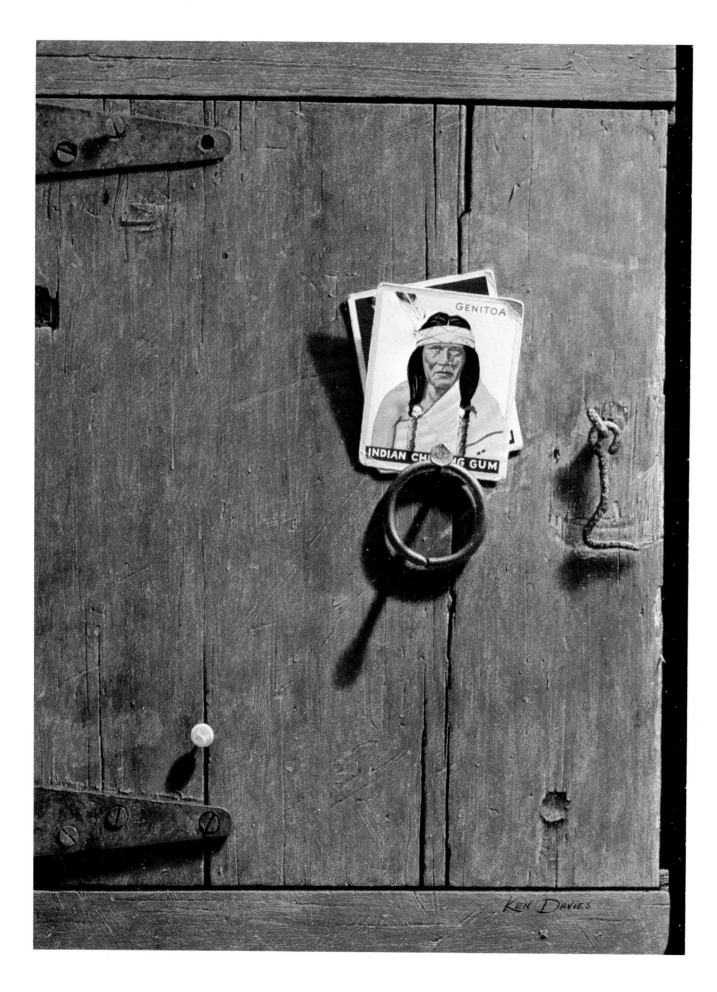

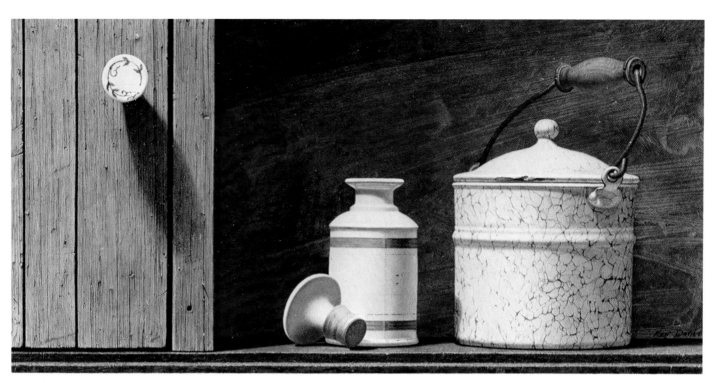

Genitoa and the Flying Horses Ring *(Left). In this trompe l'oeil I've used one of the Indian cards (the Indian's name is Genitoa) from my boyhood collection. Like so many other children, I coveted and occasionally won the gold ring while riding the Flying Horses carousel in Oak Bluffs, Martha's Vineyard. Even today the Flying Horses is still in use. The last time I returned there the attendants were still pushing the platform by hand to get it going as they did many years ago, carrying on an island institution—the oldest operating merry-go-round in the country.*

Next to the Cupboard *(Above). Two of my favorite props are used as subjects in this still life. I'm fascinated by old cupboard doors, particularly those with decorative white knobs, and I've used them and the two props repeatedly in my paintings. The blue pattern on the white knob provides an accent that suits the color harmony of the picture.*

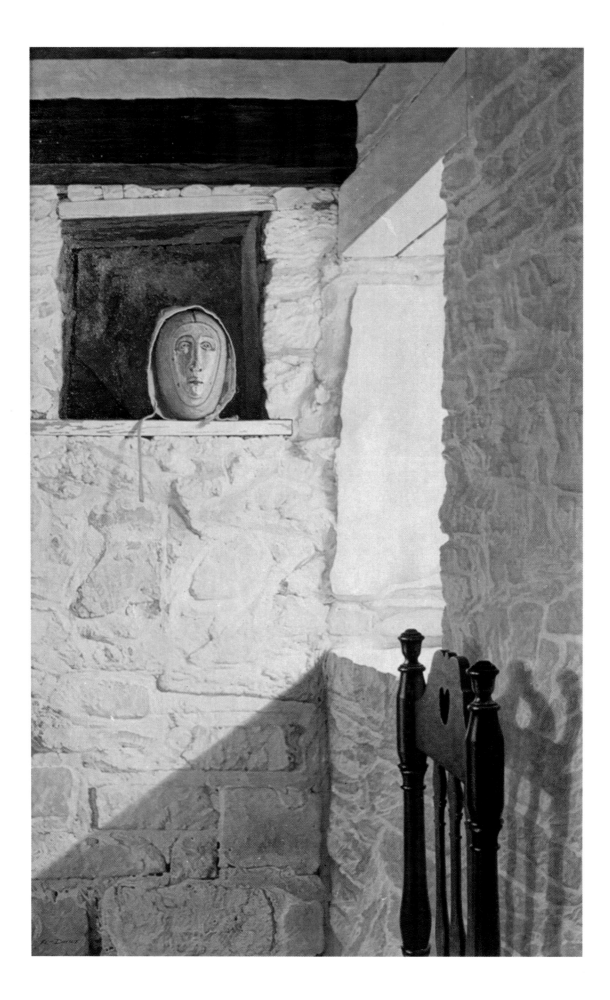

Mechanical and technical skills can be quite dogmatically demonstrated and taught, and any student, providing that she or he possesses the interest and patience, can acquire those skills by working through the first parts of this book in a dedicated way. I've said very little about *composition* until now, but from this point on more emphasis will be given to this subject.

The composition or structure of a painting, I think, is a complicated, esoteric, and problematic aspect. It's possible to make a judgment of a design for yourself, but impossible to make a definitive rule for others.

There are hundeds of books on the subject of design, and they contain hundreds of different expert opinions. Established painters are constantly involved in an intellectual struggle over how to compose their work. Students who are searching for their own "right" way may find themselves in a similar predicament. What should they do? I suggest that you start with externals: (1) read and study every available book on the theory of composition and design; (2) study the paintings of the old masters; (3) take an art history course; (4) investigate books on color and color relationships; (5) visit art galleries and museums. After a time you'll find that you've absorbed some very important information. And once you've developed an awareness of how a painting is composed, you should be ready to draw on your own internal attitudes on the design of your pictures. It is then time to ask yourself, "Where do I want the center of interest? Do I even want a center of interest? What will be the color harmony or dominance of this painting? Where shall I place my lights and darks?"

In the Whitfield House (Left). *The Whitfield House, reputedly the oldest stone house in the United States, is located in Guilford, Connecticut. I found the subject for this painting while exploring the second floor: I spotted the wooden bonnet form in the bedroom and decided to use it. The painting took more than 300 hours to complete, the longest time I've ever spent on one picture.*

BREAKING THE RULES OF COMPOSITION AND DESIGN

With the experience that comes from painting on a regular basis, your concept of composition and design will mature. Decisions will come more easily and you'll begin to use instinct more often than the rule book. I found this was especially true in my own development as a painter. Now at times I'll deliberately violate one or more of the established rules. For example, in the painting *On Peases' Point Way* I deliberately placed the focal point in dead center and made the picture almost perfectly symmetrical instead of heeding the old clichés "never put the center of interest exactly in the center; never divide a painting in half; asymmetrical is more interesting than symmetrical." And the painting worked.

SUBJECT MATTER

Many of my compositions evolve as a result of my fascination with the abstract forms of some of my subjects. This was true in *Window on Dock Street*. Several years ago, while I was on one of my many subject-searching trips on Martha's Vineyard where I've spent many summers since boyhood, I stopped for a sandwich at an outdoor lunch counter on Dock Street in Edgartown. As I turned to leave the counter, I glanced at the tiny building directly across the street and saw a window. It was one of those wonderful, unexpected moments when a complete subject for a painting suddenly appears. The abstract shapes formed by the shadows on the torn window shade and the reflection in glass of the building across the street totally intrigued me. I knew I had a good subject. The window looked exactly as you see it in the painting except for the antique doll, which I added later as a point of interest.

I felt lucky to have found the spot, thinking that if I had stopped for lunch just an hour or two earlier or later I would have completely missed this particular pattern of shapes. From experience I know that I can always return to

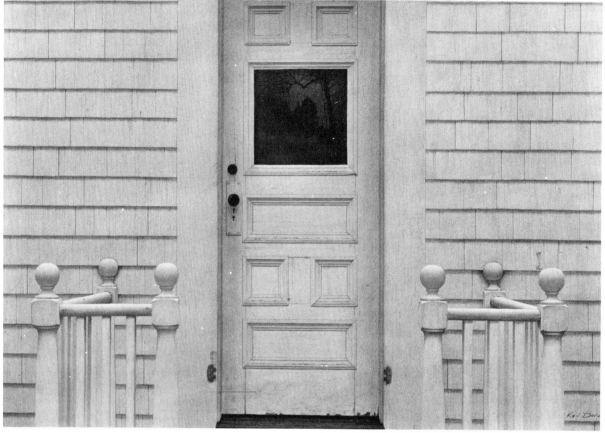

On Pease's Point Way

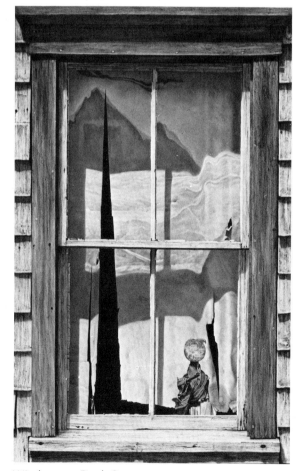

Window on Dock Street

146

the same place or subject again and again at different times of the day and find a totally new and unexpected thing happening there. Several of my paintings evolved as a result of an unexpected confrontation with the subject. Among them are, *A Spot of Red, An Abstract Trompe*, and *In the Whitfield House*, all illustrated in the Color Plates.

TROMPE L'OEIL, WHAT IS IT?

In the demonstrations that follow, I invite you to look over my shoulder and "tune in" to my own thinking on design and technical procedures while I lead you through the construction of several of my paintings from start to finish. The first demonstration will illustrate what I like to think of as my specialty, trompe l'oeil still life painting.

The French term *trompe l'oeil* translates literally as "fool the eye." For our purposes, let the definition be: *a still life painting in which the objects are so realistically rendered that the viewer is often tricked into believing they're real.* In a convincing trompe l'oeil, some of the objects seem to project themselves into the space between the flat plane of the picture and the eye of the viewer.

Trompe l'oeil painting dates back through the history of art to a legend of a Greek artist named Zeuxis of the Ionian school who painted a bunch of grapes so perfectly that birds swooped down to eat them. There are monumental examples of trompe l'oeil paintings that remain from the Renaissance period. During this time Veronese, among others, painted whole walls of rooms with decorations, false pillars, doorways, and windows. More recently Raphaelle Peale and my three personal favorites, John Haberle, William Michael Harnett, and J.D. Chalfant, established trompe l'oeil painting as a form of American folk art.

Although a trompe l'oeil is always a still life, a still life is not always a trompe l'oeil. In order to be a good trompe l'oeil the painting must have a depth that appears to be no more than a few inches.

The eye is fooled when a shallow depth is represented in the painting. Simply stated, when the human eye perceives a three-dimensional object from any distance, the eye muscles must make adjustments to focus on it. When the eye sees a painted object, the muscles no longer have to make those adjustments because the eye need only focus on the two-dimensional picture plane where illusion of depth is provided by perspective. Because the muscle adjustments are not as complicated as they are when viewing a three-dimensional scene, the depth of the painting is never really convincing. On the other hand, if the depth of the painting is extremely shallow, thereby minimizing the eye muscle activity, then the illusion of reality is enhanced.

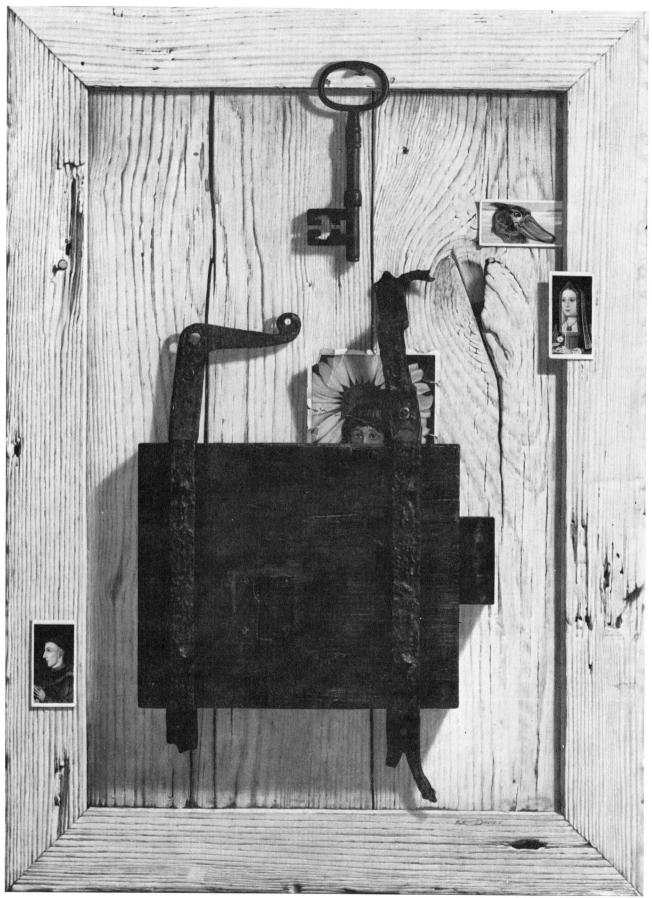

Iron, Wood, and Paper

DEMONSTRATION 1
FROM THE SKETCHBOOK

To exemplify my definition of trompe l'oeil painting, I've included several typical devices in the first demonstration painting, *From the Sketchbook*.

Setup. The background of the painting is a battered blue door with hinges (Figure 1) and a small white porcelain knob. The door and the picture plane are one and the same, which assures a minimum of depth in the setup: the depth from the tip of the white knob to the inside of the knothole is no more than an inch or so. Tacked to the door is a page from one of my sketchbooks. I plan compositional details, such as the shadows of the thumbtacks pushed in at different depths, the perforated edge of the paper, and the shadows on the door cast by the slightly curled and wrinkled page in order to heighten the eye-fooling effect in the finished painting. During the drawing I decide to show pencil sketches of three demonstrations from the book: the sketch for this painting itself is shown just behind and above the blackboard; the sketch for Demonstration 2, *Gray's Spoons*, shows to the left of the blackboard: and just barely visible to the right of the blackboard is the sketch for Demonstration 3, *A Gisler Mallard* (Figure 2).

The small blackboard, one of my favorite props bought many years ago in Williamsburg, Virginia, has been used in several of my paintings. I like it particularly because it gives me the opportunity to include painted chalk marks in a picture, and also because I can use a most startling and effective trompe l'oeil trick—a drop of water.

The Buffalo Bull Indian card tucked behind the page from the sketchbook is from a collection of chewing-gum cards I've saved since I was a young boy. The set was one of my prized possessions, and through the years I've used several cards from it in my trompe l'oeil paintings. One of them appears in *Genitoa and the Flying Horse's Ring*, which is reproduced in the Color Plates. The title of the painting was partly inspired by that card.

The final item I add to the setup is the small newspaper clipping (Figure 3), another favorite prop used by trompe l'oeil painters past and present. The clipping is part of an actual review of one of my exhibitions. The headline is quite clear, but the small typeface in the sketch is painted in illegible hieroglyphics. However at first glance the small typeface seems readable, and invariably the viewer moves in for a closer look only to find that the artist, tongue in cheek, has had his joke. Some painters have used the newspaper clipping device but have made the fine print totally readable—a most difficult feat. Notable among those are J.D. Chalfant and John Haberle, who are in my opinion two of the most skillful trompe l'oeil artists of all time.

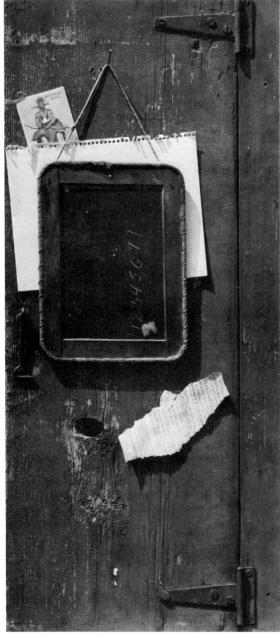

1. *Original setup*

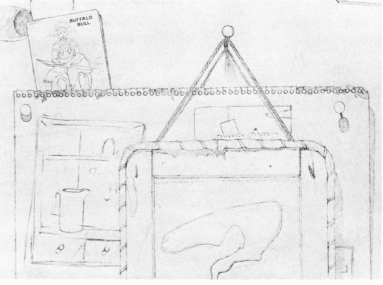

2. *Line drawing*

3. *Drawing of newspaper clipping*

Rough Sketch. For many paintings, a small rough sketch is the only preliminary drawing I make (Figure 4). The basic thinking is worked out in roughs like this before I go on to make the finished drawing on the panel. In some cases, the little pencil-rough is almost an exact miniature of the finished painting. My drawing for *The Umbrella Stand* is an example of a rough sketch with which I'm able to visualize the end result (Figure 5).

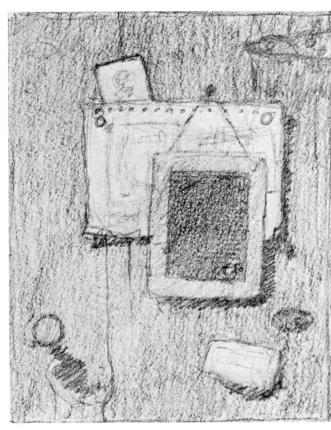

4. *Rough sketch*

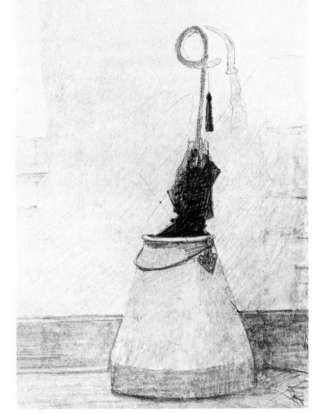

5. *Rough sketch for* The Umbrella Stand *(page 130)*

Line Drawing on Primed Panel. From the rough sketch I make a precise drawing on primed panel (Figure 6). I carefully draw the shadows in the finished line drawing. I like to use ¼" thick Masonite panels which I prime (coat) with acrylic gesso. Masonite board can be cut to the panel size you want at any lumberyard, and acrylic gesso is usually stocked by art supply stores. I apply one coat of gesso to the back of the panel and two coats to the front, using a wide, flat bristle brush. The bristle gives the gesso coat a very subtle texture, insuring against an overly smooth, slick finish. The bristle finish is also useful when developing the textures of wood or stone in a painting. Where texture is considered undesirable (in this case on the newspaper clipping and the Indian card), it can be sanded off the panel with fine sandpaper.

I take care to draw all the objects in the setup actual size. As a general rule in trompe l'oeil painting, this heightens the fool-the-eye effect. When satisfied with the drawing I spray it with a couple of coats of fixative, making sure that the whole drawing is covered.

Wash-in. I mix thin washes of pigment at the approximate values and colors I'll want them in the finished painting. I then proceed to wash in the objects and the background, brushing the thinned paint in the direction of the actual wood grain to suggest its texture. I think of the wash-in as a very valuable step. It quickly covers all of the white panel, and I can get a fairly accurate impression of the finished painting from the start.

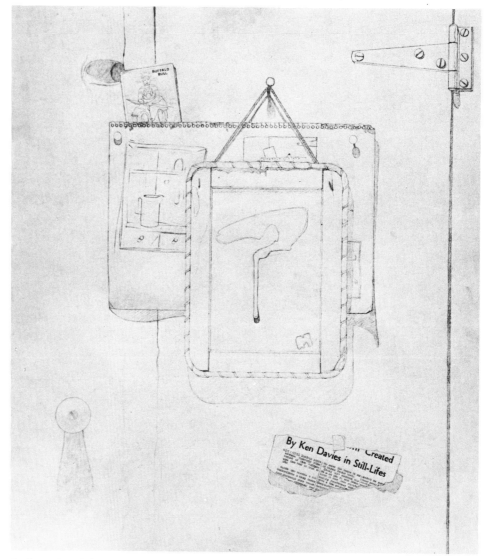

6. *Completed drawing*

Block-in and Details. The block-in is a second coat of opaque or semi-opaque paint that is applied after the wash-in is totally dry. If you've completed all the exercises, you should be quite familiar with this procedure.

In the wash-in/block-in stage in the Color Plates, the wooden door shows all three degrees of completion (wash-in, block-in, and final highlights and details). The upper left area around the knothole is finished, the middle area is blocked in with opaque color, the objects are washed in, and the lower section at the white knob and newspaper clipping is washed in and awaits a second coat.

The texture of the wood grain, created during the wash-in, barely shows through the block-in above the knob (I used some of this texture advantageously when painting the wood grain). The opaque block-in also lightens the shadows under the sketch page and the blackboard; the shadow under the white knob is still in the transparent wash-in stage and is still quite dark (Figure 7). (In the finished painting in the Color Plates the knob appears white, but it is actually several values darker to provide contrast with the highlights. Even the highlight is mixed with yellow ochre, cadmium yellow light, and white.)

I apply the paint in the wash-in and block-in just up to, yet not over, the objects. A little overlapping is acceptable, but I prefer to avoid this in order to keep the drawing intact.

Normally I'd block in the entire wood background before painting any of the texture, but to illustrate the steps involved I finish the detail on only one section of the wood before completing the block-in.

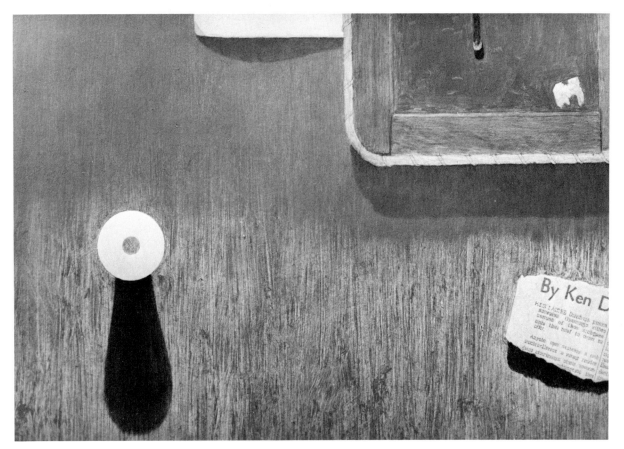

7. *Partial block-in*

Scumbling the Wood Texture. Using an old sable brush loaded with an opaque mixture of paint, I place the bristles flat against the panel (Figure 8). I dry-brush (scumble) the paint, which is slightly lighter in value than the coat beneath it. Using quick back-and-forth strokes I develop an irregular broken texture on the surface. I scumble in the shadow areas as well, making them barely discernible. This dry-brushing produces various interesting shapes.

Then, with a well-pointed sable brush, I accent the shadows and highlights of the accidental shapes produced by dry-brushing to make them look like holes, scratches, grooves, and cracks on the surface of the wood. Also, when I find an interesting shape from the original wash showing through, I make use of it for textural effects. I'd advise you to keep a piece of old, slightly battered wood around as a model to work from.

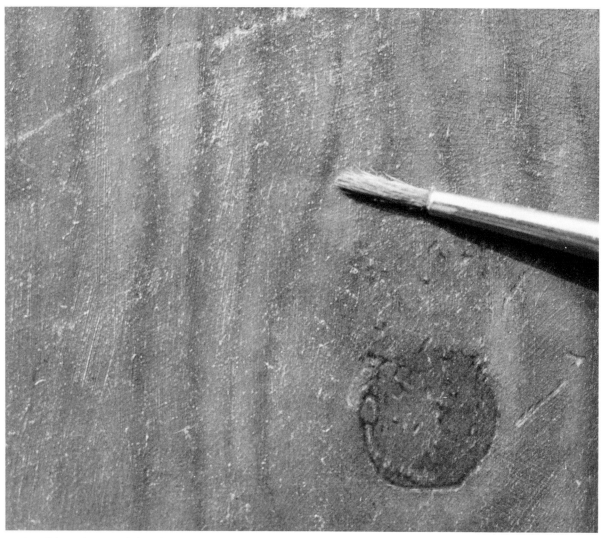

8. *Scumbling the wood detail*

Glazing the Wood Texture. After painting the texture, I let it dry thoroughly. Then I glaze the shadows as outlined in Exercise 13: (1) I wash on the glaze; (2) I daub it with a soft rag; and (3) I add one more step at this point—with an old filbert brush, I carefully dab at the edge of the finished shadow to soften it slightly. If you try this, remember that the edge of a shadow closest to the object casting it is very sharp, but the further the shadow is from the object the softer it becomes. Be sure that the shadows and the wood grain are completed before painting the objects in the setup. It's virtually impossible to glaze a shadow without running some paint over an object adjacent to the area you're glazing. This may mean repainting an already finished object; therefore, I always recommend that you paint the background first.

Before the shadows are glazed (Figure 9) you can see that the wooden door appears flat. After glazing (Figure 10), the shadows create the illusion of projecting the objects away from the wooden door and thereby begin to lend a three-dimensional effect to the picture.

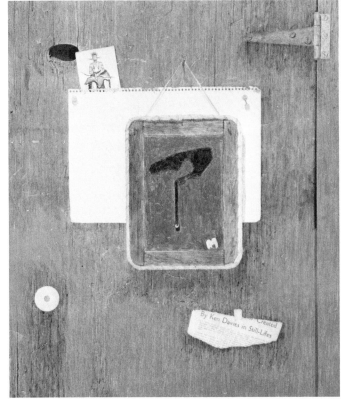

9. *Before glazing*

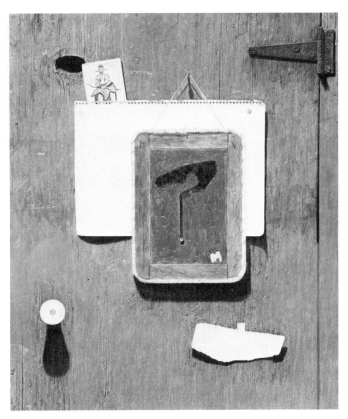

10. *After glazing*

Painting the Objects. After completing the background, the first object I tackle is the Indian card. It's painted actual size (Figure 11). My aim is to match the colors of the real card so accurately that when it's held next to the painted one it will be hard to tell which is real and which is painted. (This is a direct application of the Matching Chart assignment in Project 4.)

When the wash-in is dry (Figure 12), I block in the same area. The block-in almost completely covers the sketch, but the original pencil lines, just barely visible, still serve as a guide when it's time to add the final details (Figure 13).

After the block-in dries, I paint subtle wrinkles in the page (just as the wrinkles in the brown paper bag were drawn in Project 1). I then paint the highlights on the top perforations of the page. Just under the perforated edge I glaze the shadows down to darken them somewhat.

Next I glaze down the shadows of the thumbtacks, the right edge of the blackboard, and the strings holding it to the door. Using a pointed sable, I dry-brush the lines still visible in the pencil sketches with a mixture of raw umber, cobalt blue, and white. On completion they appear to be actual fine-penciled lines (Figure 14).

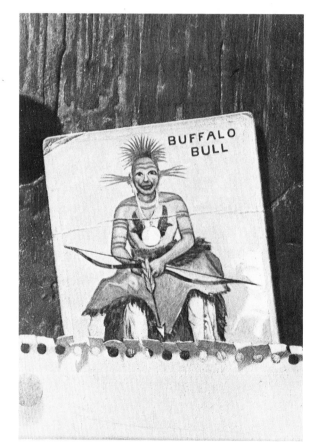

11. *Indian card (actual size)*

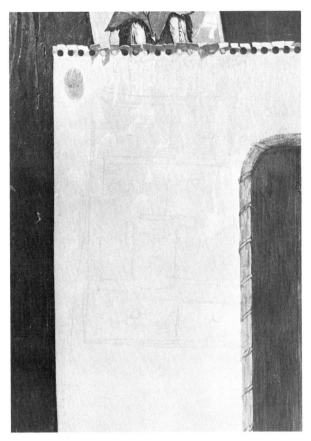

12. *Wash-in of sketchbook page*

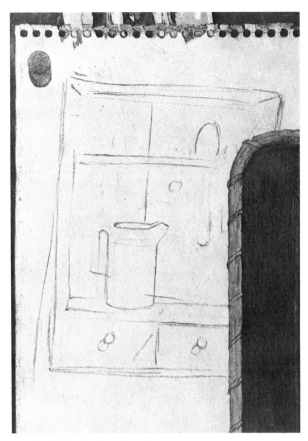

13. *Block-in of sketchbook page*

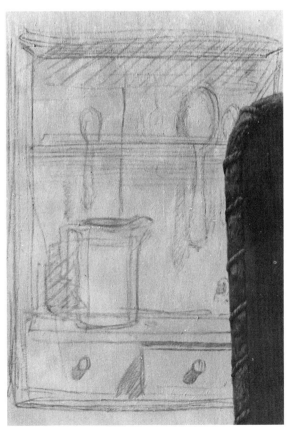

14. *Sketchbook page dry-brushed*

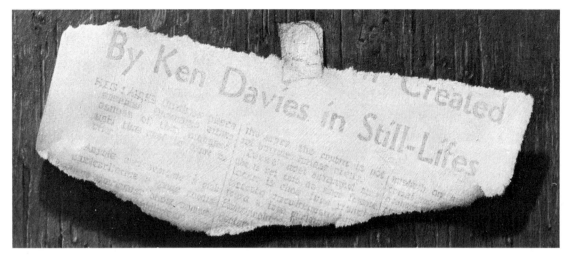

15. *Block-in of newspaper clipping*

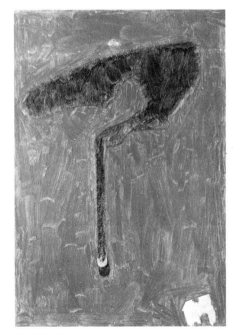

16. *Newspaper clipping completed*

By Ken Davies in Still-Lifes

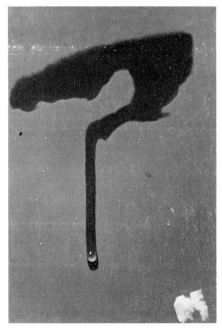

17. *Wash-in*

18. *Block-in*

19. *Completed*

The newspaper clipping is treated in much the same way as the sketchbook page. I paint the typeface with a very small sable, using a mixture of cobalt blue, raw umber, and white in place of black (Figures 15 and 16). Had I used black paint the type would have looked too dark in value to be convincing.

After painting the knob and the hinge, which are quite routine, the last object to be painted is the blackboard. After the wash-in (Figure 17) and drying period, I block it in entirely (Figure 18). Notice that in the block-in, the surface of the blackboard is not black but is a gray mixed with cobalt blue, raw umber, and white. By varying the quantity of blue and brown I can control this mixture to get different grays. (Remember the middle-value gray you painted without black on the Value Scale in Project 4?)

The wet area and the drop of water are simply darker values of the same gray mixture. The shadow under the drop is burnt umber and ultramarine blue. As I'm painting the wet spot, I keep dabbing the real blackboard with water and studying it as the drop runs down the board. I softly blend the upper edge of the wet area since the water dries there first as it moves downward on the board. A drop of water is a very effective trompe l'oeil device, yet it's actually very easy to paint. I add the shadow, the tiny light on the lower edge of the drop, and a good, sharp pinpoint of a highlight, and presto! The drop really looks wet.

While finishing the blackboard itself (Figure 19), I add some smudges and scratches with a small, pointed sable. I then carefully copy the character of real chalk letters which I had drawn on the real blackboard by dry-brushing with a slightly worn No. 8 round sable brush. Once again, although the chalk line looks white in the painting, it's actually an off-white mixture of yellow ochre, cadmium yellow light, and white.

Varnishing. I let the painting dry for about a week or so and then coat it with retouch varnish. Retouch varnish revives the areas that have dried and "gone dead." After four to six months, when the painting has dried completely, a final coating of damar and matte varnish can be applied. I've always used a ⅔ damar, ⅓ matte mixture, but I suggest that you experiment with the proportions to get the degree of glossiness you want. The professional restorers with whom I've discussed final varnishing seem to prefer the newer synthetic varnishes.

Keeping Wet Paintings Clean. I have mentioned earlier that dust is the number one enemy of the painter. I wage a constant battle with this villain, and you will, too. It's impossible to eliminate dust completely, but perhaps these tips will help: (1) when not working on the painting, lean it with its face to the wall; (2) before each painting session, lightly lift the dust from your painting with masking tape (especially before glazing or applying retouch varnish); (3) after glazing a large area, lean the painting toward the wall, leave the room, and shut the door until the glaze is dry (the less motion there is in the room, the less dust there will be to collect on your painting); (4) don't clean, dust, or vacuum your studio while there is a wet painting in it; (5) don't acquire long-haired pets that shed. I have three cats, and although I try to keep them out of the studio, they do get in from time to time. Wet paint is the perfect magnet for loose cat hairs it seems, so I keep a pair of tweezers nearby to combat this problem.

The finished painting is reproduced in color on page 56.

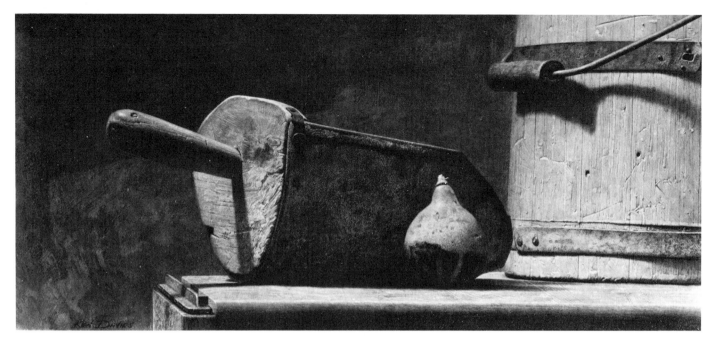

Scoop and Gourd

DEMONSTRATION 2   GRAY'S SPOONS

An old spoon cabinet that belongs to a friend was the inspiration for *Gray's Spoons*. The painting doesn't quite qualify as a trompe l'oeil because the actual cabinet is between six and seven inches deep. The depth of a trompe l'oeil setup is usually shallower (see Demonstration 1). The illusion of reality is, nonetheless, quite startling in the finished work.

Composition. To suit my proposed composition for the painting I alter the appearance of the cabinet somewhat by adding drawers at the base and reducing the number of spoons which originally hung across the top shelf to three. In the finished painting in the Color Plates you can see that the white knob on the right-hand drawer is slightly larger than the one on the left. Since the drawer is slightly open, the right-hand knob is brought closer to the viewer's eye. By the rules of perspective, then, this knob must be larger to give an illusion of closeness.

For contrast and interest I add the white pitcher to the setup. Most of the final decisions on composition are made in a small rough sketch which I use as a preliminary to the line drawing. (The rough sketch for this painting is included in Figure 2 of Demonstration 1, *From the Sketchbook*.)

Line Drawing. After making the final decisions on the placement of the objects, I make a line drawing using simple one-point perspective (Figure 1). The eye level, or horizon line, is just under the shadow of the upper shelf of the cabinet, and the vanishing point (indicated by a small dot) is in the center of the cabinet. All receding lines of the sides of the cabinet and drawers converge at that dot. This is a practical application of one-point perspective, which was discussed in A Lesson in Perspective presented earlier in this book.

After sketching the outlines, I rough-shade some of the shadows in the drawing to get an early effect of light and shade areas.

Drawing the Spoons. In sketching the spoons, I use the approach to drawing symmetrical objects outlined in Project 1, Line Drawing. I draw the center line, and I outline half of the spoon. Then I trace it, flip the tracing over, and bringing the center lines into register, I transfer the tracing to the opposite half of the spoon. Finally, I add the outlines of the reflections on the handles and the bowls (Figure 2).

Drawing the Pitcher. The floral border along the top of the pitcher is a particularly important detail to retain (Figure 3). I foreshorten the tiny roses as they follow the curve of the pitcher to enhance the illusion of roundness. (This is the same principle as foreshortening a circle into an ellipse discussed in A Lesson in Perspective). Also, I use a very dark pencil line to draw the border so that the details will show through during the wash-in and block-in stages. If detail like this is lost during the painting procedure, two undesirable things happen: (1) you've wasted time drawing it in the first place, and (2) it's far more difficult to reshape the details with paint or pencil over the oil block-in.

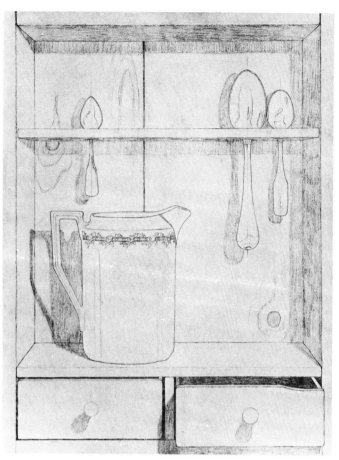

1. *Line drawing*

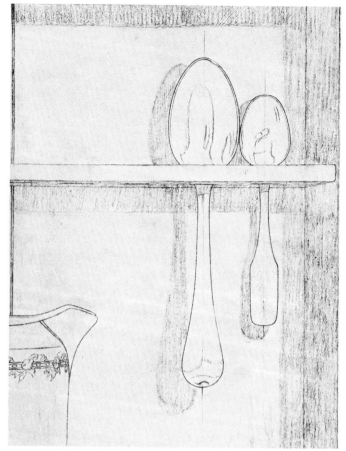

2. *Drawing of spoons*

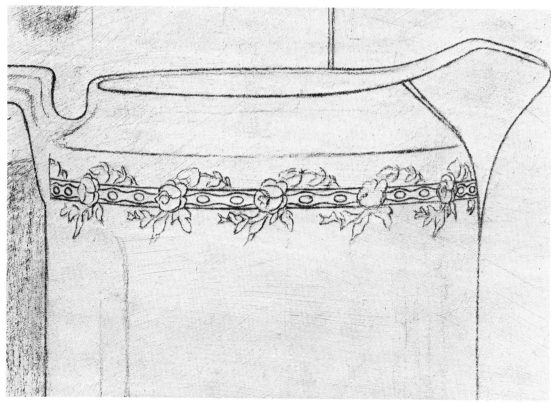

3. *Foreshortening the roses*

Wash-in and Block-in. I take great care (by using adequately thinned transparent paint) not to lose the drawing in the wash-in stage. (See the wash-in stage of *Gray's Spoons* in the Color Plates.) I paint all the wood and surface textures according to the procedure outlined in Demonstration 1 under Wash-in. Then, to reproduce the wood grain of the back wall of the cabinet, I block in the back wall with a flat layer of paint (Figure 4). When the painting is completely dry, I paint each line of wood grain with a thin coat of raw umber using a pointed No. 8 sable brush. To soften the grain and make it appear to blend in with the wood surface, I dab at each line of the grain with the flat side of a No. 7 filbert.

Scumbling. After allowing the painting to dry, I scumble the entire surface with a light, opaque mixture of raw sienna, raw umber, and white (Figure 5). As much as possible I try to keep the objects intact and avoid overlapping the paint onto the spoons, knobs, and pitcher. The scumbling technique makes the wood grain more believable. A common error in beginners' work is to paint wood grain too dark, thereby giving it an artificial look.

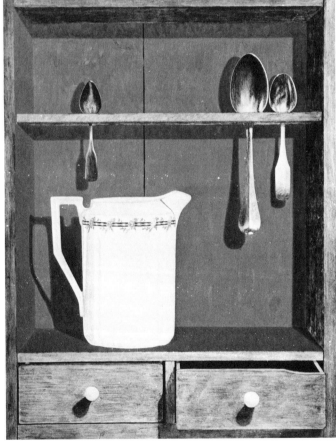

4. *Block-in of back wall of cabinet*

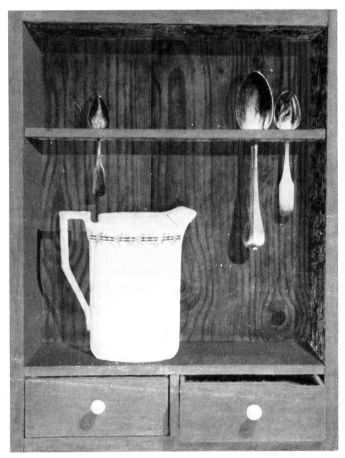

5. *Scumbling*

Final Details and Glazing. I next add all the tiny scratches and pinholes in the wood with a very small, pointed sable (No. 1). While painting the block-in I am especially careful to paint all edges of the shadows slightly softer than I eventually want them. This is important because if edges are too sharp in the block-in stage it's virtually impossible to soften them with the glaze. Yet the opposite is true; it's easy to sharpen up an edge when glazing. When all the details are thoroughly dried, I glaze the shadows. To make allowances for the reflected light I paint the inner right side and inner top of the cabinet lighter in value than the shadow on the back wall (Figure 6).

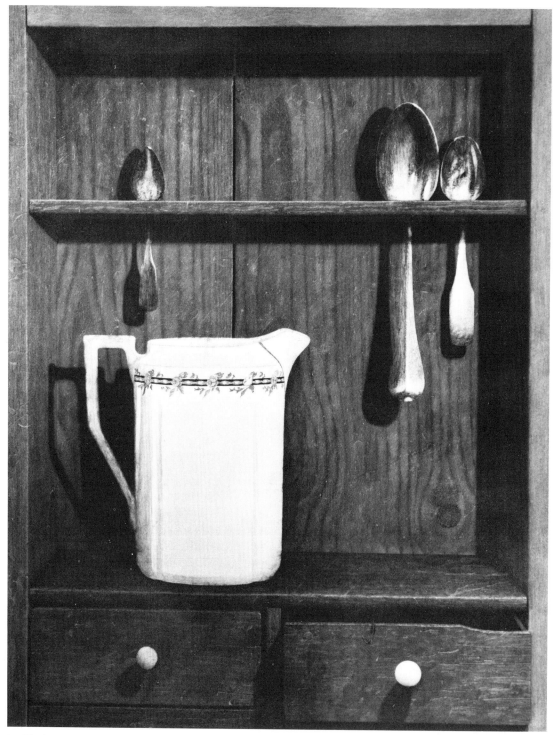

6. *Glazing*

Detailing the Spoons. In the close-up you can see that the silver spoons are completed except for the handle of the small one at the right. If you compare the details of the highlights and reflections in the bowls of the spoons to the drawing, wash-in, and block-in, you see that they remain virtually unchanged throughout. (See Exercise 5, Painting Glass and Metal.) The highlights are very light in value and appear white (Figure 7), but you can see from the finished painting in the Color Plates that the highlights are slightly tinged with yellow ochre and cadmium yellow light. This coloring is the standard result of lighting indoor setups with incandescent light.

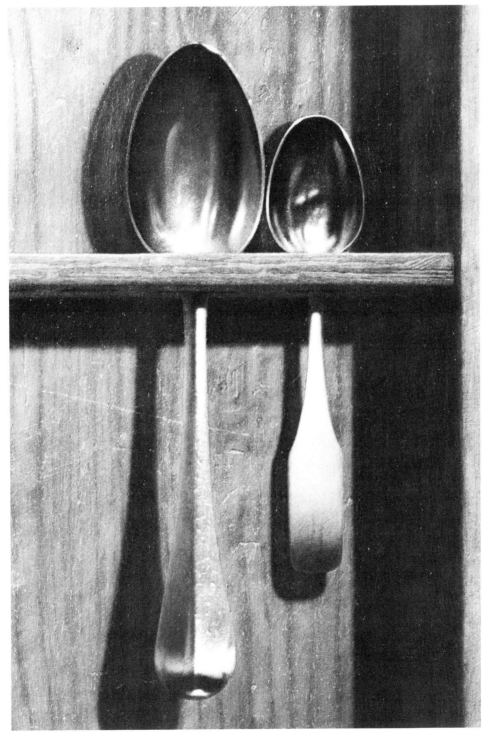

7. Detail of spoons

Painting the Pitcher. In the finished block-in of the white pitcher the lightest values appear to be white, but they are actually painted a darker value than white to offset the final highlights. The dark value of the wood around the pitcher further heightens its white appearance. (This principle is presented in Project 2 where the two gray squares seem to change in value when surrounded alternately by black and white borders.)

I blend the area where there is transition from light to shadow areas on the curve of the pitcher by dabbing and brushing with a filbert. Part of the detail on the floral border is almost, yet not completely, lost during this stage. This is unavoidable since I want a uniform transition from light to dark. However, it's very important for me to see the original detail through the blend. The floral decoration on the right side of the pitcher is relatively easy to see because there is little or no blending in that spot (Figure 8).

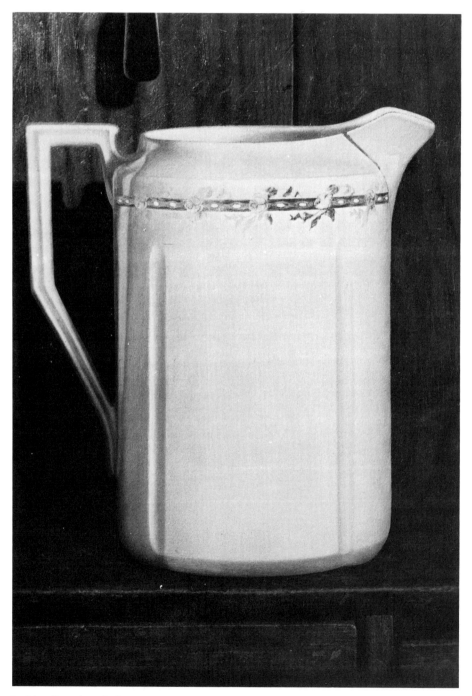

8. *Blending the pitcher*

Turning the Edges. I darken the floral border in the shadow area on the left and add final highlights, cracks, and surface details to complete the white pitcher. I glaze the shadows with a mixture of cobalt blue and raw umber. Often there is a danger that a white object against a dark background will appear to have been cut out of paper and pasted down on the painting. To avoid this I "turn the edges." By this I mean that I paint an extremely thin, dark line along the edge of the object. While the line is wet, I dab it carefully with an old, worn filbert brush, blending it very slightly into the object. I feel that this extra step makes a tremendous difference to the painting and is well worth the time and patience it takes.

The finished painting is reproduced in color on page 58.

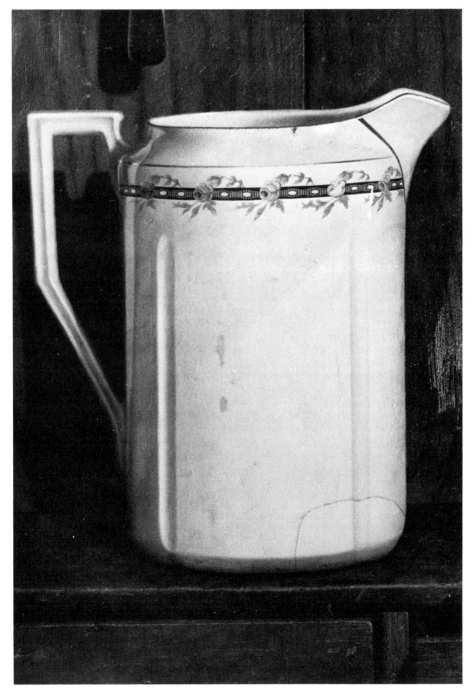

9. *"Turning the edges" on the pitcher*

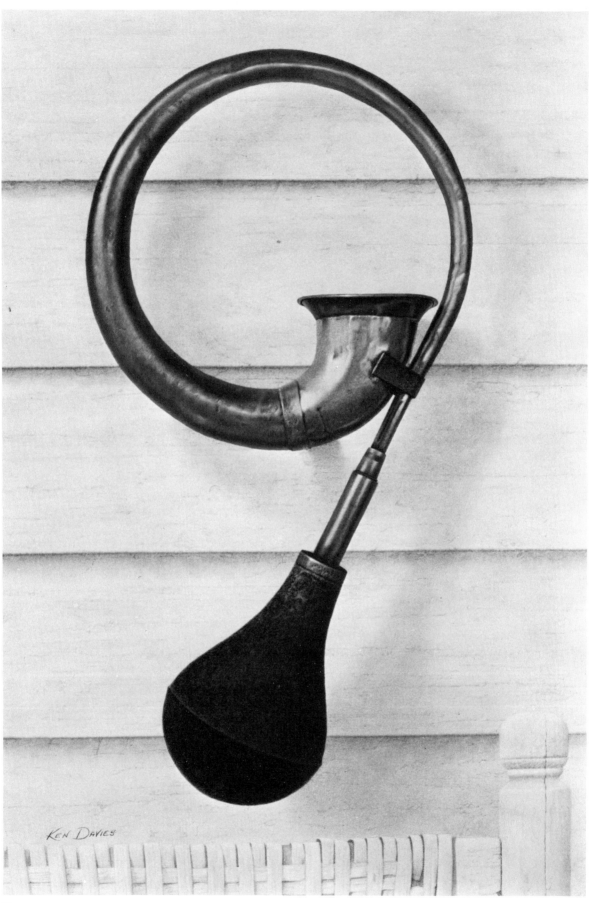

Horn

DEMONSTRATION 3 **A GISLER MALLARD**

The two wooden decoys that inspired *A Gisler Mallard* were spotted in a northern Connecticut antique shop by a fellow faculty member. (The mallard decoy was named after the man who made it and in duck-hunting circles his name is well known.) I bought the pair sight unseen from my colleague's vivid description and hearty recommendation. When the two decoys arrived I saw that they were everything he had described, and I began to think about painting them right then and there.

Composition. Because the decoys are dark in value, I decide they will look best set against a light background. The old, white clapboard of the house where I live has a wonderfully mellow quality that comes from years of weathering. I've used parts of the house for details in several paintings, and this seems like another perfect opportunity to use it as a backdrop. After a few strolls around the house, I finally decide on a section of wall outside the kitchen window on which are fastened cleats and ropes used to raise and lower the awnings.

My next problem is to set the decoys up against the house just below eye level. Since I don't have a table that seems just right, I invent one by combining real and imaginary parts of an old workbench.

Then I feel that the composition will need a thin, vertical shape at the left. Rummaging around at the back of my garage, I find just the prop I want—an old scythe handle—and with this the composition is complete.

While I'm putting together the setup, I develop the rough pencil sketch (Figure 1). The finished painting is almost identical to the pencil rough.

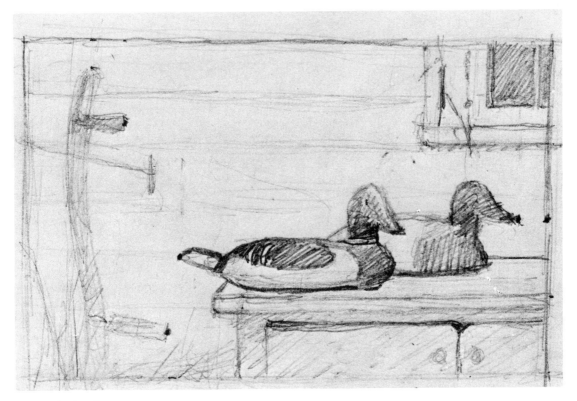

1. *Rough sketch*

Line Drawing. I make the line drawing on a Masonite panel primed with gesso (Figure 2). As I pencil in the setup, I add the stone foundation that shows slightly at the lower left corner. Before this impromptu addition, I found I had three isolated dark shapes—the window, the decoys on the workbench (as a unit), and the scythe. The foundation relates the scythe to the decoys and table, making the darks much more interesting. Moreover, I think the composition as a whole becomes more pleasing and solid-looking.

In the drawing the eye level is at the bottom of the clapboard that passes just behind the decoy's head. In the center of the picture a black dot marks the vanishing point. Upon examining the clapboards you can see a little of the under edges of those above the horizon line. The higher they are above the horizon line the more of the under edge you can see.

In the close-up of the decoy in the forefront (Figure 3), most of the subtle shapes on the darkest part of the back were sketched to serve as a kind of map during the wash-in. In the detail of the cleat and the rope (Figure 4), the twisted fibers of the ropes are darkened so they will also be visible after the wash-in and block-in. (See the wash-in stage of *A Gisler Mallard* in the Color Plates.)

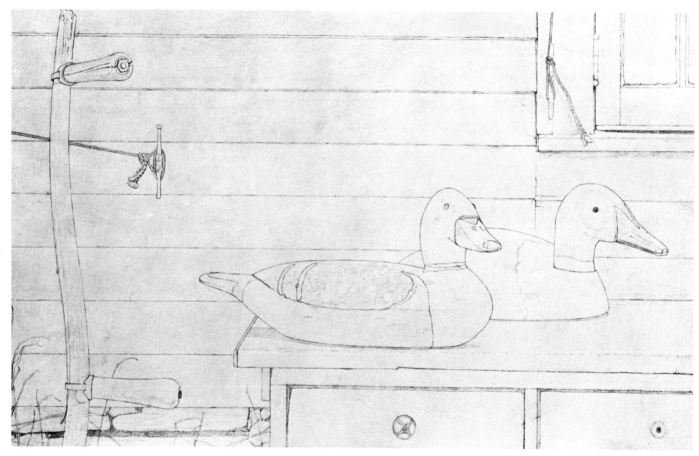

2. *Line drawing*

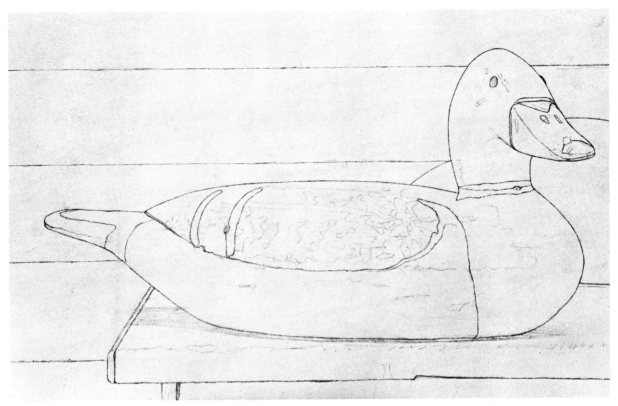

3. *Drawing of front decoy*

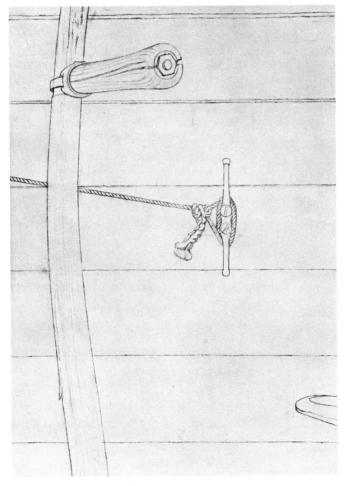

4. *Drawing of cleat and rope*

Painting the Clapboards. I paint the clapboards in various stages of completion (Figure 5). The lowest one is washed in. The next has been washed in and a first coat of rough texture created by dragging the side of an old round sable brush lengthwise over it has been added. The same brush technique was used to paint details on the wood surfaces in the first two demonstrations. But this time I add darker accents and details to the rough texture on the third clapboard, which has already received the first two steps. I paint the final and darkest accents on the topmost board. Each clapboard is painted in these four steps, and each one takes approximately three to four hours from start to finish.

When I work on this type of wood detail, I'm careful not to overdo the texture. I try to strike a happy medium by keeping details subtle. Wood surfaces should entertain the eye upon close examination, yet not distract the viewer from looking at the painting as a whole.

Painting this kind of texture can become rather monotonous, and the general tendency is to get fed up and rush through the procedures just to get them over with. Try to resist the temptation to hurry the job; it can ruin an entire painting. After a couple of hours of steadily painting details, I get that feeling myself. At that moment, I put the brush down, pick up my golf club, and hit a dozen or so balls. It doesn't necessarily help my golf score, but it does break the tension and monotony of painting.

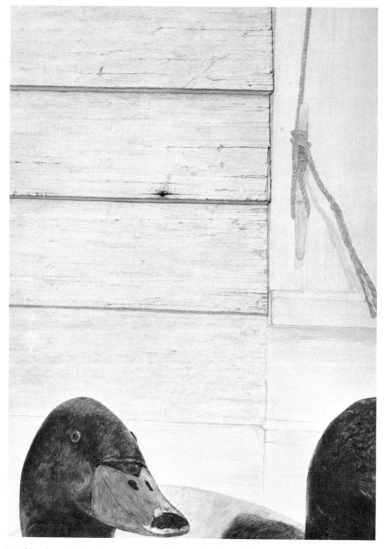

5. *Clapboards in four stages of completion (bottom to top) wash-in to finish*

Painting the Scythe and Rope. I wash in part of the scythe handle and the rope attached to the cleat with thinned paint (Figure 6). The texture created by the wash-in on the scythe handle will be utilized in painting the detail of its grain.

The close-up of the rope next to the window shows it in all three stages of completion (Figure 7). The uppermost part of the rope is finished, the middle part, which is wound around the cleat, is blocked in, and the lowest part is washed in.

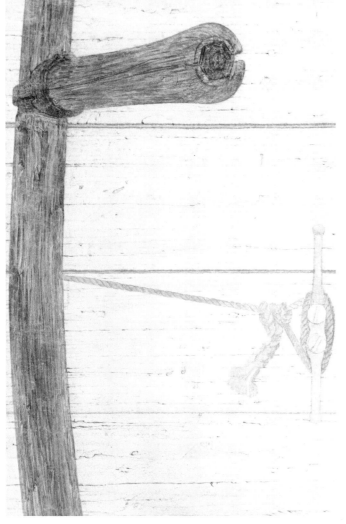

6. *Wash-in of scythe handle, rope, and cleat*

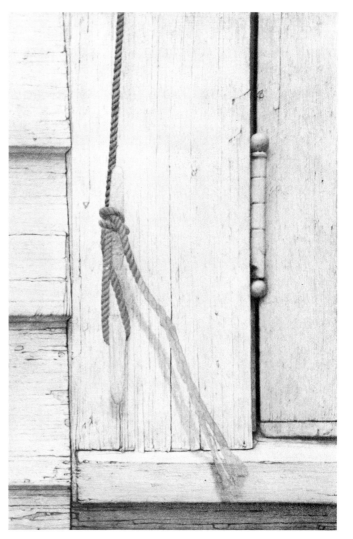

7. *Rope in three stages of completion (bottom to top) wash-in, block-in, and finish*

Part of the workbench is washed in, and its brushstrokes indicate the direction of the wood grain even at this preliminary stage (Figure 8). It will next be blocked in and glazed and scumbled as part of the detailing step.

Painting the Decoys and Workbench. The wash-in of the decoys has been completed; the block-in and detailing of the workbench are almost finished (Figure 9). The top of the workbench is made up of horizontal, elongated shapes. These shapes are important because they flatten the top surface and make it recede from the viewer.

I block in the decoys (Figure 10) and glaze down the shadow under the edge of the workbench to give it a three-dimensional look. The decoys, although now blocked in, are hardly changed from the wash-in stage.

The close-up of the mallard decoy, the central object of the painting (Figure 11), has been completed by what I call *selective rendering*. By that I mean I don't try to duplicate each and every crack and groove on its surface. Instead, I take advantage of what are, to my way of thinking, the most attractive details. I copy these quite faithfully and disregard the others. Occasionally I replace the unused details with my own invented shapes suggested by the wash-in. Which shapes to retain and which to discard are a matter of personal taste, and I believe that experience helps in making the best choices.

The finished painting is reproduced in color on page 60.

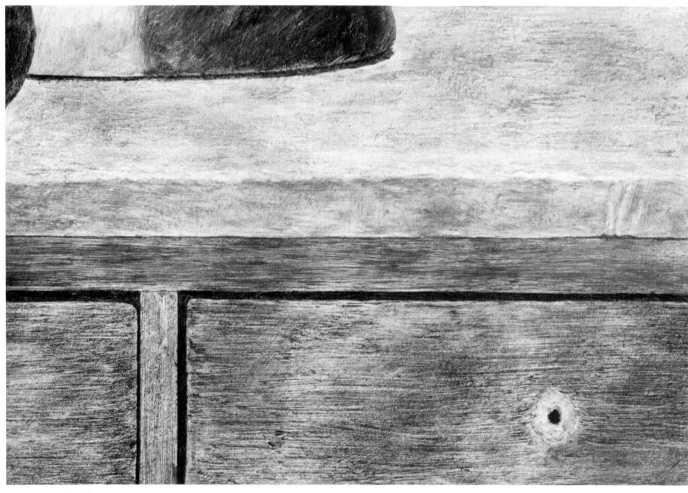

8. *Wash-in of workbench*

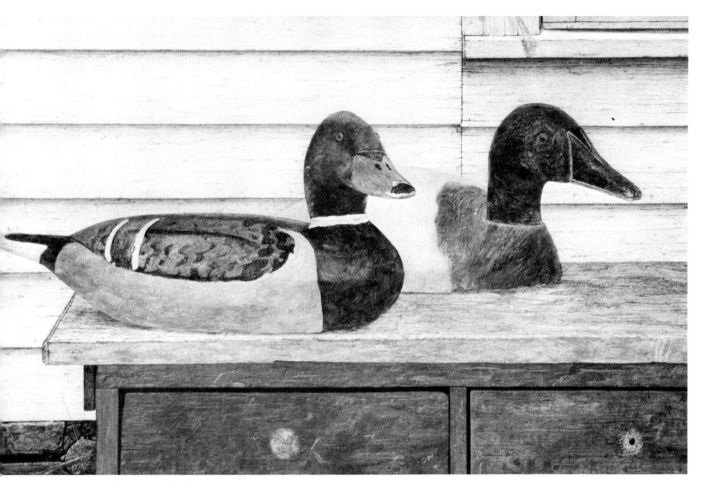

9. *Wash-in of decoys; block-in of workbench*

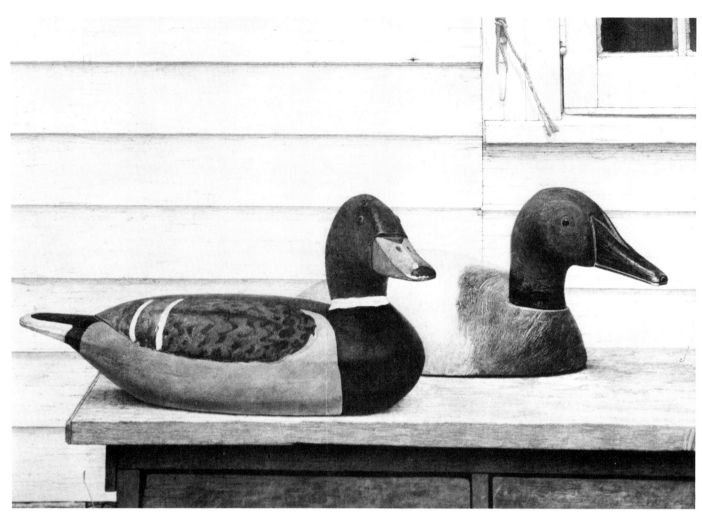

10. *Block-in of decoys; workbench shadow area glazed*

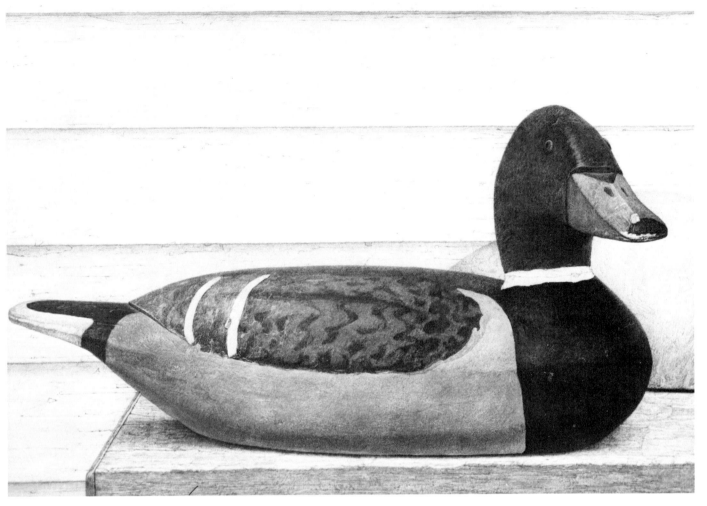

11. *"Selective rendering" of front decoy*

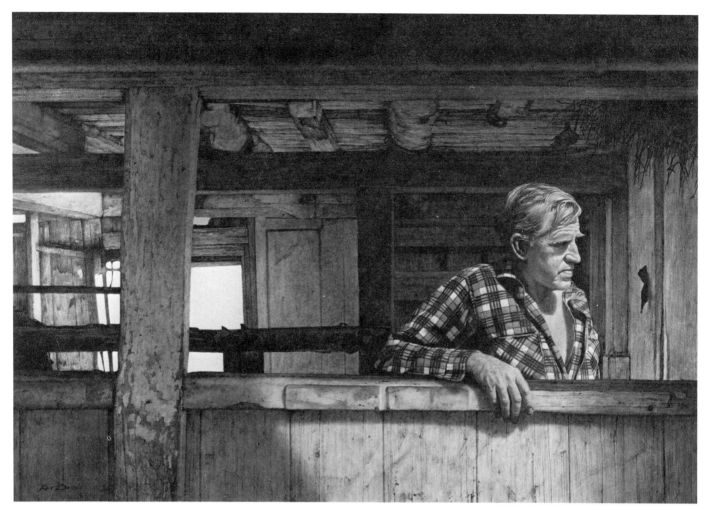
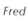

Fred

DEMONSTRATION 4 ON 139 NEAR 80

You may wonder why I include a painting of a barn in a book devoted totally to still lifes. The reason is that I consider the subject of this painting a still life. I don't believe there's a great difference between using the wooden wall of a barn as the backdrop for a trompe l'oeil still life and painting the entire barn in its own setting. Each entity can be part of a still life—the barn building, the tree, the pump, and the logs can be considered separate setups within the whole. There is no formal decree disputing my claim that a still life does not have to be restricted to the area of a tabletop. So if you enjoy painting buildings, barns, stone walls, or fences, call them landscapes or still lifes, but go ahead and paint them!

My own reason for painting barns stems from a long-standing affection for typical New England barn buildings. As subjects for paintings, I consider them ideal. Their shapes, colors, and sizes are limitless. Decidedly rich in source material, their aged wood exteriors are studded with shingles, latches, and hinges, while inside they are treasure chests bursting with irresistible trappings. It's not at all unusual for me to find subjects for a dozen or more paintings in a single barn.

I remember the sheer pleasure with which I explored the interior of a deserted barn one day and found an abstract pattern of lights and darks set off by wood beams glowing with age, their surfaces rich in detail. The scene truly took my breath away, and I used it soon after as the setting for the painting entitled *Fred*. The interior was recorded exactly as I saw it; not one detail was changed. Yet I felt that a human figure was needed for enlivenment. Soon after, I persuaded Fred, a friend for many years, to pose for me, and it was one of the the very rare instances when I've used a human figure in a painting.

I came upon the barn that inspired the painting in this demonstration accidentally while driving on Route 139 near Route 80 in North Branford, Connecticut, four years ago. It instantly caught my attention but didn't stir enough excitement to warrant a stop to investigate further. About five months later, just after a snowfall, I drove along the route again, and this time the sight of the barn dusted with snow set off a reflex. Blindly ignoring the road conditions, I jammed on my brakes to take a better look. The shape of the snow on the roof and the wood siding of the barn attracted me. The contours of the sloping eaves set the wheels in motion, and I was impatient to paint the barn still life.

Composition. Using the barn and the large tree as focal points, I begin to develop the composition. The barn, I think, will be placed in the upper right corner of the panel, fronted by a broad expanse of snow. I rough in the main shapes of the foreground and middle ground with charcoal pencil. I'm mainly interested in the major shapes rather than what they will contain. And when their places are established, I stop work to search for the appropriate coordinates to fill the voids and create perspective. I find most of what I need in my yard. For instance, the weeds shown poking through the snow were the result of my lack of enthusiasm with the lawn mower the previous fall, and the logs were the result of a burst of enthusiasm with the saw the previous day. The composition becomes whole with the addition of an old pump and a Connecticut snowfall.

Line Drawing. I make the line drawing directly on Masonite panel primed with gesso (Figure 1). The emphasized lines drawn on the silo represent the deepest cracks and the changes of color on the vertical slats. I sketch in only the largest branches of the trees; I'll add the smaller ones directly with a brush in the final step. In keeping with my usual painting procedure, the branches and weeds are drawn heavily so they won't be lost under the wash-in and block-in. I shade the rocky outcropping at the left of the barn to divide and clarify its different faces and prevent a jumble of lines from spoiling the whole shape.

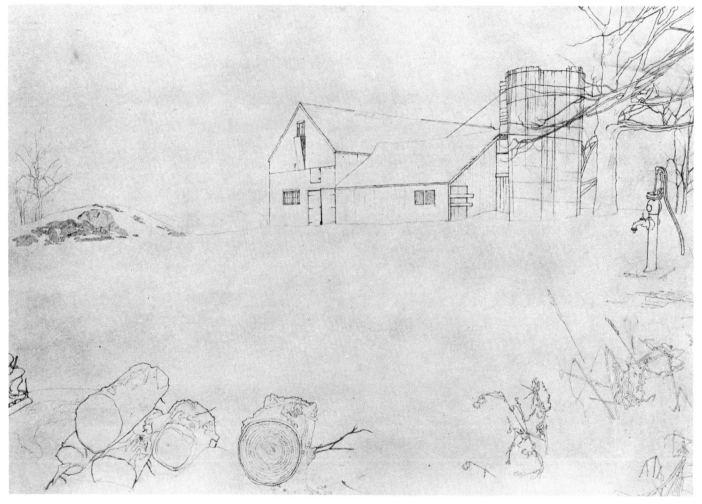

1. *Line drawing*

Wash-in. I reverse procedure and wash in the barn before painting the sky. (See the wash-in stage of *On 139 Near 80* in the Color Plates. Although I usually recommend painting backgrounds first, in this instance I want to key the value of the sky with the barn and snow. The sky, I feel, has to be darker than the snow on the roof, but at the same time light enough to offset the superimposed patterns of the body of the barn and the tree.

While the silo is still wet, I scratch out the thin, small branches of the tree with an old, stiff filbert brush. Although I plan to include puffy cumulus clouds, I wash in the entire sky area (with the exception of the slightly oblique cloud line running from the upper left edge to the barn) with a relatively flat, even color to establish its value. The oblique line suits the composition. It simply feels right and I'm instinctively comfortable including it. I rough-sketch the shapes of the clouds after the barn is dry (Figure 2).

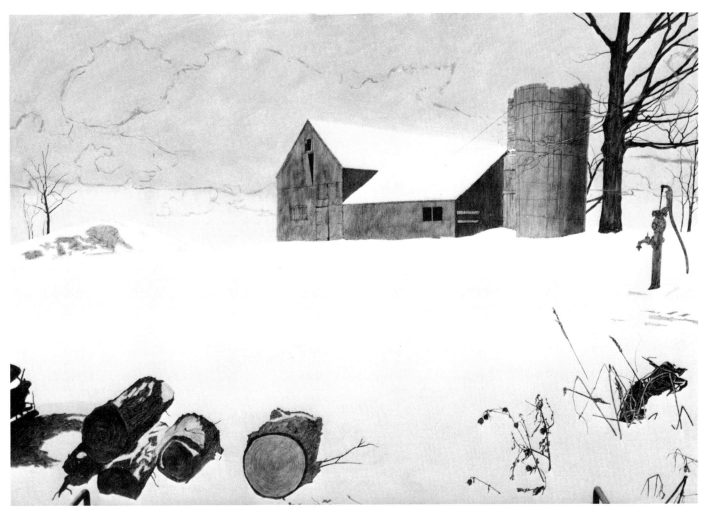

2. *Wash-in with rough-sketched clouds*

Painting the Background. The second coat of paint on the sky slightly overlaps the trees and parts of the barn (Figure 3), yet I take great care not to lose the drawing. At this critical point I run into unexpected trouble. Ideally, I prefer to be in complete control of a painting from beginning to end, to know exactly which effects I want and how to achieve them. But this time proves to be a bit different. It's late afternoon when I finish blocking in the sky, and just afterward I quit for the day. Upon resuming work the next morning I take a fresh look at the painting in progress, and it's immediately obvious that the clouds are all wrong for the picture. I was evidently carried away with their shapes, but now they look busy, with too much contrast, and they detract from the painting. I wanted the sky to be interesting, yet subtle, a backdrop for the barn rather than an aggressive passage. I correct the problem by painting a semi-opaque coat of light-value gray over the entire sky. After the paint dries, I can just barely see the cloud shapes through it (Figure 4). Remembering the mistake I made, I block in new cloud shapes to make them less overpowering in value and contrast.

The most interesting part of the sky is the open space to the left of the barn. Behind the tree the sky becomes very simple: almost flat. The corrected sky and an added stand of distant trees complete the background (Figure 5). At this point I block in the snow with a flat off-white.

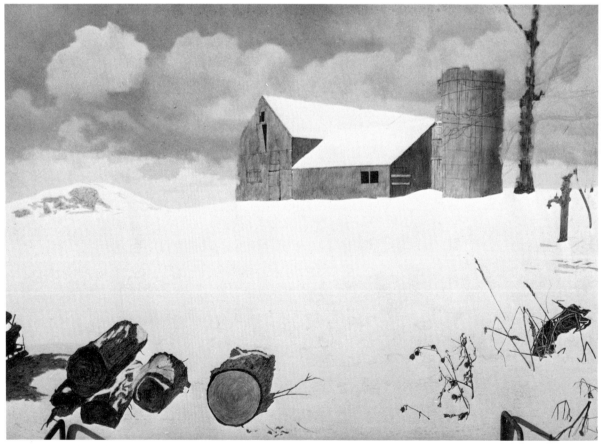

3. *First cloud block-in*

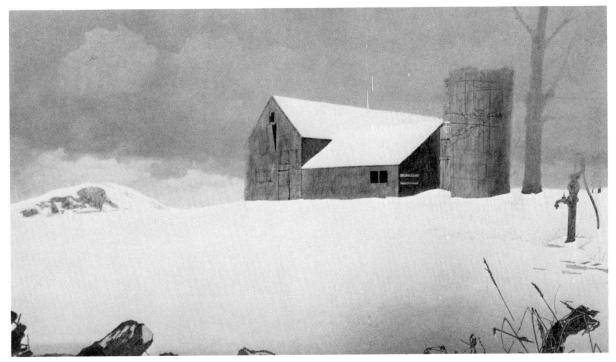

4. *Clouds corrected*

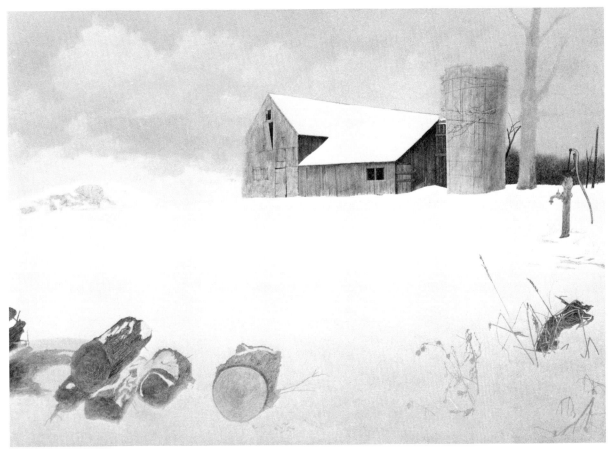

5. *Completed sky and block-in of snow*

Painting the Barn. In the close-up of the barn (Figure 6) the finished center section is a bit duller and grayer than the gaudy red color I applied during the wash-in (see the wash-in stage of *On 139 Near 80* in the Color Plates). To tone down the color of the first coat, I lightly dry-brush it with a coat of burnt umber and cobalt blue. While this second coat is still wet, I dry-brush light values of cerulean blue and raw sienna into it using vertical strokes to describe individual boards. Methodically, I apply the colors in combination and separately by turns over the surface. The layered colors slowly begin to resemble the aged barn siding.

After a drying period, I paint dark cracks and light accents on the siding of the barn. My aim is to present detail as it would be seen at a distance rather than painting each board in the fine detail reserved for objects at close range.

I finish the remainder of the barn body (Figure 7) and block in the silo. Through the paint I can just barely see the tree branches I've scratched out of the wash-in. I paint them with opaque color using a pointed sable brush.

Painting the minute branches of the trees is a complicated job, and by comparison the water pump is easy going, taking only a few hours to paint (Figure 8).

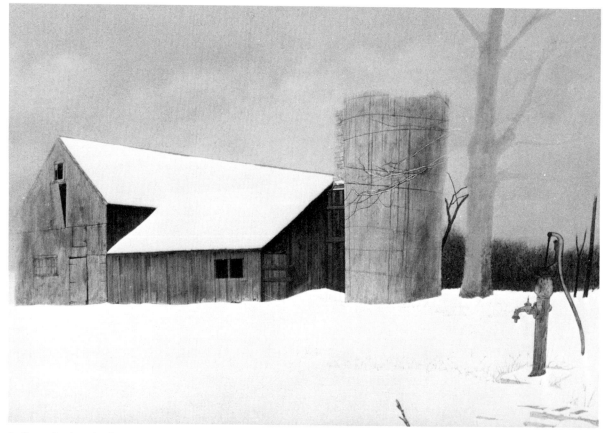

6. *Barn dry-brushed*

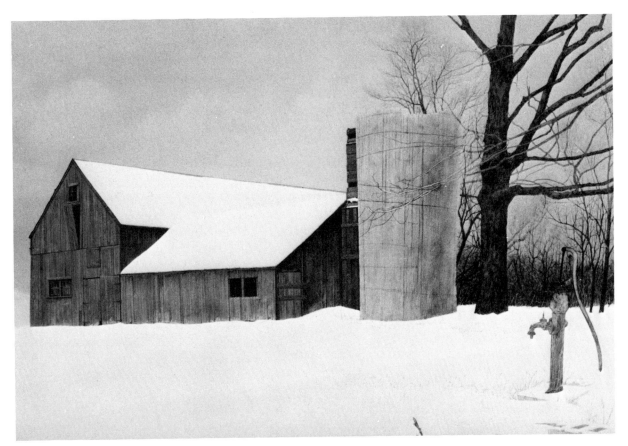

7. *Barn completed; silo blocked in*

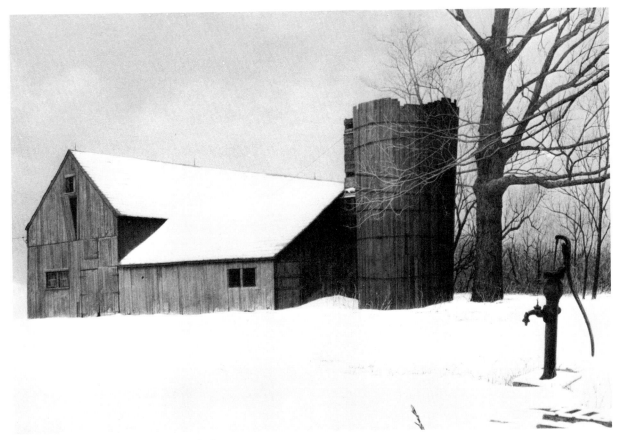

8. *Branches and water pump detailed*

Painting the Foreground. I glaze down the large shadow across the foreground with my favorite color mixture—cobalt blue, raw umber, and white. The glazed shadow painted across the snow in the foreground lightens the value of the logs (Figure 9). My reason for glazing over the logs rather than around them is to coordinate the value and color of the snow lying on their tops to the snow on the ground.

I darken areas of the logs on the left and block in the final coat. The remaining logs will be painted similarly.

To complete the weeds in the foreground, I simply darken them with opaque paint—an easy matter since they are still visible through the wash-in, block-in, and glaze. (See the completed painting in the Color Plates.)

The overhead wire leading from the barn off to the left is an afterthought. The curve of the wire is a challenge to paint without a drawing beneath to guide the brush. My solution is to draw the precise curve I visualize on a thin piece of cardboard and cut the cardboard at that line with a mat knife to make a template. I place the guide on the painting and follow it very lightly with a sharp pencil. It's then a simple matter to paint the wire with a small, pointed sable brush keeping my wrist steady with a mahlstick.

The finished painting is reproduced in color on page 62.

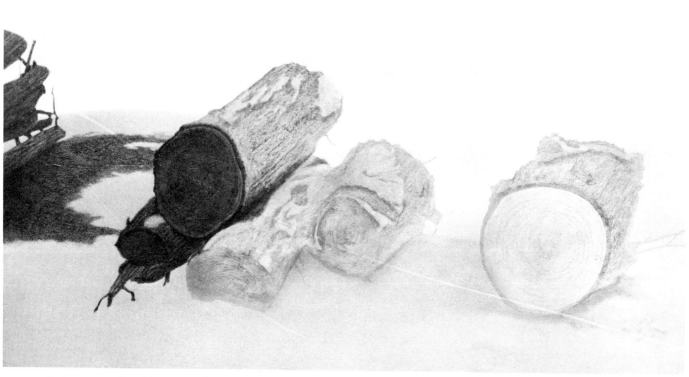

9. *Foreground and logs glazed*

LIST OF PLATES

BLACK AND WHITE

page

COLOR

page

*Information on signed, limited editions of the color reproductions
of Ken Davies paintings available from: Box 902, Madison, Conn. 06443*

CREDITS

Photographers: E. Irving Blomstrann

Eugene Brenwasser

Richard Chamberlain

Geoffrey Clements

Helga Studios

Monroe Vaughn

Student Work: Lynne Hudak   Project 2: Assignment 1, Figure 4

Ric La Terra   Project 2: Assignment 2

Roger Woronecki   Project 2: Assignment 3

Jim Laurier   Project 3

Mark Keigwin   Value Scale, Matching Chart, and
Color Exercises 1,2,4,6,10,12,13

Michael Mariano   Color Exercises 3,5,7,8,9,11

GLOSSARY

Analogous colors. Colors adjacent to each other on the color wheel; colors of the same family which have the same base.

Binder. A material which holds together particles of pigment in a continuous film.

Blending. Applying color gradations to the painting surface to gradually merge areas of different value.

Chroma. The degree of intensity or brilliance of a color.

Color temperature. The warm or cool quality of a color; for example, Prussian blue is a cool color and cadimum red is a hot color.

Complementary colors. Colors placed directly opposite each other on the color wheel: orange and blue, red and green, yellow and violet.

Composition. The structure of a picture made by the artist that coordinates shapes, values, and colors.

Crosshatching. Shading a drawing by making two sets of parallel lines that cross each other.

Direct painting. Laying down paint on the painting surface without underpainting (wash-in).

Dry-brushing. Applying a layer of opaque pigment with a semi-dry brush to get a rough or broken effect.

Feathering. A method of blending with a brush by using quick, light strokes to pull one color into another.

Fixative. A chemical lacquer that is sprayed on a drawing to prevent the lines from smudging.

Genre painting. A painting in which the artist depicts everyday objects realistically.

Gesso. A white liquid plaster or acrylic mixture that is applied to a surface in preparation for painting.

Glazing. Brushing a dark, transparent layer of paint over a lighter layer. This allows the undercoat to show through.

Graying down. Reducing the strength of a color by mixing it or glazing it with its complement, thereby neutralizing it.

Highlight. The point of greatest light intensity on a represented form.

Line. The edge of a shape that describes its boundary or form.

Matte. A dull finish.

Medium. A substance added to pigment to make it more fluid; materials used for artistic expressions, i.e., oil paint, watercolor.

Monochrome. A color scheme in which a single color of various shades is used.

Opaque. Nontransparent.

Palette. An oblong board or pad on which an artist mixes colors; sometimes used to mean the range of colors used by an artist.

Pigment. A powdered coloring matter mixed with a binder, linseed oil, to make oil paints; informally, the whole paint substance itself.

Primary colors. Red, yellow, and blue.

Priming. Preparing the painting surface with gesso or paint.

Scumbling. Brushing opaque color over an already painted and dried surface, sometimes allowing part of the undercoat to show through.

Stump (tortillon). A narrow, tightly packed roll of paper, pointed at one end, used for rubbing and/or blending drawings.

Stippling. Painting or drawing small dots rather than lines to create a form, shadow, or highlight.

Taboret. A low table with drawers and cabinet to hold drawing and painting supplies.

Trompe l'oeil. A French term meaning "fool the eye"; a painting rendered so realistically that the viewer is temporarily convinced the objects are real.

Value. The relative lightness or darkness of a color.

Wash-in. A transparent layer of thinned paint; usually a first coat.

INDEX

Edited by Sarah Bodine
Designed by Bob Fillie
Set in 11 point Zenith by Publishers Graphics, Inc.
Printed by Parish Press, Inc., New York
Bound by A. Horowitz and Son, New York

THE ENCYCLOPEDIA OF
ORNAMENTAL
GRASSES

*How to Grow and Use Over 250 Beautiful
and Versatile Plants*

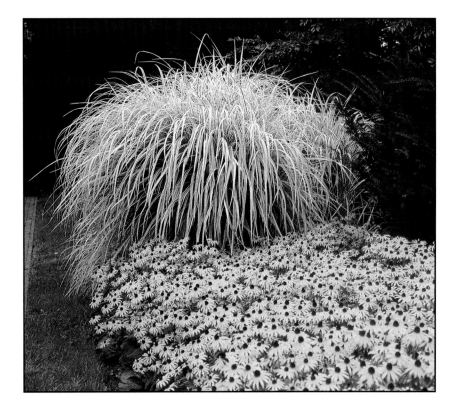

Text by John Greenlee • Photography by Derek Fell

Foreword by Wolfgang Oehme

Rodale Press, Emmaus, Pennsylvania

A FRIEDMAN GROUP BOOK

Copyright © 1992 by Michael Friedman Publishing Group, Inc.

If you have any questions or comments concerning this book, please write:

Rodale Press
Book Readers' Service
33 East Minor Street
Emmaus, PA 18098

Library of Congress Cataloging-in-Publication Data

Greenlee, John.
    The encyclopedia of ornamental grasses : how to grow and use over 250 beautiful and versatile plants / John Greenlee; photographs by Derek Fell; foreword by Wolfgang Oehme.
        p.   cm.
    Contents: Includes bibliographical references and index.
    ISBN 0–87596–100–2 (hardcover)
    1. Ornamental grasses.   2. Ornamental grasses—Encyclopedias.
I. Title.
SB431.7.G74   1992
635.9'349—dc20   92–10833
                                                           CIP

THE ENCYCLOPEDIA OF ORNAMENTAL GRASSES:
How to Grow and Use Over 250 Beautiful and Versatile Plants
was prepared and produced by
Michael Friedman Publishing Group, Inc.
15 West 26th Street
New York, New York 10010

Editors: Sharyn Rosart and Sharon Kalman
Consulting Editors: Ellen Phillips and Barbara W. Ellis
Copy Editors: Candie Frankel and Barbara M. Webb
Art Director: Jeff Batzli
Designer: Lynne Yeamans
Layout: Tanya Ross-Hughes
Photography Editor: Christopher C. Bain

Typeset by Bookworks Plus
Color separations by United South Sea Graphic Art Co.
Printed in Hong Kong and bound in China by Leefung-Asco Printers Ltd. on acid-free ∞ paper.

Distributed in the book trade by St. Martin's Press

2   4   6   8   10   9   7   5   3   hardcover

All photographs © Derek Fell, with the following exceptions: © C. Colston Burrell 78, 162; © Monika Burwell 87; © Rick Darke 29a, 37, 85a, 140, 155; © S.W. Edwards 156; © John Greenlee 15, 23a, 28a, 30, 30a, 31, 33a, 34a, 37a, 40, 50, 52a, 53a, 56, 56a, 58, 59a, 60, 61, 68, 69, 69a, 71, 75, 76, 79a, 82, 83, 87a, 95a, 96, 98b, 99, 106, 111, 112, 116, 117, 125, 143, 150, 151, 152, 156a, 162a, 163; © Michael Lewis 146; © Robert Lyons 29, 65; © Charles Mann 33, 146a, 159a; © Scott Ogden 78; © S.W. Snyder; © Cynthia Woodyard 167; © Lewis Yarlett 168.

The grasses pictured on the front jacket are:

(clockwise from top left) *Cortaderia selloana* (Pampas grass), *Helichtotrichon sempervirens* (Blue oat grass), *Typha angustifolia* (Narrow-leaved cattail), *Miscanthus sinensis* 'Graziella' ('Graziella' Japanese silver grass), *Miscanthus sinensis* 'Variegatus' (Variegated Japanese silver grass), *Imperata cylindrica* 'Red Baron' ('Red Baron' blood grass), *Miscanthus sacchariflorus* (Silver banner grass), *Calamagrostis acutiflora* 'Stricta' (Feather reed grass), and center, *Miscanthus sinensis* 'Variegatus' (Variegated Japanese silver grass).

Grasses pictured on the back jacket are:

(left) *Typha angustifolia* (Narrow-leaved cattail) and (right) *Miscanthus sinensis* 'Gracillimus' (Maiden grass).

To my teachers; especially Jack Catlin, Jim Degan, David Lennom, Kurt Bluemel, Ryan Gainey, and my parents.

And most of all to Carol Hoffman, who has endured above and beyond the call of duty. My eternal thanks.

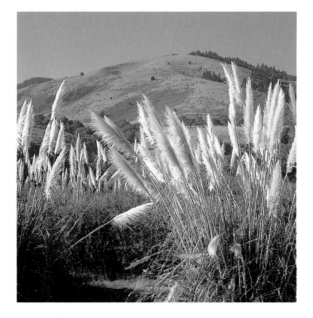

ACKNOWLEDGMENTS

Any work of this nature is not possible without the assistance and support of others. Some helped in technical ways, others provided photography or a quiet space to write. My sincere gratitude to all: David Amme, Randy Baldwin, Mr. Bean, Craig Bennett, Carol Bornstein, Colston Burrell, Monika Burwell, The Klingers, Jackie Coburn, Rick Darke, Don Davis, Neil 'Prairie' Diboll, Rick Diebold, Marcia Donahue, David Douget, Edith R. Eddleman, Steve Edwards, Roger Gettig, Angus Gholson, Sam Flowers, Dave Fross, Gary Hammer, Kim and Bruce Hawks, Dale 'Wildman' Hendricks, Don Herzog, Carolyn Hoffman, Ted Kipping, S. Kitters, Robert Kourik, Steve Lelewer, Judith Lowry, Doris Martin, Pat McNeal, Matt Moynihan, Cathy Musial, Bart O'Brien, Scott Ogden, Wolfgang Oehme, Rodger Raiche, Steve Schmidt, 'Lord' John Snowden, Scott Stewart, Peter Streklow, Wilbur Ternyik, Barton Warnock, Bill Welch, Cynthia Woodyard, and Lewis L. Yarlett. A special thanks to the crew at the Friedman Group, whose tireless efforts made this book a reality: Sharon Kalman, Chris Bain, Tanya Ross-Hughes, and Sharyn Rosart.

Derek Fell wishes to thank the following people and institutions for permission to photograph their garden designs:
Kurt Bluemel, Kurt Bluemel Inc., Baldwin, Maryland
Chicago Botanical Garden, Chicago, Illinois
Robert Fletcher, Pacific Palisades, California
Denver Botanical Garden, Denver, Colorado
Norm and Phyllis Hooven, Limerock Ornamental Grasses Inc., Port Matilda, Pennsylvania
Hershey Gardens, Hershey, Pennsylvania
Longwood Gardens, Kennett Square, Pennsylvania
Hiroshi Makita, Collegeville, Pennsylvania
Wolfgang Oehme and James van Sweden, Oehme, Van Sweden Associates, Washington D.C.
J. Liddon Pennock, Meadowbrook Farm, Meadowbrook, Pennsylvania
Thomas A. Reinhardt, Martina Reinhardt, Mark Moskowitz, Creative Landscaping, Long Island, New York
Carter van Dyke, Doylestown, Pennsylvania
Western Hills Nursery, Occidental, California

CONTENTS

Foreword

As a longtime enthusiast of ornamental grasses, I feel
heartened by the way they are finally sweeping the North
American landscape. I am seeing more nurseries wanting
to grow them, more clients asking about them, and a
greater receptivity for their use in corporate landscaping.
Could it be that North America is returning to its great
prairie heritage?

Whatever the reason for this greater acceptance, I wish to
credit two pioneers in growing grasses: Richard Simon, of
Bluemount Nursery, and Kurt Bluemel, of Kurt Bluemel,
Inc. (both near Baltimore). Richard, Kurt, and I, beginning
in 1957, were the first in this country to propagate and use
grasses on a larger scale.

We were building on the knowledge of the late Karl
Foerster (1874–1970), the famous horticulturist and author from Potsdam, Germany, who said, "Grass is the hair
of the earth." Foerster was a visionary who realized early
the function of grasses in softening the garden and giving it
a more natural look. From the time they thrust their green
spiky heads through the soil in the spring, through dramatic summer and fall lushness and the brownish, feathery
maturity of winter, grasses make a distinctive statement
each season. As Foerster noted, "How terrible a garden
without grasses."

Now the garden world is fortunate to have this new
reference by John Greenlee, with photography by Derek
Fell, *The Encyclopedia of Ornamental Grasses*. It contains a
most comprehensive list of grasses and describes each
plant in detail, including cultural requirements, propagation, and landscape use. Additionally, it describes all the
cultivars and named selections currently available. For all
those people who often ask for a book about grasses, at last
there is a major work to which I can happily refer them.

Wolfgang Oehme

A note from the author

I can remember when grasses first started to intrigue me. We had a garden to design and my associate Mike Sullivan had the notion to use ornamental grasses. Grasses? I thought. My training in ornamental horticulture had never taught me anything about grasses, except as lawns or weeds. I had never considered them as individuals, and certainly not as exceptional or beautiful "ornamentals." I was curious—just what were these ornamental grasses?

At first, teasing tidbits came to light. A snippet of information here, from Carol Bornstein at the Santa Barbara Botanic Garden; a taste of a few there, at Gary Hammer's nursery in Sunland, California. And then, pay dirt: Seems there's a nursery near Baltimore. A Czechoslovakian gentleman named Kurt Bluemel.

I shall never forget the summer I flew to Baltimore to see Bluemel's nursery. The grasses were rippling in a gentle breeze and I couldn't keep my eyes off them. I felt like a child in a toy store. Look how many grasses! Just look at them move! I had had no idea. Where had these plants been throughout my horticultural career? I hadn't seen them in gardens or books. The images of Kurt's nursery were never to leave me. They remain clearly in my head as though it were only yesterday.

That was almost six years ago, and much has happened since. As I plunged into these plants, I found myself continually drawn to learn more about them. Traveling across the country and to England, I began to see grasses in gardens and in nature that I had never dreamed existed. With each successive trip, I learned more about them. By now my professional focus had changed from landscape contractor to grass grower. Trained as a nurseryman at California Polytechnic, then falling into garden construction, I now found myself in a nursery growing and learning about grasses. Somewhat an expert by default in California, I lectured around the country on the beauty and utility of ornamental grasses.

When I was asked to write this book, I had no idea what I was getting into. It became a classic example of the trite but apt phrase "The more I learned, the less I knew." This encyclopedia marks only a brief passage in my pursuit of grasses. Because, in researching this book, I have only come to discover how much more there is to know.

So I offer this book as a beginning, not an end. I hope it will open the eyes of others to the magic and beauty of ornamental grasses. Whether you garden in Seattle, Miami, St. Louis, San Diego, or Toronto, a world of ornamental grasses awaits. Let me introduce you to a few of my new friends.

John Greenlee

INTRODUCTION

Grasses are found throughout the world, in nearly every habitat. Wherever you happen to be, with few exceptions, there are grasses. Grasses knit together on the sandy beaches of Florida and cling to the rocky cliffs of Maine. They flourish in the shady depths of Appalachian forests, and hold their own on the windswept peaks of the Rockies. Even in the humid swamps of Mississippi and around the cool Great Lakes, grasses find their niche. Nature has equipped these plants with rugged adaptability and wide tolerance of climatic fluctuations, making grasses extremely successful competitors.

Man has had a long association with grasses. Our ancestors are believed to have evolved in the grasslands of Africa. Our civilization is built on the domestication of grasses and grassland animals. Most of our most important food crops—corn, wheat, rice, oats, barley, sorghum, sugarcane, and rye—are grasses.

American sodbusters built their houses of grass, using the thick turf of the prairie. So, too, the Japanese use grass—bamboo, that is—to construct elegantly simple teahouses. Thatched roofs or walls are still a popular choice in many countries. Peoples around the world have fashioned grasses into fences, worked them into mats, crafted furniture, hats, sandals, even musical instruments, from these valuable plants. Fragrant vetiver is used in perfumes and cosmetics, and lemon grass is a favorite with cooks. The fisherman's favorite bamboo pole and the reeds for the orchestra's woodwind section would not exist in a world without grasses. Grasses are tightly woven into almost every aspect of our lives, and yet we rarely think of them.

Although grasses grow just about anywhere, most of our great grasslands are found on well-drained fertile soils in full sun and near water. These also happen to be ideal areas for farms, cities, highways, and just about any other center of human activity. As a result, human development has overtaken the grasslands, destroying native habitat and threatening species with extinction. The situation is especially grim in regard to fragile ecosystems like wetlands. The mix of grasses and other plants found in wetlands is important to the ecological health of the land, filtering and holding water. Even small pockets of wetlands are vital, yet these areas remain threatened today. Ecologists have long known that the grasslands and wetlands of this country are being irreparably altered, yet this natural vegetation is still undervalued and endangered.

The North American continent is home to what was once one of the world's greatest grasslands, the prairie. Originally, this sea of grass was a thousand miles wide and over three thousand miles long, occupying the center and interior of the continent. Today, very little of this grassland remains. In California, the great Central Valley was also once a thriving grassland, teeming with elk and other wildlife. In Florida, the incredible Everglades are grasslands, too.

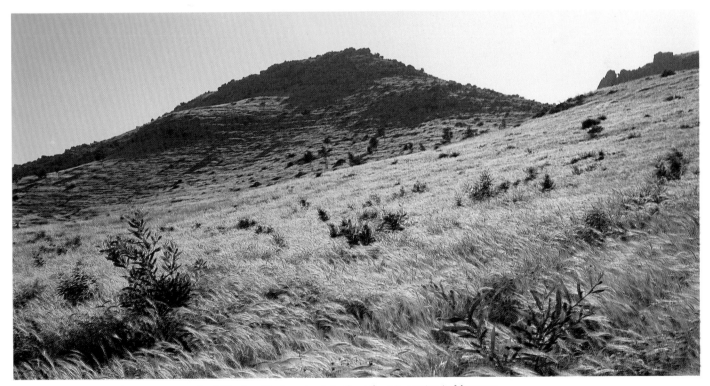

Sunlight plays on the glistening awns of wild barley, *Hordeum* spp., in the Atlas Mountains in Morocco.

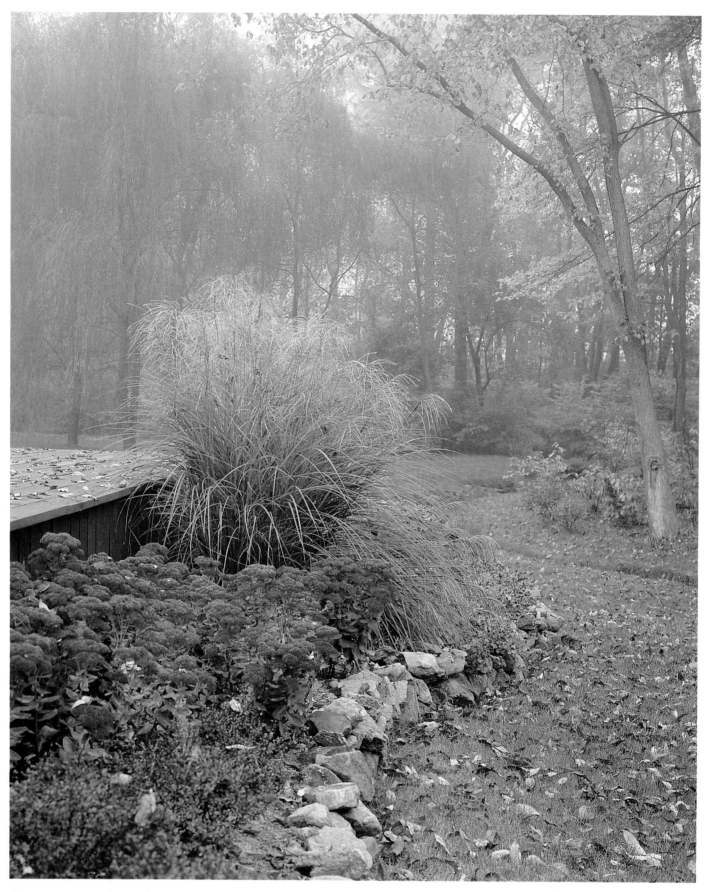

On a misty autumn day, maiden grass adds a graceful accent to the garden.

The native grasslands around the world have retreated—turned under by the plow, grazed by domesticated animals, drained into land that is usable for building or farming. The tallgrass prairies of the United States are still covered with tallgrass—only now it is corn instead of the native species that once stretched from Canada to the Gulf of Mexico. Wide-ranging buffalo and elk have been replaced by large, sedentary flocks of steer and sheep, and the grasslands were overgrazed and damaged. Wetlands everywhere are still being destroyed, just as the Everglades were misguidedly "improved" decades ago.

Our reliance on grasses is indisputable. And in our landscaping, too, grasses have proved to be our most valued ornament: the American lawn, by far the most popular ornamental grass planting. Mowed turf accounts for the largest percentage of gardened land—50,000 square miles by some estimates. Americans spend an estimated thirty billion dollars per year planting, maintaining, and promoting the mowed lawn. Michael Pollan, in his book *Second Nature,* noted that "lawns ... like the interstate highway system, like fast food chains, like television [have] ... served to unify the American landscape." Until recently, no one seemed to question a lawn's value and its impact on the environment.

Of course we will always need turfgrass for recreation and enjoyment. But, as in other aspects of American life, we are rethinking our priorities and values about lawns in a changing and ever more fragile environment. As houses are pushed closer and closer together, gardens get smaller. Our maturing "urban forests" create shadier, less favorable conditions for the mowed lawn. Changing needs provide changing perspectives. Does a family with no small children still need a big lawn? Do we want to devote hours of precious time to lawn care? Might several neighbors with small yards share a single mower? Can we add easy-care, well-suited groundcovers and learn to kiss the lawnmower goodbye?

A growing environmental awareness has uncovered flaws in America's most popular ornamental. The pollution created by turfgrass culture—combustion of fossil fuels necessary to mow, edge, and blow clean turf—has become an important issue. Commercial crews driving to and from lawn areas add to the pollution. Grass clippings often end up in landfills, contributing to our waste disposal problems. And, as if all this were not enough, Americans continue to add deadly poisons and chemical fertilizers to the soil. These nitrates and poisons are increasingly finding their way into our groundwater and, from there, into our rivers, lakes, and bays.

In arid western climates and hot southern climates, the green sward of turf has other ecological consequences. For every neighborhood of green lawns in Southern California,

there is a drained wetland or a dammed wild river in the north. Grasses that require 40 to 60 inches of rainfall a year, planted in climates that provide only 10 to 12 inches per year, can exist only with additional water. The water has to come from somewhere, and as our population grows, our water resources are shrinking. There are too few wild rivers left to dam.

All of these concerns are responsible for a new and growing movement toward ecologically sensitive American gardens, dubbed "the new American garden" by some proponents. These new gardens are appropriate for their climate and ecology, and they are not chemically dependent. They're less demanding of our water supplies and more self-sufficient.

The philosophy behind these gardens combines horticulture and ecology in harmony. The unimaginative, sterile green rug of lawn is being replaced by more dynamic and more interesting plantings. The new American garden means a return to our native grass heritage, with free-growing grasses used as they appear in nature. Now we are learning a new appreciation for the beauty and grace of these captivating plants.

The arrival of the ornamental grasses onto the American horticultural scene has transformed our gardens. Offering freedom from the drudgery of turf, these grasses give us a chance to preserve a bit of the past. And they work well with other plants in the garden. Their great variety of sizes, shapes, and colors adds texture, motion, and grace to the landscape.

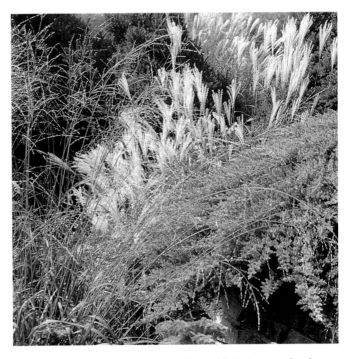

Moor grass, left, and flame grass combine with junipers and sedums to create a naturalistic setting in Kurt Bluemel's garden.

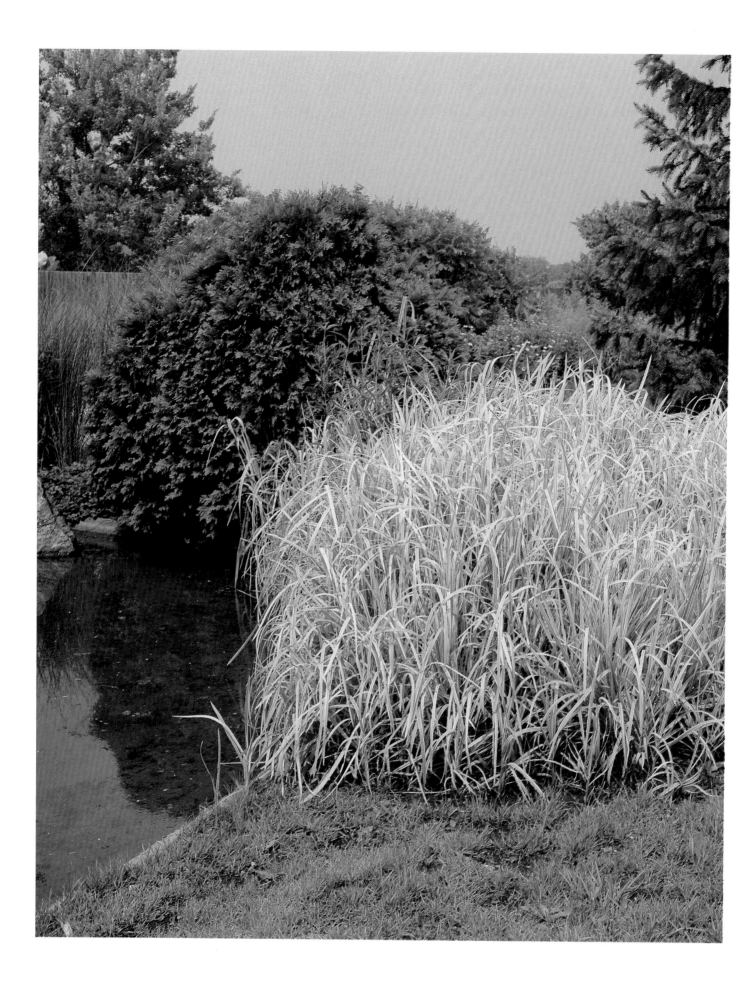

PART I

INTRODUCTION TO ORNAMENTAL GRASSES

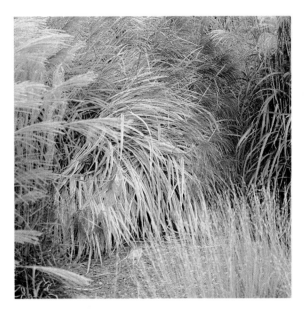

Opposite: Grasses come in many colors besides green, such as the creamy white foliage of variegated manna grass, *Glyceria maxima* 'Variegata.' Above: *Miscanthus* cultivars differ in foliage color, size, and flowering times. In this October scene, *Miscanthus sinensis* 'Zwergelefant', with green foliage on right, has been in flower since July, while white-foliaged *Miscanthus sinensis* 'Variegatus' has flowers just now emerging.

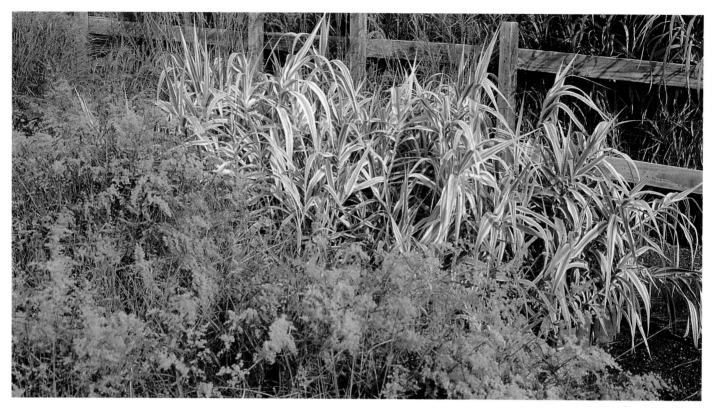

The creamy yellow foliage of *Arundo donax* 'Variegata' makes a pleasing combination with the pale pink flowers of natal grass, *Rychelytrum repens.*

What Are Ornamental Grasses?

The term *ornamental grass* is somewhat confusing because this label is applied not only to true grasses, but to close relatives of grasses and to grasslike plants in general. In a strict sense, true grasses are members of Gramineae, the grass family, but many of the plants we think of as grasses are actually sedges and rushes, which belong respectively to Cyperaceae, the sedge family, and Juncaceae, the rush family. Together, these three families comprise the bulk of the plants we call ornamental grasses.

Other plants are also grass look-alikes. These we call grasslike plants. The genera *Ophiopogon* (mondo grasses), *Liriope* (lilyturfs), *Hemerocallis* (daylilies), *Phormium* (flax lilies), and *Yucca* all have members with grasslike foliage. These plants are not covered in this book. Neither are plants from the lily and iris families, such as wandflowers or fairy wand (*Dierama* spp.) or bear grass (*Xerophyllum tenax*). Fairy wand is an iris relative with delicate grasslike leaves. Bear grasses, members of the lily family, are popular in the florist trade and are grasslike in appearance. The list goes on.

Many bulbs have grasslike foliage, too. Examples are alliums and amaryllis (*Hippeastrum* spp.). These grass mimics have great appeal when used in combination with the grasses. Not surprisingly, many of these plants are native to grassland ecologies, so they grow naturally with the grasses. In fact, many of our most prized bulbs and wildflowers need grasses and grassland ecologies to thrive. In California, the native grasslands are home to many bulbs. Among the most treasured of these are the mariposa or butterfly tulips (*Calochortus* spp.). Revered by English gardeners and ignored in America, these bulbs once flourished in California grasslands composed chiefly of needlegrasses (*Stipa* spp.). The disappearance of the grasslands also meant the destruction of what were once extensive populations of these magnificent bulbs. Grassland wildflowers were also decimated. California poppies (*Escholtzia californica*) and lupines (*Lupinus* spp.) were said to be so brilliant in their display that ships at sea could set their course by the blaze of flower color. By growing ornamental grasses in our gardens, we can reclaim a part of our horticultural heritage.

In summary, ornamental grasses are grasses and grasslike plants that are used chiefly for ornament. They are a large and complex group of plants with wide ranges of habitat and culture. You don't need to know the complicated botanical differences between true grasses and sedges or the similarities of sedges and rushes to appreciate their grace in the garden. (Readers who are interested in complex botany may pursue further botanical references, listed on page 179, for detailed information.) This book will focus on the beauty of ornamental grasses and their uses in the garden.

How Grasses Grow

Few people understand how grasses grow, perhaps because our most popular use of grass is mowed lawn. We never really see how a grass behaves when left untouched. To use ornamental grasses successfully, you need an understanding of just how grasses grow.

Annual, Biennial, or Perennial

Grasses fall roughly into three major groups: annuals, biennials, and perennials. *Annual grasses* live a complete life cycle in one year or one season. They emerge from seed, grow roots, stems, and leaves, flower, and die in one season. Most of our important food grasses are annuals. Annual ornamental grasses are often overlooked, but many of them are decorative and easy to grow. Some seed companies offer "sampler" mixes of annual ornamental grasses, which will give you a taste of what's available. Annual grasses are not included in this book.

Biennial grasses sprout from seed, grow through the season, overwinter, and continue to grow into the next season, when they flower and die. Their life cycle is completed in two seasons. Relatively few grasses fall into this category, and none of the grasses in this book are true biennials.

Perennial grasses live and grow for more than two seasons. The most important ornamental grasses are perennials. Many perennial grasses are extremely long-lived, persisting for decades. They can be herbaceous, woody, or semi-woody. The largest group of woody grasses also happens to be the largest group of true grasses: the bamboos. Too large and too complex to be adequately dealt with here, the bamboos are not included in this book.

Many grasses are perennial in one climate and annual in others. Tender fountain grass (*Pennisetum setaceum*), for example, is a perennial grass in the mild Mediterranean climate of Southern California, yet it is considered an annual in the Pacific Northwest. Each grass has its own tolerance to cold and heat and reacts differently from one climate to the next. The encyclopedia section of this text indicates the longevity of each grass in a given climatic zone. Often, as little as 20 miles may separate a climate in which a certain grass could only be considered an annual from a climate in which the same species is perennial.

Seasons of Growth

Grasses are classified as either warm-season or cool-season species, depending on when they are in active growth. *Warm-season grasses* grow when temperatures begin to warm in spring. They flower and set seed in summer and fall, and become dormant with the onset of winter. *Cool-season grasses* begin growth in late winter or early spring. They flower from winter into early summer, and become dormant or slow-growing in summer. These grasses resume active growth when cooler temperatures return in fall. In areas with mild winters, cool-season grasses often continue growing all winter.

A grass's seasonal habit of growth is often related to the climate in which it originated. Species that are native to areas with dry summers, for instance, often become dormant during the hot months and resume growth when temperatures cool and fall rains begin. Those grasses that are natives of areas with cold winters go dormant in fall, waiting for the warmth of spring to begin growing.

These seasonal patterns can change, depending on different climates or conditions. Under normal conditions, a cool-season grass is dormant during the summer, an inherent defense against drought. But if you water regularly, some plants will continue to grow.

WARM-SEASON GRASSES Warm-season grasses grow best at temperatures between 80°F and 95°F. They grow vigorously from spring to summer, then flower and begin dormancy in fall. Most warm-season grasses, like the leaves on trees and shrubs, turn a different color in autumn. Every wonderful fall color imaginable can be found in these grasses. As winter approaches, warm-season grasses continue to change color, becoming completely dormant. The past season's growth—leaves, flowers, and stems—dries and blanches to tan, wheat, or white. These

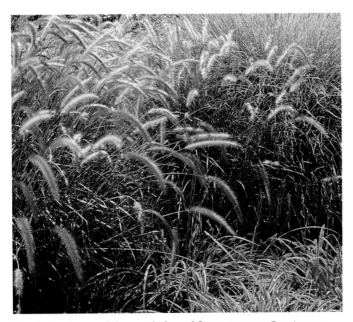

The fluffy plumes of the purple-leaved fountain grass, *Pennisetum setaceum* 'Rubrum', in the foreground contrast with the green foliage of *P. alopecuroides*, still yet to bloom.

winter colors have their own subtle beauty and purpose in the garden. Many warm-season grasses are useful for attracting winter wildlife into the garden.

Dormant winter foliage of warm-season grasses usually persists throughout the winter. Often the combination of snow, wind, and rain knocks the dormant foliage to the ground, but some grasses are better at standing up to winter weather.

With the spring thaw, warm-season grasses once again begin growing. New shoots rise from the base, and the cycle is repeated. The emergence of the grasses truly announces the arrival of spring.

COOL-SEASON GRASSES   Cool-season grasses grow best at temperatures of 60°F to 75°F. They begin new growth in fall and are some of the first perennials to bloom in the garden. Some are even winter-blooming. Cool-season grasses are often more moisture-loving than warm-season species. Their leaves are usually evergreen, and in winter may be highlighted with red, plum, purple, yellow, or brown. Many of these winter colors disappear when temperatures begin to warm and later spring growth overtakes the earlier foliage.

THE EFFECT OF CLIMATE   The classification of cool-season and warm-season grasses is somewhat arbitrary, because many grasses grow quite differently from climate to climate. Some cool-season grasses that are evergreen in South Carolina go completely dormant in Philadelphia—the previous year's growth freezes to the ground, and the plant resumes growth later in spring. How well a grass maintains its winter color also depends on winter temperatures and exposures. In the comparatively mild Southeast, the grass may be completely evergreen and actively growing all winter long.

To determine how a particular grass will grow in your climate, check the entry in the encyclopedia section. Then refer to the USDA Plant Hardiness Zone Map on page 181 to see if the plant is hardy in your area.

Growth Habit

Two types of growth habits characterize grasses. *Running grasses* spread by creeping stems, forming dense mats. Many running grasses can be invasive. *Clumping grasses* grow in tufts, slowly increasing in girth. Both types have their place in the garden.

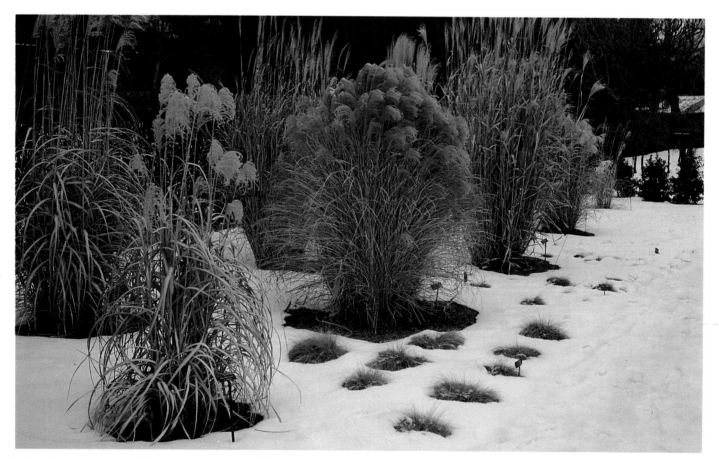

Winter-dormant grasses still erect against a mantle of snow at Longwood Gardens in Pennsylvania.

RUNNING GRASSES   Running grasses are also called spreading or creeping grasses. They spread by means of aboveground stems called stolons or underground stems called rhizomes, structures that can be delicate and hair-like or thick and hard. (When running grasses are spread by rhizomes, they are also called rhizomatous grasses.) Given years of growth under ideal conditions, the mature rhizomes of grasses like prairie cord grass (*Spartina pectinata*) can require a backhoe to remove.

   Many running grasses can be invasive. Those that spread by means of stolons root along the stems as they grow, forming a dense turf. Such grasses are often used as lawns. Ornamental grasses such as variegated St. Augustinegrass (*Stenotaphrum secondatum* 'Variegatum') and buffalo grass (*Buchloe dactyloides*), which grow by stolons, can colonize large areas.

CLUMPING GRASSES   Clumping grasses, which grow in tufts, are often called bunch grasses, especially by ranchers and range management specialists in the West, where these species are important forage grasses. Clumping grasses vary from the delicate little 2-inch mounds of bearskin fescue (*Festuca scoparia*) to huge plants like pampas grass (*Cortaderia selloana*). Some clumping grasses or sedges, such as Berkeley sedge (*Carex tumuicola*), can appear like a sod or turf if they are planted close enough to grow together.

Grass Form

Grasses come in many shapes and sizes. There are six primary categories used to define the shapes of grasses. These categories describe the form of the foliage, not of the flowering stems, or inflorescences, and apply regardless of the plant's height.

TUFTED   Usually spiky foliage or fine-textured with upright leaves arising from a basal clump. Example: Blue fescue (*Festuca cinerea*).

MOUNDED   Somewhat weeping; mounding foliage. Top growth covers lower leaves. Example: Black-flowering pennisetum (*Pennisetum alopecuroides* 'Moudry').

UPRIGHT   Erect. Foliage grows vertically in a uniform or even columnar form. Example: Cattail (*Typha latifolia*).

UPRIGHT DIVERGENT   Foliage grows up and out in an erect or stiffly ascending manner. Example: Blue oat grass (*Helictotrichon sempervirens*).

UPRIGHT ARCHING   Foliage ascends vertically then becomes fountainlike at the top. Example: Silver feather maiden grass (*Miscanthus sinensis* 'Silberfeder').

ARCHING   Foliage arches up and out, in somewhat equal proportion. Example: Palm grass (*Setaria palmifolia*).

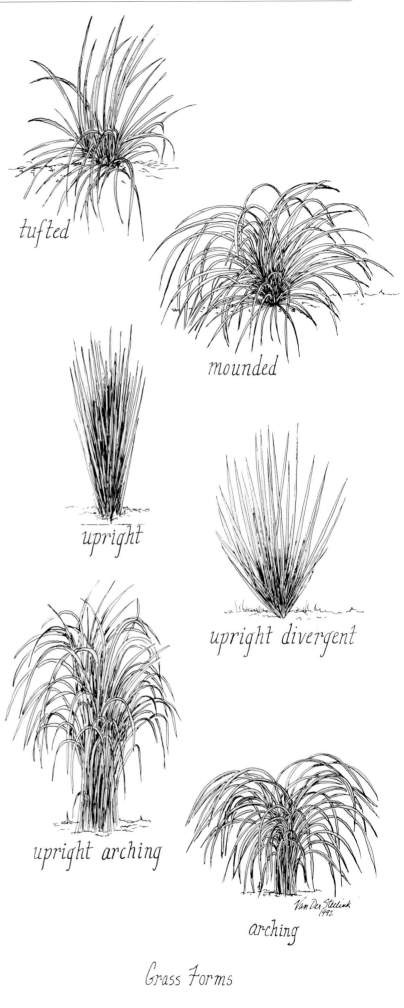

tufted

mounded

upright

upright divergent

upright arching

arching

Van Der Steelink
1992

Grass Forms

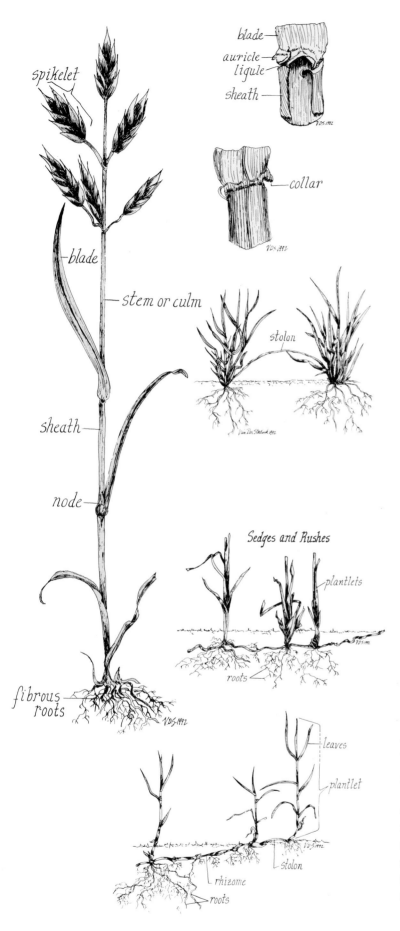

Grass Structure

The Life of a Grass

When a grass is left uncut, unmowed, and untouched, it becomes a plant entirely different from the grass that makes up the familiar lawn. The great majority of grasses are easy to grow and quick to bloom when liberated from constant mowing or grazing. Following a grass as it grows reveals its amazing vitality.

Most grasses are capable of growing to their mature size in one or two seasons. Mature can mean 12 inches tall, as in the case of large blue hairgrass (*Koeleria glauca*), or 12 feet tall, as in the case of giant Chinese silver grass (*Miscanthus giganteus*). Pampas grass (*Cortaderia selloana*) shoots up so fast that on a hot summer day you can hear the plant growing. Sugarcane (*Saccharum officinarum*) grows at a rate that exceeds that of most plants because it has accelerated photosynthetic abilities. In fact, many grasses have this ability; given ideal conditions they will take their place quickly in the garden.

From a seedling or a small plantlet, grasses begin to produce roots, shoots, and leaves. Like other perennials, the amount of foliage a grass produces depends directly on the establishment of a good root system: Once grasses are firmly rooted, they generally are quick to produce foliage and flowers.

Perennial grasses can be extremely long-lived, and some persist for decades without division. Others are weakly perennial: They may die out in the center after a few years and need dividing for rejuvenation. Some short-lived grasses are quite showy and worth replanting. It's important to know whether a grass will be suitable for the use you intend. Remember to carefully read the encyclopedia entry for each grass you want to plant.

Leaf and Stem

Grass leaves—fine and wiry, flat and broad, folded, curly, or anything in between—fill our gardens with texture and motion. But all those shapes have a practical side, too, evolved in response to climate and conditions. Rolled or folded leaves, for instance, slow down the evaporation of water and are often found on grass species from dry areas. Razor-sharp edges and wickedly pointed tips help protect grasses from foraging animals.

The foliage of ornamental grasses comes in every shade of green, from lime to dark forest green, and in colors of red, yellow, blue, purple, and brown. Some species are soft and downy to the touch, others are shiny or pleated, and some can slice skin like a razor. Grasses that are spotted or striped with white or yellow add a feeling of light and movement.

The stem of a grass, called the *culm*, bears leaves, flowers, and seeds. Culms vary from thin and flexible to woody and rigid. Leaves form on the culm, and flowers are borne at the top of it.

Culm and leaf arrangements differ from grass to grass. In tufted and mounded forms, culms remain hidden at the base of the grass, becoming visible only when flower spikes begin to emerge. The culms of upright-growing grasses are often a visible and noticeable part of the plant throughout the growing season. Grass culms are usually similar in color to the foliage, but these stems can have contrasting colors. 'Pele's Smoke' sugarcane (*Saccharum officinarum* 'Pele's Smoke') has polished burgundy red canes and translucent purple leaves.

Many sedges and rushes appear identical to true grasses, but others have a completely different arrangement of culms and leaves. Some members of the sedge family (Cyperaceae) form tubular stems with greatly reduced leaves. A good example is Egyptian papyrus (*Cyperus papyrus*), which has bare stems 6 to 9 feet tall, topped with a large umbel-like cluster of drooping leaves, up to 2 feet wide. The culms of rushes, members of the Juncaceae family, are almost always cylindrical, and leaves are greatly reduced or absent. But woodrushes (*Luzula* spp.) have grasslike leaves and flowering stems, and look more like sedges or true grasses.

Flowers and Seed Heads

What most people refer to as a grass's flower is in fact an inflorescence, a group of flowers. Each tiny, individual flower, held in a structure called a spikelet, remains hidden until flowering time. Grass inflorescences have three basic forms: spike, raceme, or panicle. A spike is the simplest arrangement: The individual flowers are attached directly to the main stem, with no branches. In a raceme, the spikelets are held on branches directly attached to the main stem. A panicle is the most complex arrangement, bearing spikelets on branches or stalks off a main stem. A panicle may include flowers arranged in racemes on its branches. The flowers on spike, raceme, or panicle may be arranged loosely, giving an open, airy feel, or they can be dense or even one-sided.

Spikelets usually emerge one-color, then mature to another color. On newly emerging inflorescences, spikelets can be shades of green, red, pink, silver, or bronze. As they mature, they mellow to tan, gray, gold, and brown. Some spikelets appear hairy or bristly, thanks to a pronounced needlelike awn that extends from the spikelet. The silky awns of feather grass (*Stipa* spp.) capture the light and sway in the slightest breeze.

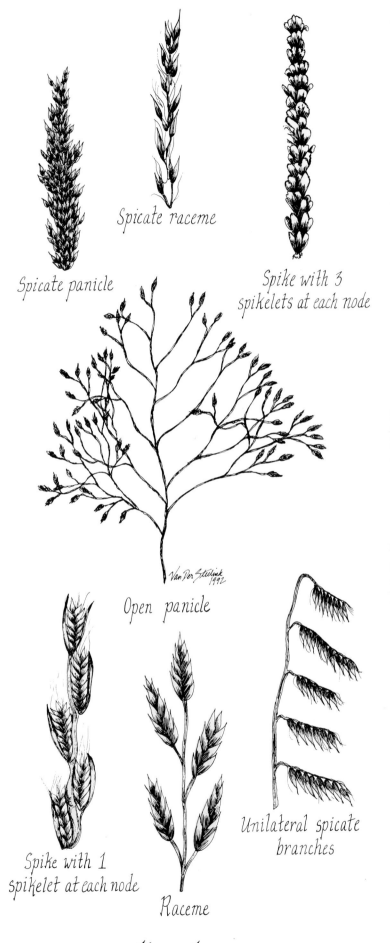

Spicate raceme

Spicate panicle

Spike with 3 spikelets at each node

Open panicle

Spike with 1 spikelet at each node

Raceme

Unilateral spicate branches

Flower Forms

When grasses go to seed, the flowers often take on a completely different form and color. The silky plumes of maiden grass (*Miscanthus* spp.), red, purple, or white on emergence, become fluffy and puff up like cotton candy, maturing to creamy tan or brown whisklike plumes. Grass seeds are usually dispersed by the wind and fall to the ground. Light seeds may float in the breeze. After the seeds have dispersed, flower heads usually remain erect until wind, rain, or snow knock them to the ground. Often, these old flower spikes remain decorative in the garden through the winter.

The vast majority of grasses bloom May through July. However, there are grasses that bloom into November, and some that bloom in winter.

Fall, Winter, and Spring Again

As fall approaches and the days become shorter, grasses again begin to change. Warm-season grasses now assume their autumn colors. By late fall, their colors are blanched to the soft hues of winter. Next year's growth, the living buds, lie dormant at the crown of the plant, ready to emerge with the coming of spring. Cool-season grasses begin to grow again in fall, long after flowering.

In late winter or spring, depending on the grass, new shoots begin to emerge through the dried remnants of last year's growth. In gardens, we often cut grass back to keep the plantings tidy. In nature, grasses grow up through last year's growth until they have grown past this old growth, which has begun to decompose. With the emergence of new growth, the cycle has come full circle and another season is under way.

The Basics of Ornamental Grass Gardening

Whether you are looking for an unassuming filler or a dynamic accent, grass is a wonderful addition to the garden. The strong vertical or fountaining form of ornamental grasses combines with their feathery flower heads and soothing neutral colors to make a unique contribution to the landscape. But designing with ornamental grasses is both exciting and overwhelming—there are so many choices and possibilities.

Grass foliage moves in a breeze and catches light like few other plants. It adds texture and color: metallic blues, coppery browns, and every shade of green imaginable. As grasses grow and the seasons change, so does their foliage color. Many grasses have dazzling fall colors—red, orange, yellow, and purple. Other seasons can also affect the colors of grass foliage. Many have showy coloring as they flush with their new spring growth; others make fabulous winter accents, especially in snowy climates.

Grasses offer an impressive array of plumes and seed heads for interest throughout the year. Many grasses are in full glory when little else is showy in the garden.

Using Grasses in the Landscape

Beauty alone is reason enough to include ornamental grasses in your landscape. You'll enjoy creating interesting combinations of grasses and flowers or other ornamentals. They take their place in the border easily, setting off neighboring plants with their presence. Try bold-leaved foliage plants with grasses, or add a jolt of bright color in front of that graceful green. Some combinations, such as coreopsis and tall sedums, are already becoming classics.

These adaptable plants can work hard, too. Tall grasses divide the garden into distinct spaces, or provide a backdrop to borders or other plantings. They're effective as hedges or screens, and many, including vetiver (*Vetiver zizanioides*) and giant reed (*Arundo donax*), can serve as windbreaks. Fast-spreading running grasses are indispensable as groundcovers. They colonize an area quickly, reducing dust and erosion and stabilizing soil. A host of new grasses can function as lawn, offering a beautiful and ecologically appropriate alternative to turfgrass. Some newer lawn grasses don't even need mowing!

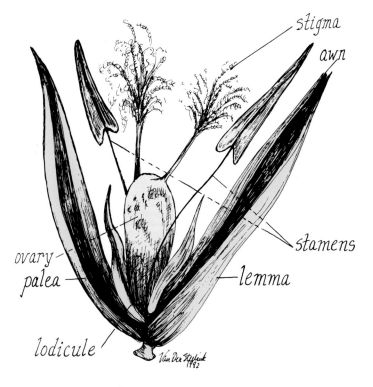

Flower or Spikelet

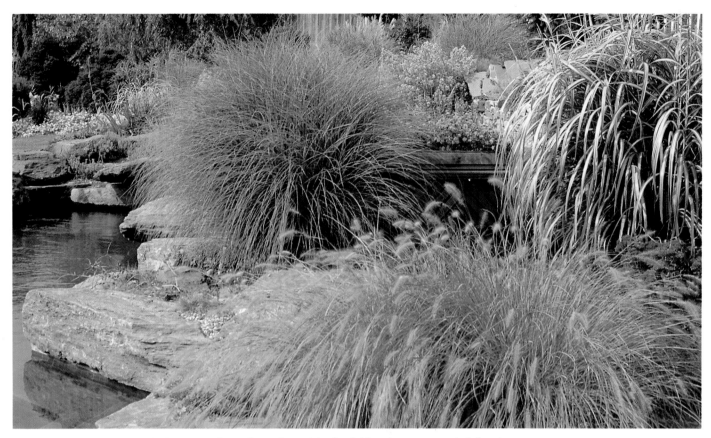

An assortment of grasses poolside at Kurt Bluemel's garden in Maryland. Most grasses are at their best in or near water.

Ornamental grasses can fill difficult garden niches, too. Many species excel where other plants might struggle to grow. Many tolerate extremes of temperatures, climate, and soil, thriving even in salty, alkaline, or acid soils. Found in almost every kind of natural habitat, from coastal dunes to alpine meadows, grasses are a good choice for gardeners everywhere.

GRASSES IN SPECIAL GARDENS Even if your only garden is a clay pot on the balcony, you can enjoy the pleasures of ornamental grasses. They lend themselves beautifully to all kinds of special gardens.

Container gardens.
If you garden in pots or on city rooftops, discover how versatile these tough, beautiful plants are. Many species are suitable for shallow containers and exposed sites.

Rock gardens.
Miniature grasses are effective in rock gardens and trough gardens. Some skill is required to grow many alpine grasses, but enthusiasts are experimenting with more varieties all the time.

Water gardens.
Grasses unlock a whole new world of ideas for water plant enthusiasts. If you're a water gardener, you can choose from over a hundred species that thrive in or near the water.

Wildlife gardens.
Birds and other wildlife are attracted by grasses in your garden. The seed heads are eagerly sought for winter food, and the foliage supplies shelter.

Craft gardens.
The showy flowers and graceful foliage are appealing in fresh or dried arrangements. And you can use grasses for weavings and basketry, too.

Cooks' gardens.
Try grasses for flavorings and food. Lemon grass (*Cymbopogon citratus*) soup is a popular Thai dish. Indian rice grass (*Orysopsis hymenoides*) was an important food source for southwestern Native Americans, and wild rice (*Zizania aquatica*) is still enjoyed today.

MEADOW PLANTINGS It seems obvious, but grasses are unsurpassed for creating meadows. Until lately, most "meadow mixes" have been sold without any grasses included. These seed mixes tend to unravel after the first season because a true meadow is composed of a balance of grasses and flowers. Without grasses there is no balance, and the flowers are quickly overtaken by weeds. But if grasses are included, they become the main fabric of the tapestry, with annuals and perennial meadow flowers woven through.

Selecting and Buying

Choosing the right grass for your garden may seem overwhelming at first, so let's make it simple. The same decisions you make in choosing any other perennial must be made with grasses. Here are some guidelines to start you thinking.

- Choose a grass that's right for your climate. Consider both your hardiness zone (see page 181) and any local conditions such as wind, salt air, alkaline soil, or drought cycles. Your local Cooperative Extension office can provide you with some general ideas.
- The grass must fit into your landscape plan—it must be the right size and shape, be the right color, and bloom in the right season. Think about the neighboring plants before you add grasses to a bed or border. Will they complement each other, or will the grass overpower them?
- If ease of maintenance is important to you, you'll want to keep that in mind as you read through the encyclopedia entries.
- Consider, too, the growth habit of the plant. Running grasses with invasive tendencies must be confined by physical barriers; grasses that self-sow readily will require vigilant weeding.

Planting ornamental grasses calls for some additional thought. Be sure you understand a grass's habit before you plant. Is it a clumping grass or a running grass? Is it evergreen in your climate? Are you counting on cold weather to keep an invasive grower under control? Plan ahead to avoid serious gardening mistakes.

Invasive Grasses

Invasiveness is a vital consideration, especially if your garden is near undisturbed native plant communities. But even urban gardeners need to be concerned. Birds and other animals and the wind can spread grass seeds far and wide. An escaped grass may come to dominate a natural system, just as the escaped garden flower purple loosestrife (*Lythrum* spp.) has taken over much ground across the Northeast.

Only a small percentage of grasses are potentially weedy. It's tempting to plant them because they often have great horticultural value and great beauty. Sometimes a grass that reseeds itself readily in one climate does not exhibit this tendency in another. Many Mediterranean and subtropical grasses—tigers in their native habitats—are pussycats in cold northern climates, where their seed fails to overwinter and germinate. Similarly, many moisture-loving northern and European grasses have no chance of escaping into dry

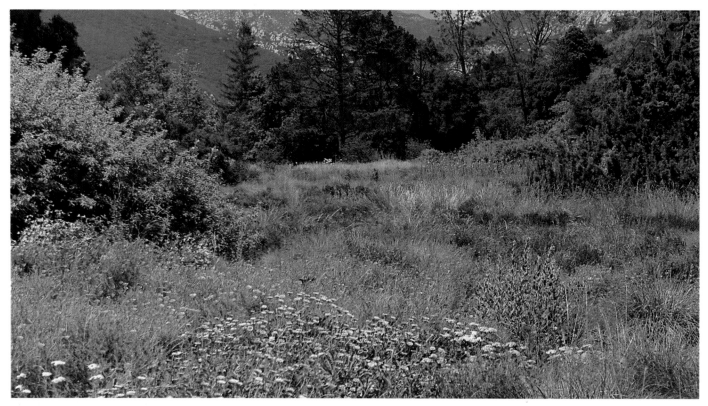

The meadow at the Santa Barbara Botanic Garden in California artfully demonstrates how to use grasses and wildflowers.

chaparral or southwestern prairie, where rainfall is scant. Grasses known to be weedy in certain climates or under certain conditions are noted in their listings in the encyclopedia section of this book.

We are just now beginning to understand the complicated relationships of disturbed ecosystems. Many ecologists argue that exotic grasses invade only areas that are already disturbed in some way. But the fact remains that many of our native grasses continue to decline, while exotic species make increasing inroads into natural areas. You, as a responsible gardener, must be aware of potentially invasive grasses.

Using Native Species

Today's gardeners are more aware of their own impact on the environment. Restoration, the process of returning the land to its former habitat, usually as it was before man's influence, is gaining popularity. If you want to use grasses native to your area, contact your local or regional plant societies and botanic gardens. Your local Cooperative Extension Service may have this information or may be able to direct you to seed sources.

Many restorationists urge the selection and use of locally collected seed and plants whenever possible. Wide-ranging grass species such as little bluestem (*Schizachyrium scoparium*), which can be found from Canada to Florida and Maryland to Utah, may have many naturally occurring genetic variations, each more suited to one particular region. A community of this grass in Maine would probably be better adapted to cold winters than a community of the same species in Georgia. Likewise, a blue gramma (*Bouteloua gracilis*) from a region of high rainfall and summer rain like Iowa might be less suited for an Arizona garden than a grass of the same species from a community growing in the California desert. Many of these differences and adaptations are not well understood, yet it makes sense to use plants that are thriving in an area with climate and conditions similar to yours.

In trying to prevent erosion, stabilize dunes, improve stock ranges, and reseed after fires, misguided governmental agencies in the past have aided foreign species. Cooperation between ecologists, botanists, and horticulturists in various government agencies is resulting in more emphasis on using native grasses. It is an unfortunate reality that once native grasses have been replaced by foreign species, reestablishing the natives may be exceedingly difficult.

This encyclopedia contains the largest number of native American grasses of any gardening book to date. We hope that many more native grasses will find their way into gardening plans.

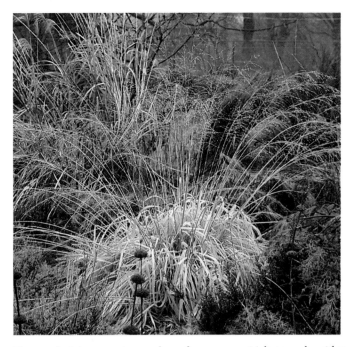

The wonderful warm-winter colors of moor grass, *Molinia,* and maiden grass, *Miscanthus,* brighten a dark winter day in the garden.

Evergreen or Deciduous?

Determining whether a grass is evergreen or deciduous is not a cut-and-dried process, because many grasses behave differently in different climates. The question is important especially to southern and western gardeners, who see more of their garden more of the time due to a lack of snow cover. It's also an important consideration in arid western climates, where dormant dried grasses can pose a serious fire danger.

In general, warm-season grasses tend to go dormant in winter; these plants are called deciduous. Cool-season grasses are more apt to be evergreen. But a hard freeze will often affect even "evergreen" grasses, burning or damaging the foliage. Depending on local conditions, new foliage may be quick to emerge. You will note grasses described as semideciduous or semi-evergreen in the encyclopedia section, if they are prone to behavior one way or the other depending on climate conditions that year.

Often, many cool-season grasses flower in spring and shut down new growth for the summer. No new foliage is produced, and dried seed heads cover the plant, making the grass look gold or brown rather than green. In some cases, cutting back foliage and shearing off old flower stems stimulate new growth. If this is the case, it is noted in the encyclopedia.

Some grasses that go dormant in dry summers will remain evergreen if you supply regular summer water. This tendency is mentioned in individual plant descriptions.

If fire is a consideration in your area, take care when planting grasses near buildings. Some grasses provide more fuel than others. Controlled burning is one way to reduce the danger, and most grasses can withstand being burned. If preventive burning is not feasible, cut back your grasses once they become dormant. New growth is less of a fire hazard than dry dormant foliage.

How to Buy Grasses

You can purchase grasses potted in soil, barerooted without soil, or as bareroot divisions. Mail-order nurseries have a large selection. Grasses are easily shipped and often are sent by delivery services or air freight.

Because ornamental grasses are a relatively new phenomenon, many local garden centers do not yet have large selections. Also, many grasses are somewhat difficult to maintain in container cultivation, and so they look unattractive in the garden center. However, the way they look in the garden center may not reflect their appearance once they are planted. Garden centers offer grasses in a variety of container sizes. Specimens and slower-growing grasses are often offered in traditional 1-gallon and 5-gallon pots. Groundcovers and low-growing plants are usually available as flats or plugs. Grasses such as moor grass (*Molinia* spp.) and some feather grasses (*Stipa* spp.) often do not bloom until their second season, so buying a larger plant is generally a good idea.

Bareroot plants are usually shipped with a 3- to 4-inch root ball, depending on the individual nursery. First-time mail-order customers are often dismayed by the appearance of their newly arrived grass. This dormant plant, often without visible signs of growth, is met with skepticism by the buyer, who cannot imagine that the dead-looking piece of sod will soon be 3 feet tall and as wide. But most grasses fill in very fast, and that 3-inch root ball may indeed be a nearly mature plant only one season later.

Grasses, especially dune grasses and large-scale groundcover plantings, are sometimes sold as bareroot divisions. Plants such as wild rye (*Elymus* spp.) are often sold by the culm. The catalog usually specifies the size, length, and thickness of the shoot. Bareroot divisions are usually packed without soil around the roots; plants must be from 1 to 2 feet long in order to bury them deep into sand.

Order grasses in fall and winter to assure availability in the spring. Rare and unusual cultivars and varieties may require considerable effort to locate. The list of nurseries on page 180 will help you find the grasses you need. If you are unable to locate the grasses you are interested in purchasing, local wholesalers may be able to provide you with a list of retail nurseries or garden services from which you can buy.

Most mail-order nurseries ship from early spring to late spring, with limited shipping in summer and fall. Many grasses cannot be shipped as barerooted plants in the hot summer months, and the weight of potted plants discourages most nurseries from shipping this way. In addition, by summer the foliage has emerged and can be damaged in shipping. These reasons keep most mail-order nurseries from shipping during the summer. Subtropical grasses are the biggest exception to this. Many of these grasses ship just fine in the warm summer months, because they do not begin growth until late in the spring. Often, they are not even available for early spring plantings. Some cool-season grasses can be barerooted in the fall and shipped with success, and some nurseries offer limited fall shipping.

Planting Ornamental Grasses

When to Plant

Most grasses are best planted in early spring so they will be established before the heat of summer. In addition, a better selection of grasses is usually available in the spring. In mild or southern climates, grasses can be planted year-round. Container-grown grasses can be planted in summer as long as adequate moisture or shading is provided to allow plants to get established.

Cool-season grasses can be planted in the fall, and they enjoy the early start. Though top growth may be marginal, fall plantings let roots become established prior to spring's burst of growth. This pays off with stronger, faster-growing plants in the spring. Fall planting carries the risk of winterkill. Protect new plantings from desiccating winter winds and keep them adequately moist to prevent the

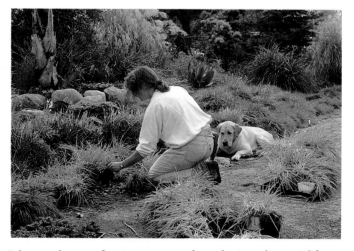

February planting of spring grasses in the author's garden in California. Dormant grasses in the background are still erect.

plants from drying out. Late fall plantings of some grasses may require winter protection (see page 18). To be safe, plant early in the fall.

Planting in the summer can be risky, because heat spells can catch new grasses before they have had enough time to establish. Cut the foliage back by one-fourth to one-third when you plant in hot summer, to prevent foliage damage until plants are established. New foliage is quick to return. During heat spells, plants may need constant moisture to avoid drying out.

Seeding grasses directly in the garden is best done in early spring, so the plants can become established before the heat of summer. Summer seeding is possible, but new plantings may require constant attention and watering, and you may need to overseed bare spots. Fall and winter seedings are slow to establish and are usually not advised, though in mild climates some grasses do just fine.

Soil Needs

Most grasses aren't fussy at all. They require little or no soil preparation or special care. This does not mean that plants do not grow better in improved soils. Most grasses readily reward any improvements with increased vigor and growth.

Soil

In general, grasses appreciate a soil rich in organic matter. But you must strike a balance between adequate care and overstimulation. Too much nitrogen may contribute to weak, floppy foliage, and a lowered resistance to insects and disease. Give your grasses an extra boost of nitrogen by applying well-rotted manure or compost. But once new grasses are established, cut down on fertilizers and let them adapt to a leaner soil.

Grasses are quick to adapt to their existing soils, so traditional soil preparation is often unnecessary. In some circumstances, however, special soil preparation is required for good growth. The art of garden-making lets you modify the soil, so you can grow almost any plant. More basic improvements are sometimes necessary, too. Grasses requiring good drainage, such as alpine grasses, benefit from the addition of sand or gravel. In many hot southern climates and southern clay soils, good drainage is essential to prevent rot in cool-season grasses that are more at home farther north.

Eliminating Noxious Grasses

The worst enemy of an ornamental grass planting is a noxious perennial grass. In the South and West, Bermuda grass (*Cynodon dactylon*) is one of the worst weeds in an

ornamental grass planting. Quack grass (*Agropyron repens*) often plagues gardeners in other parts of the country.

Eliminate perennial pest grasses long before planting. Organic control of running grasses can be difficult. Hand-pull as much of the pest grass as you can. Be sure to remove any broken bits of roots or stolons, which can reroot. Take your time and do a thorough job. When you are sure all the grass is removed, loosen the planting area with a garden fork and water the soil well. Wait two weeks for the pieces of grass you missed to rejuvenate and sprout. Weed out all traces, then let the prepared area sit for another two to four weeks to make sure all noxious grass is gone.

In the event of severe infestations, it may be nearly impossible to eradicate an undesirable grass. This is often solved by planting a more aggressive, taller grass that will shade out and dominate the lower weedy grass.

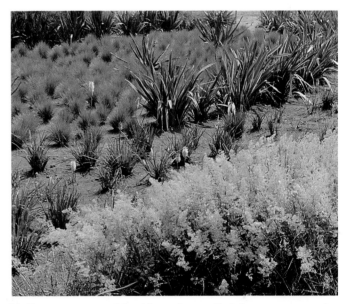

Mediterranean perennials with natal grass, *Rychelytrum repens,* and blue oat grass, *Helictotrichon sempervirens,* in the nursery ready to be dug and shipped.

Spacing

Determining the spacing of grass plantings can be a function of several factors: budget, aesthetics, and how fast you need cover.

Spacing is more often a matter of personal taste than of rules. There is no real right or wrong. Spacing clumping grasses farther apart gives a hummocky look preferred by some gardeners. Others like closer spacing, which creates a massing effect. As a general rule, place plants as far apart as their eventual height. Grasses that mature at 3 feet tall, for instance, may be planted 3 feet apart from center to center. On slopes or where a quick cover is desired, plant closer to help hold a steep bank or grade.

One of the most common mistakes to avoid when planting ornamental grasses is failing to realize just how big a plant will grow. Another common error is planting large grasses too close to a walkway. Remember to keep the eventual girth of the plant in mind.

Close spacing is a luxury that requires a large budget. If your budget is limited, it will just take a little more time for your planting to fill in.

Planting

Planting grasses is a relatively easy process; you just need to apply the same principles used in planting any perennial garden. Keep these guidelines in mind when planting grasses.

- Always try to match the original soil line of the plant.
- Avoid planting too high or too low below the crown. Many grasses, especially when small, will not tolerate being planted too deep.

- Water newly planted grasses immediately, and remember that newly planted grasses are particularly susceptible to drying out. On a hot summer day, young grass plants that have not been properly watered and are exposed to the sun can be killed in less than an hour.

Mulching

Once your newly planted grass has been watered deeply, mulch it to get it off to the best possible start. Mulching is an important step in ornamental grass gardening: It cools the surface temperature of the soil in hot climates, preserves moisture, keeps down weeds, and provides necessary soil nutrients. Mulching also provides a measure of winter protection, insulating both plant and soil. And a mulched surface provides an attractive backdrop while newly planted grasses are filling in. Wood chips, bark, compost, leaves, and grass clippings all make suitable mulches. Most grasses grow better with a 2- to 3-inch layer of mulch over the soil surface.

An accent grass, dwarf pampas grass, *Cortaderia selloana* 'Pumila', rises above a groundcover of side oats gramma, *Bouteloua curtipendula.*

Maintaining Ornamental Grasses

If they're properly selected and placed, most ornamental grasses need very little care or maintenance. However, some grasses do best with extra attention at various times of the year; these are noted in the encyclopedia section.

Watering

Once the plants are rooted, adjust watering to individual needs. In hot, dry climates, newly planted grasses may need water several times a day to be kept sufficiently moist. Keep the foliage cut back to one-fourth or one-third to reduce transpiration. Renewed, vigorous foliage will soon return. If newly planted grasses do get scorched or suffer dried foliage, simply cut back to force new growth.

In most gardens in the East and Midwest, grasses need little or no supplemental irrigation once they are established. Native, locally adapted grasses in all regions of the United States need no supplemental water. Many ornamental grasses, once established, are reliably drought-tolerant and will need additional water only in extreme periods of drought. Even if you don't water them, most grasses can weather a drought with little damage.

The growth of grasses can be regulated by watering or withholding water, especially in dry southern and western climates. Water the plant regularly and it will grow lushly and copiously; ration the water and the plant may be tight and slow-growing. In dry climates, water can literally be used as a growth regulator. On a dry slope, for example, the foliage of dwarf pampas grass (*Cortaderia selloana* 'Pumila') may reach 3 to 4 feet tall and 4 feet wide with flowers 2 to 3 feet above the leaves. But, on an irrigated golf course in rich soil, its foliage can reach 6 feet tall and 7 feet wide with flowers 3 to 4 feet above the foliage—hardly a dwarf!

Avoid extreme watering regimes. Grasses used to growing with lots of water will scorch easily if water is withheld. If this should occur, renew foliage by cutting back to the crown and resuming regular watering. Cool-season grasses can be cut back one-third, but most warm-season grasses need a hard chop. Warm-season grasses that have suffered drought stress may need to be cut to within several inches of the ground so that all-new foliage reemerges. It is surprising how fast new growth returns—many grasses can grow ½ inch per day.

Watering grasses can pose an interesting challenge to the homeowner. Water is most efficiently supplied if it can get directly to the roots; thus, overhead spray irrigation is not as efficient as drip irrigation. In some cases, watering from above also causes a more rapid decline of the flowers. The rapid growth in height of some grasses may defy overhead irrigation as well. How do you spray over a 6-foot grass? The best way to water is at the base of the plant. Drip hoses or bubblers are efficient ways to irrigate. One note of caution: If you install sprinkler heads, remember where you have placed them, or you may inadvertently cut them when you are cutting back the foliage.

Cutting Back the Foliage

The single most important maintenance rule for growing healthy, attractive grasses, with few exceptions, is to cut back the foliage at least once a year. New plantings of cool-season grasses may not need clipping until the end of their second season. In mild climates, some cool-season grasses may not require yearly cutting back, unless the foliage is unattractive or thick with old leaves. Some people do not cut back their grasses at all. The combination of old growth and new growth may look messy, but it doesn't affect the health of the plant.

Cutting back is a substitute for the natural processes of periodic burning and grazing that take place in natural grassland ecology. Spring burning removes last year's growth and exposes the soil to the warming rays of the sun, a boost for newly emerging grasses. While many grasses prefer to be burned, it is dangerous and often not possible for the home gardener. In many prairie plantings, however, burning is a recognized method of range management. Always check with the authorities to find out if burning is allowed in your area.

Cut back ornamental grasses just before or as the new season's growth begins to appear. It's best to cut most grasses back in late winter—generally, late February or early March, depending on climate. This timing allows you to enjoy the glories of winter foliage.

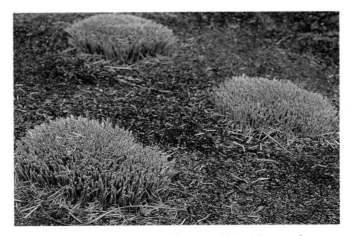

Dormant grasses, cut to the ground, are usually quick to send up new foliage. These *Miscanthus* clumps, cut to the ground in February, will be 7 feet tall and 6 feet wide by August!

As winter deepens, warm-season grasses take on their winter look. Many grasses have pale parchment or ruddy winter foliage that appears warm and bright under overcast skies. They hold this color well into the season, and are lovely when contrasted with a white blanket of snow under dark skies. Cutting in the fall would eliminate these grand winter effects.

Dormant grass left standing keeps the garden alive in winter with sound and movement. Graceful leaves and seed heads bend and rustle in the wind, adding interest even if admired through a window. Birds and wildlife visit the winter garden, seeking seeds and shelter. On the practical side, dormant foliage above the plant helps insulate it from cold and rain, and old foliage directs water away from the clump and helps prevent rot. Cutting back early will remove this protection. Still, some gardeners prefer a tidy look and cut back their grasses in the late fall, after fall color has left the foliage. Institutional gardens on tight budgets often cut their grasses back in the fall, because there are many early-spring chores and their staffs are small.

In mild climates, fall cutting can provide early renewal. The new season's growth begins to emerge in early winter, sometimes even in late fall. In these cases, cutting back early means a more attractive plant earlier in the season. In dry southwestern climates, dormant foliage may pose a fire hazard, and the removal of dormant foliage may be the law.

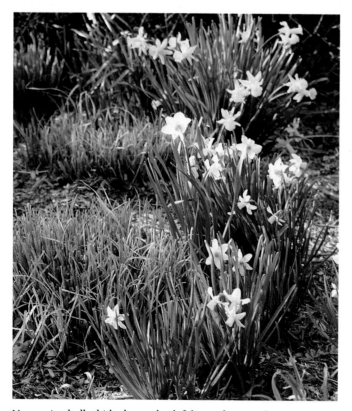

New spring bulbs hide the cut-back foliage of winter-dormant grasses.

HOW TO CUT BACK   How far to cut back grasses and how to do it are the two big questions. The answers depend on what grass it is and how big your garden is.

Most grasses should be cut back to within a few inches of the ground. Some grasses, usually cool-season grasses, do not like to be sheared too closely. Many feather grasses (*Stipa* spp.), for example, resent a close cut. Often, plants shorn too closely will not recover. To be safe, unless you have been successful in the past, cut back cool-season grasses to two-thirds of their full size.

Cutting old foliage before the new foliage arises is easier than trying to work around newly emerging shoots. Avoid damaging new shoots, but don't despair: A new crop will usually replace any that you accidentally slice off.

In a small garden, a sharp pair of hand pruners will work well for most cutting. Grasses with soft foliage can be cut with a string trimmer (like a Weed Eater), though this often leaves a ragged appearance. Tough, tall perennial grasses are most easily cut by a weed trimmer with a sawblade attachment. Keep all blades sharp. Some grasses develop thick canes with lots of silica in the foliage, which can quickly dull a blade.

Some grasses, usually spring bloomers, have spent flowers by midsummer that can look tattered and unattractive. Remove them once they have finished blooming. Cut the stems below the top of the foliage so the old stalks aren't visible.

A few grasses, especially wild ryes (*Elymus* spp.), can be sheared several times in the same season to force new growth. Shearing this grass in midsummer forces fresh, new metallic blue foliage for the late season.

In mild climates, some warm-season grasses like kangaroo grass (*Themeda* spp.) are sheared in September to force new growth for the fall. Although the flowers are sacrificed, the fall foliage is particularly showy. More experimentation is being done with this method to help sharpen and improve fall color on warm-season grasses in mild climates. While not as many flowers form on the new growth, still some will often appear. The trade-off is richer fall color later in the season.

Staking

Floppy grass foliage and flower stems are usually caused by insufficient light, over-fertilization, or excessive amounts of nitrogen. If you have a large, floppy grass, secure strong metal pipes in or near the clump, sinking them close to ground level. As the grass grows, insert smaller-diameter pipe into the tubes, and discreetly cover the supports with foliage. Remove pipes before cutting back the grasses. Support smaller grasses with wire loops, twiggy brush, or other holders as you would perennials or vegetables.

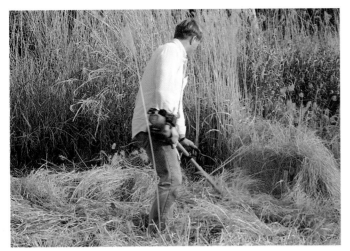

A weed trimmer fitted with a blade attachment is useful for cutting back tall grasses.

Dividing and Transplanting

Grasses are divided and transplanted to propagate more plants, to renew older existing plants, and to relocate existing grasses. (Propagation is discussed in detail below.) Many grasses require thinning or dividing to keep them looking their best. Older clumps may flop or grow too large for the space they occupy, or they may die out in the center and require rejuvenation. Growing trees and shrubs may provide too much shade for older grasses, requiring their removal and replacement with more shade-tolerant grasses. Large grasses that have been improperly placed may need to be moved to a more suitable location.

Divisions and transplantings are done at different times of year, depending on the type of plant and the plant's condition.

Warm-season grasses are best divided in late winter and early spring, and cool-season grasses in fall, winter, and early spring. A good method of gauging when to divide a grass is to watch for signs of active growth. Grasses may tolerate division at other times of the year, but the best time to divide is usually as new growth begins. Subtropical and tropical grasses can be divided even when actively growing.

Digging and dividing large clumps requires a strong back, a sharp axe, a saw, a shovel, and lots of work. Though many grasses tolerate being completely bareroot, it's always best to keep some soil on the roots of the plant you are digging. First divide the plant into fairly good-sized divisions. Most grasses can be divided further, into small shoots, if you want lots of divisions, but it will take them longer to reach full size than larger divisions.

When dividing grasses, cut the foliage back one-fourth to one-third to reduce loss of moisture through transpiration. Always keep newly divided plants moist and in the shade until they are in the ground.

Propagating Ornamental Grasses

Grasses are propagated mainly by division and seed. Some species can be grown from cuttings or from plantlets that form on certain grasses. Division is the only way to reliably propagate grasses and to perpetuate a plant's unique characteristics. Propagate named cultivars of ornamental grass by division only, to ensure uniformity: Many grass cultivars do not come true from seed, so a particular seedling may or may not be identical to its parent. But most seed-grown grasses are reasonably like the type.

Seed

While volumes of information have been published on growing cereal grasses from seed, little data exists on growing ornamental grasses from seed. Germination rates, times, percentages, and the feasibility of planting ornamental grasses from seed are all open to experimentation. Consult with a local grass grower before attempting a large-scale seeding of an ornamental grass. Many grasses are not available from seed, and some that are prove considerably expensive.

Some grasses can be directly seeded into the garden, but others must be grown from seed in the greenhouse. Often the seed is extremely fine, capable of blowing away in the slightest breeze. Other grasses can be directly seeded if drilled or placed beneath the soil. Seeding of some grasses has been tested, but much more needs to be learned.

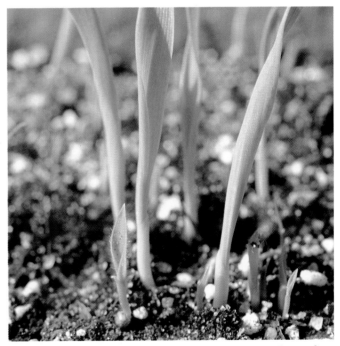

Emerging grass seedlings should be allowed to form several sets of leaves before transplanting.

In general, those grasses that can be grown from seed germinate in 10 to 20 days. Sometimes foliage emerges in 3 to 5 days; other times it may take 100 days or more to germinate. Some grasses prefer stratification of some kind prior to planting. Presoaking in warm water or chilling in damp sand are two seed treatments that have been practiced with ornamental grasses. Experiment with a small amount of seed rather than an entire crop. If little is known about direct seeding, it is better to start seedlings indoors and transplant them once they are established.

Despite apparent drawbacks, growing grasses from seed can often be rewarding and exciting. Many of the fine varieties and cultivars of ornamental grasses currently available were seedling variations themselves. If all grasses were grown from division, we would lose out on yet-undiscovered individuals. Some grasses are extremely variable from seed, but others are reasonably like their parents. Often, it is not important for all the plants to be exactly identical. Many botanists and ecologists feel that seed-grown plants create a stronger plant community in the garden than do large populations of a single cultivar. They feel that plants grown from seed are hardier and can fight off insects, diseases, and environmental changes better than divided or asexually propagated plants.

Division

As previously discussed (see page 21), different grasses are divided at different times of the year. Grass culms may separate easily by hand or may require a knife, a saw, or clippers to pry apart. Grasses with rhizomes, or underground stems, can be propagated by sprouting new plants from pieces of rhizome. Grasses with stolons, or above-ground runners, can be multiplied by rooting pieces of stolons. Always keep newly divided grasses from drying out. Protect them from hot sun and drying winds.

Cuttings

Some grasses will grow from cuttings of stems or other plant parts. Grasses that form thick culms or canes will often root from cuttings. Sugarcane (*Saccharum officinarum*) roots easily from cuttings of the cane. Successful cuttings have also been made from lemon grass (*Cymbopogon citratus*), fountain grass (*Pennisetum* spp.), and maiden grass (*Miscanthus* spp.). Because division is so easy, little work has been done with cuttings to date. However, research in this area is increasing, and new successes are being reported all the time. Grasses are being rooted with and without hormone applications. I hope that more research will soon be done in this area; the promise lies with grasses that have been difficult from division.

Plantlets

Some grasses and sedges, such as umbrella sedges (*Cyperus* spp.), will form new plants from buds held in the terminal bracts. Simply cut the terminal heads and float them upside down in water. Provide high heat and humidity for fast results. New plants will form in the axils of the bracts. Take newly rooted plants out of the water and place in soil.

A few grasses are viviparous, meaning that plants, rather than flowers, form on their flower stalks. Propagate these plantlets by detaching them and placing them in soil, where they will take root. A good example of a viviparous grass is 'Fairy's Joke' tufted hairgrass (*Deschampsia caespitosa* var. *vivipara* 'Fairy's Joke'), which produces loaded stalks of plantlets. It is not uncommon to see the occasional odd plantlet on most grasses.

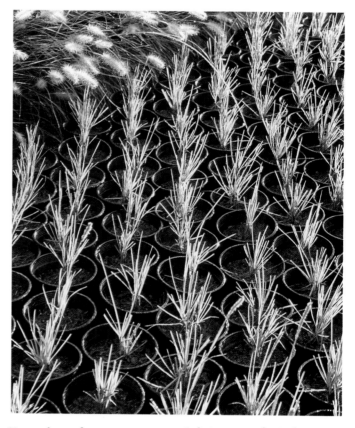

Young plants of autumn moor grass, *Sesleria autumnalis,* in the nursery.

Pests and Diseases

As a group, grasses are remarkably free of pests and diseases. When properly selected and placed in the garden, they are generally disease- and insect-free. Though some grasses are more prone to problems than others, most are easy to grow and undemanding.

Mealybugs and Aphids

Most grasses are rarely affected by insects. Some larger grasses can become hosts to mealybugs, but such infestations are rare. These white, cottony insects are usually found down in the leaf sheath, where the leaf connects to the stem. If the infestation is severe, dab the mealybugs with cotton swabs dipped in alcohol. Good air circulation will help prevent problems.

Aphids can sometimes be found on the succulent new growth. In most cases, treatment is unnecessary because the plants will quickly outgrow the insect-damaged foliage. However, you can wash aphids off foliage with a high-pressure hose, or treat with insecticidal soap.

Snails and Slugs

Snails and slugs can do far more damage to certain grasses than insects do. Most grasses are not affected by slugs and snails, and no treatments are necessary. Succulent-leaved grasses, subtropical grasses, and sedges are most susceptible to damage. A strip of copper edging or diatomaceous earth will deter slugs. Handpick at night, dropping slugs in soapy water, set out beer traps, or sprinkle with salt.

Gophers

For gardeners in the West, gophers are the greatest menace of all to ornamental grasses. A single gopher can raise havoc with a grass planting. Gophers tend to eat the roots right at the crown of the plant, often shearing it off at ground level. In areas where gopher infestations are severe, use wire baskets to prevent gophers from reaching the crown. Place grasses in large baskets made of chicken wire or a smaller mesh. A 2- to 3-foot basket is ideal.

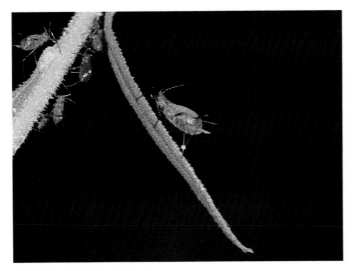

Aphids, a common grass pest.

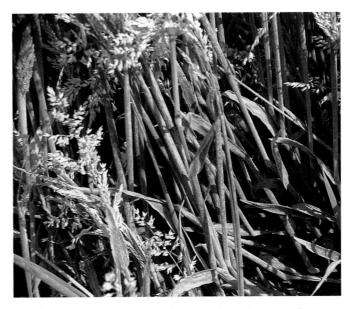

Rust disease on *Holcus lanatus*, velvet grass. Rust disease is often prevalent in wet, humid, spring-like conditions. It will usually disappear on its own as the season progresses.

Rabbits

Rabbits are another major problem for grasses. Certain grasses are like dessert for rabbits. Often, rabbits do not bother grasses with wiry, fine-textured, or sharp leaves. If natural food is available, rabbits will usually not prove a problem. Use a fence to keep rabbits out of your garden.

Deer

Deer are rarely a pest of grasses. Sometimes they will lightly browse succulent new growth; however, once the grass has toughened, deer will leave it alone.

Deer will generally try any new plant in the garden once, if not twice. Usually they do not like sharp-edged leaves and so will leave most grasses alone. In areas where deer are a problem, stick to growing sharper-leaved grasses, and consider erecting a deer-proof fence.

Rust

Rust is a fungal disease that shows up on ornamental grasses as orange spots, which can spread to cover the leaves. Remove infected leaves as soon as you see them. Clean up the garden at the end of the season, removing and destroying rust-infected plant material. If your grasses were troubled by rust last season, prevent its return by making periodic applications of wettable sulfur, starting several weeks before the disease normally strikes. Water the ground, not the foliage, and space susceptible grasses far enough apart for good air circulation.

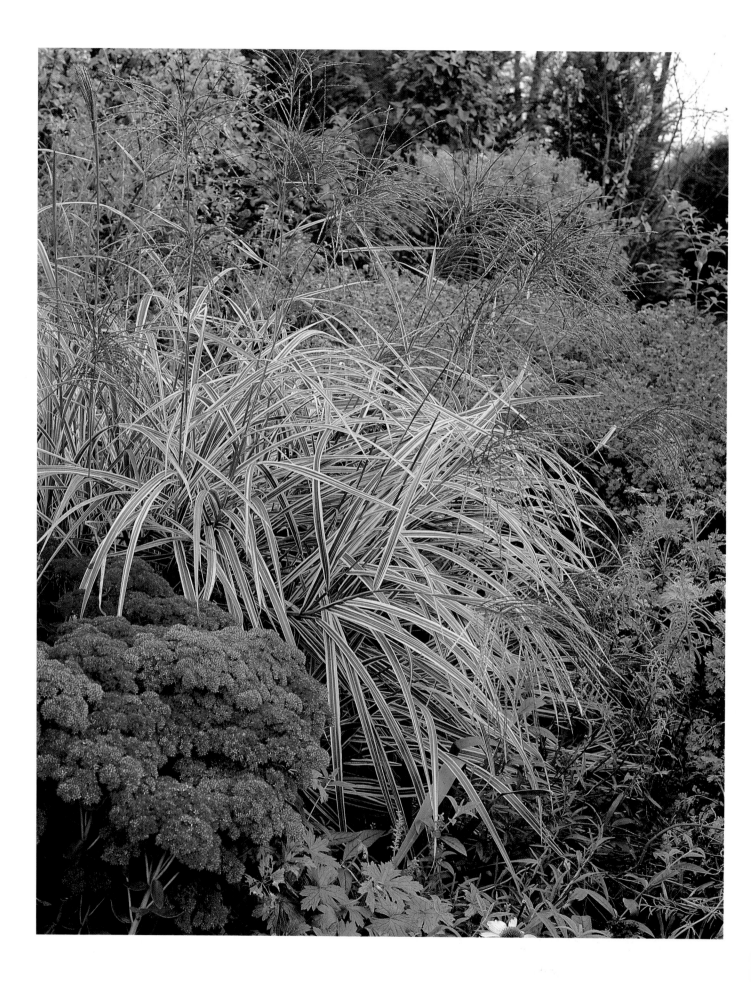

PART II

ENCYCLOPEDIA OF ORNAMENTAL GRASSES

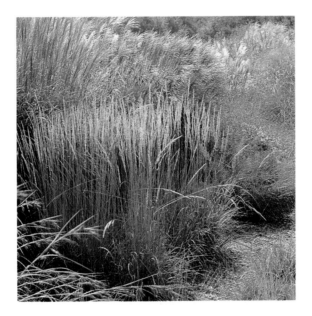

Opposite: The rich foliage of variegated Japanese silver grass spills forward under the weight of newly emerging flowers in this autumn border. Above: The pinkish plumes of various *Miscanthus* cultivars, background, dwarf the erect spikes of Foerster's feather reed grass, *Calamagrostis arundinacea* 'Karl Foerster', center, in Kurt Bluemel's demonstration garden.

BOTANICAL NAME	***Achnatherum calamagrostis* (also known as *Stipa calamagrostis*)**
PRONUNCIATION	ack-NATH-er-um kal-uh-muh-GROS-tis
COMMON NAME	Silver spike grass, spear grass
USDA HARDINESS ZONE	6 to 9
ORIGIN	Mountains of southern Europe
PREFERRED SITES	Warm sites in forest openings

DESCRIPTION: Cool-season, moderately spreading silver spike grass is distinguished by showy, long-lasting flowers and attractive foliage. Its medium green to grayish leaves, ¼ to ⅜ inch wide, grow 8 to 12 inches long on moderately spreading rhizomes. The foliage, 1½ to 2½ feet high, forms dense colonies that spread rapidly in light-textured, moist soils. The flowers bloom in June and are held on 2- to 3-foot upright spikes that bend gracefully under the weight of the flowers. The fluffy panicles grow 12 inches long and 2 to 3 inches wide, emerging a silky yellowish white and becoming a pleasing cream color at maturity. They are long-lasting and showy well into winter, especially in mild climates. The foliage turns orangish yellow with the onset of fall, becoming wholly dormant in cold climates and semidormant in mild climates.

LANDSCAPE USES: Silver spike grass is best in masses or drifts, where it has room to show off its silvery flowers. It is good on slopes, near stream banks, as a background for perennial borders, and along woodland edges. Its spreading habit makes it useful for erosion control and naturalizing. The flowers are stunning in fresh or dried arrangements.

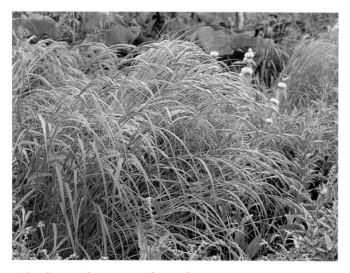

Achnatherum calamagrostis, silver spike grass.

CULTURE AND PROPAGATION: Silver spike grass grows best in fertile, moist soil in full sun or partial shade. It will tolerate some drought but grows poorly in hot, dry southwestern soils. In the West, it does best with regular water. Silver spike grass will languish and bloom poorly in too much shade. It is tolerant of moist soils if plenty of sun is present, and is tolerant of a wide range of soils if sufficient moisture is present.

Propagation is best by division, in the fall or spring. Propagating from seed is possible but difficult.

PESTS AND PROBLEMS: Not usually invasive, silver spike grass may creep into adjoining plantings under optimum conditions. Unwanted plants are not difficult to remove.

ACORUS
SWEET FLAG, ACORUS, CALAMUS

Acorus is neither a true grass nor a sedge, but actually a member of the Araceae, the arum or philodendron family. The two species and many cultivars of this grassy perennial are valuable additions to plantings along ponds or water gardens, or in any boggy area. Sweet flag contains the essential oil calamus, which imparts a sweet fragrance to all parts of the plant.

The roots and rhizomes of sweet flag have long been a source of perfume. Its foliage is often used as a strewing herb and in potpourri, and has been added to gin and beer as a flavor smoother and enhancer.

"Calamus" is derived from the Greek word *kalamos,* meaning "reed." The name describes its grassy, reedlike foliage which, depending on the species or cultivar, ranges from 1-inch miniatures to 6-foot giants. Sweet flag species of Europe and Asia are typically found in boggy places or in shallow ponds. Introduced into the United States during colonial times, sweet flag has naturalized in marshy places throughout the East.

It has a typical philodendron-like flower that, fresh or dried, is beautiful in floral arrangements. The yellow-green spathes are borne in clusters on short, spiked branches that arch upward directly out of the reedlike foliage. Often, flowers will appear only when plants are grown in water and may be insignificant in some cultivars.

Sweet flag takes on many garden roles, from groundcover to accent plant. The sweet-scented foliage can be enjoyed in pots, tubs, ponds, and water gardens. Sweet flag will even grow indoors in good, strong light. There are currently six different species and cultivars of sweet flag available from nurseries, and more are sure to follow.

Sweet flag prefers fertile, constantly moist, acid soil in full sun to partial shade, but it will tolerate a wide range of conditions as long as moisture is constantly available. It resents drying out and will show its sensitivity by producing brown tips and burnt foliage. It will grow in shallow water or boggy soils. In hot inland climates, plants do best in light shade or half-day sun. However, too much shade will stunt plants and cause taller plants to flop.

Sweet flag propagates easily by division. Propagating by seed is also possible with the species, but all cultivars must be propagated by division.

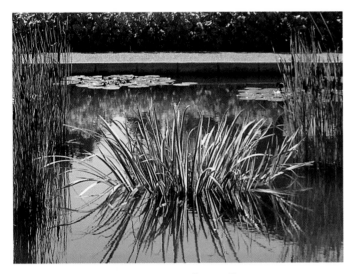

Acorus calamus 'Variegatus', variegated sweet flag.

BOTANICAL NAME	*Acorus calamus* 'Variegatus'
PRONUNCIATION	ah-KOR-us KAL-ah-mus var-ee-uh-GAH-tus
COMMON NAME	Variegated sweet flag, variegated calamus

DESCRIPTION: Variegated sweet flag is similar to sweet flag in all respects except that its foliage has vertical creamy yellow-white stripes. Foliage usually grows 3 to 4 feet tall.

LANDSCAPE USES: Variegated sweet flag makes a dramatic foliage accent in or around water. The yellow foliage will brighten a dark corner of a pond and provide a pleasing reflection on the water's surface. An excellent subject for pots or tubs, variegated sweet flag is dramatic when planted singly or in groups. It is particularly beautiful if planted where early morning or late afternoon sun can backlight its foliage.

BOTANICAL NAME	*Acorus gramineus*
PRONUNCIATION	ah-KOR-us gra-MIN-ee-us
COMMON NAME	Japanese sweet flag, grassy-leaved sweet flag
USDA HARDINESS ZONE	7 to 10
ORIGIN	Japan, China
PREFERRED SITES	Moist or boggy soils, wet areas

DESCRIPTION: Japanese sweet flag is an evergreen grasslike plant with glossy, dark green, fragrant leaves ½ inch wide and 6 to 12 inches tall. The foliage arises from slowly spreading, non-invasive rhizomes. It will grow in full sun or light shade but must be kept moist. Its flowers are small and inconspicuous. Japanese sweet flag has many cultivars, and certainly more will follow. Those currently available from nurseries and garden centers are listed below. Some are more readily available than others; miniatures usually command a high price.

LANDSCAPE USES: Japanese sweet flag is effective as a groundcover or as a pond or path edging. The crushed or bruised foliage emits the sweet calamus scent that is a welcome addition to any garden. Compact cultivars are excellent planted between stepping stones or in the cracks of paving. Good fillers, they are somewhat slow to establish but will tolerate heavy, constant traffic. Compact cultivars can be interplanted with the species or with dwarf sedges to make a fragrant lawn, with the source of the perfume a mystery and a delight to the untrained eye.

Dwarf and miniature variegated cultivars are good pot and bonsai subjects. Miniatures are useful as groundcovers under bonsai specimens. In rock gardens, Japanese sweet flag makes a good groundcover and accent plant. Its noninvasive habit lets it combine easily with other moisture-loving plants. It can be planted directly in a shallow pond.

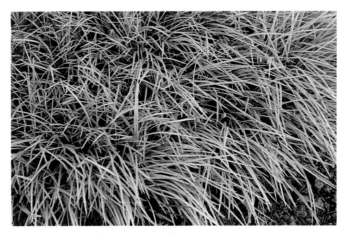

Acorus gramineus, Japanese sweet flag.

CULTURE AND PROPAGATION: Japanese sweet flag will produce burnt tips and yellowed foliage if it is allowed to dry out. Miniatures will quickly die if allowed to dry out. Alleviate this problem by setting pots on shallow trays with gravel and water underneath. In hot inland climates, grow Japanese sweet flag in light shade. With good light and sufficient air circulation, it makes an excellent indoor plant. The soil should be well drained but constantly moist.

PESTS AND PROBLEMS: Japanese sweet flag may be subject to spider mites. Watch for stippling on the foliage and listless growth, and treat immediately if detected, by washing the spider mites off with a steady spray of water.

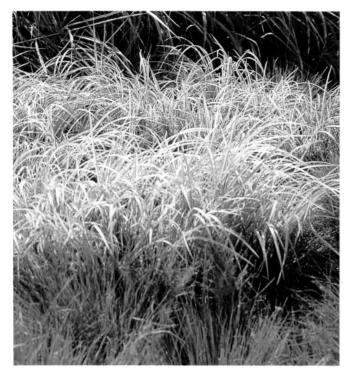

Acorus gramineus 'Ogon', golden variegated sweet flag.

BOTANICAL NAME	***Acorus gramineus* 'Ogon'**
PRONUNCIATION	ah-KOR-us gra-MIN-ee-us OH-gon
COMMON NAME	Golden variegated sweet flag

DESCRIPTION: The rich golden yellow foliage of golden variegated sweet flag grows ⅛ to ¼ inch wide and 10 inches tall. This superb cultivar is a fine addition to any garden. One of the best sweet flag cultivars, the golden foliage of golden variegated sweet flag makes a good pot and tub subject, edging, or groundcover, and brightens a garden path or pond.

BOTANICAL NAME	***Acorus gramineus* 'Pusillus'**
PRONUNCIATION	ah-KOR-us gra-MIN-ee-us pyoo-SILL-us
COMMON NAME	Dwarf grassy sweet flag

DESCRIPTION: Dwarf grassy sweet flag has dark green foliage ⅛ inch wide and 3 to 5 inches tall. It is slow-clumping and excellent planted between stepping stones because it will tolerate light foot traffic. It is effective but expensive for mass plantings.

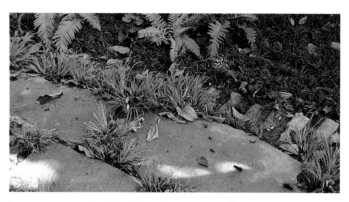

Acorus gramineus 'Pusillus', dwarf grassy sweet flag.

BOTANICAL NAME	***Acorus gramineus* 'Variegatus'**
PRONUNCIATION	ah-KOR-us gra-MIN-ee-us var-ee-uh-GAH-tus
COMMON NAME	White-striped Japanese sweet flag

DESCRIPTION: An old garden cultivar with green and creamy white variegated foliage, white-striped Japanese sweet flag grows ⅛ to ¼ inch wide and 6 to 12 inches tall. This cultivar grows best in light shade. In full sun it will look unattractive. It is attractive planted in masses along pond edges or streamsides.

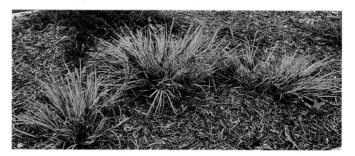

Acorus gramineus 'Variegatus', white-striped Japanese sweet flag.

OTHER *Acorus gramineus* CULTIVARS AND VARIETIES ARE:

'Masamune' ('Masamune' sweet flag): white-striped variegated leaves; grows to 6 inches tall; rare.

'Oborozuki' ('Oborozuki' sweet flag): yellow-striped foliage; grows to 8 inches tall.

'Pusillus Minimus' (Miniature Japanese sweet flag): leaves grow to 2½ inches; very slow-growing; rare.

'Pusillus Minimus Aureus' (Miniature variegated Japanese sweet flag): foliage bleached golden yellow; quite rare.

'Tanomanoyuki' ('Tanomanoyuki' sweet flag): occasional stripes of yellow foliage; grows to 9 inches tall.

'Yodonoyuki' ('Yodonoyuki' sweet flag): green foliage bleached yellow along the midrib; rare.

ANOTHER SWEET FLAG SPECIES IS:

Acorus calamus (Sweet flag): a tall-growing, green-leaved species; grows 4 to 6 feet tall.

BOTANICAL NAME	**Agropyron magellanicum (also known as Elymus magellanicus)**
PRONUNCIATION	ag-roh-PEYE-ron ma-jel-LAN-ih-cum
COMMON NAME	Blue wheat grass, Magellan blue grass
USDA HARDINESS ZONE	5 to 9
ORIGIN	South America
PREFERRED SITES	Well-drained soil, coastal slopes

DESCRIPTION: Clumping, blue-foliaged blue wheat grass is arguably the bluest of ornamental grasses. It is often listed under different names, and several cultivars may be available, but all are graced with metallic blue foliage. Quite similar in leaf texture to blue Lyme grass (*Elymus arenarius* 'Glaucus'), blue wheat grass forms dense clumps 1 to 1½ feet tall and as wide. Its smooth leaves, ¼ to ½ inch wide, are 8 to 12 inches long. In June, its flowers erect a wheatlike bluish green spike that matures to a straw color. Though noticeable, the flowers are secondary to the striking color of the foliage. Blue wheat grass is evergreen in mild climates. It may go dormant in cold climates.

LANDSCAPE USES: Blue wheat grass makes a fine accent or specimen in perennial borders. The blue color is almost iridescent and easily becomes a focal point. It is good in combination with purple flowers and bronze foliage, and combines well with dwarf conifers. Though not spectacular, the flowers are attractive in fresh or dried arrangements.

CULTURE AND PROPAGATION: Blue wheat grass grows best in moist, well-drained soil in full sun. It resents hot, dry sites or soggy, wet soil. It needs excellent drainage and half-day sun to survive hot inland climates, but does well in coastal gardens. Largely untested in California, it is a fine plant in the Pacific Northwest.

Propagate by division or seed.

PESTS AND PROBLEMS: A recent introduction to the United States, blue wheat grass may be difficult to find in nurseries.

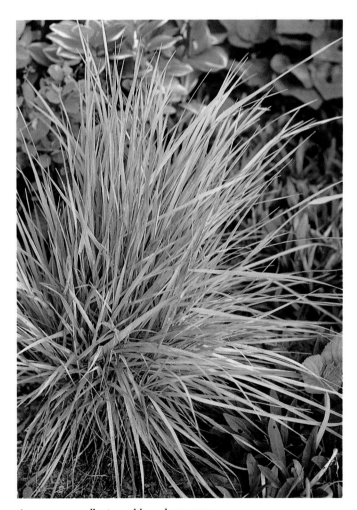

Agropyron magellanicum, blue wheat grass.

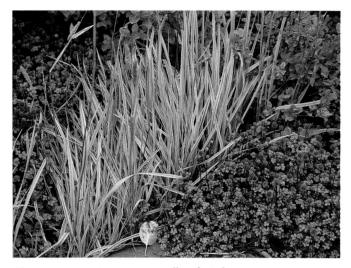

Alopecurus pratensis var. *aureus,* yellow foxtail grass.

BOTANICAL NAME	*Alopecurus pratensis* var. *aureus*
PRONUNCIATION	al-o-PEK-u-rus prah-TEN-sis AW-ree-us
COMMON NAME	Yellow foxtail grass
USDA HARDINESS ZONE	6 to 9
ORIGIN	Eurasia
PREFERRED SITES	Meadows, woodlands

DESCRIPTION: This mostly evergreen grass has bright yellow-green linear stripes along light green leaves, giving the plant an almost lime green cast. A cool-season grass, yellow foxtail is a slowly spreading grass with a low-growing, matlike habit. The leaves are ¼ to ⅛ inch wide and 4 to 6 inches tall, and flop along the ground. This plant has a slender flower spike that emerges in the spring and rises 6 to 12 inches above the foliage. Although noticeable, it is not particularly showy. The "foxtail" is a cylindrical panicle soft to the touch. Noninvasive, yellow foxtail grass grows best in full sun, except in hot climates, where light or afternoon shade will keep the plant looking more attractive.

LANDSCAPE USES: Yellow foxtail makes a good filler and spiller. Evenly moist soil is preferred; it seems to resent either boggy or dry soils. Plant it alone or in masses. It is an excellent grass for planting with spring bulbs, which contrast or blend with its yellow-green foliage.

CULTURE AND PROPAGATION: Yellow foxtail grass excels in cooler climates and doesn't grow well in hot temperatures. Because of this, it is probably not a good plant for dry, desertlike climates.

Propagate by division in the spring or fall. It does not naturalize from seed.

PESTS AND PROBLEMS: In warm climates yellow foxtail grass is subject to rust, a fungus disease, at the times of the year when rust is prevalent. Treat with an appropriate fungicide (see page 23), or simply cut back the foliage to within 1 inch of the ground and fertilize.

BOTANICAL NAME	*Ammophila arenaria*
PRONUNCIATION	am-AH-fil-la ayr-en-AYR-ee-ah
COMMON NAME	European beach grass, European dune grass
USDA HARDINESS ZONE	5 to 10
ORIGIN	Europe
PREFERRED SITES	Coastal sand dunes

DESCRIPTION: This spreading, warm-season grass forms thick colonies along sandy beaches and dunes. It has an American counterpart, American beach grass (*Ammophila breviligulata*), native to the shores of the Great Lakes and sandy areas in the Northeast. European beach grass was introduced to the United States by the Army Corps of Engineers to stabilize dunes, effectively establishing European beach grass along most of the Gulf and West Coast. It is now the dominant coastal grass throughout Oregon and Washington. While its sand-binding abilities are legendary, European beach grass has taken over the habitat of native dune grasses such as Pacific dune grass (*Elymus mollis*) and sea oats (*Uniola paniculata*).

European beach grass has long, leathery, gray-green leaves that are ⅛ to ¼ inch wide with rolled edges, making the leaves look cylindrical. Spreading foliage grows 2 to 3 feet tall. The grass forms thick rhizomes that hold sand in place, preventing loss from wind and erosion. Plants tend to form dense hummocks that collect windblown sand.

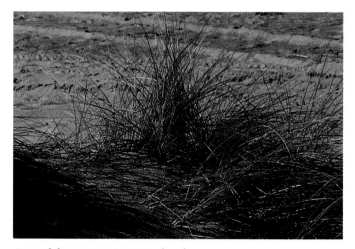

Ammophila arenaria, European beach grass.

Flowers emerge in June in a simple spike borne 1 to 2 feet above the leaves. Leaves and flowers tend to flop, so the plant remains only 2 to 3 feet tall. Flowers are not particularly showy.

LANDSCAPE USES: European beach grass is used primarily as a large-scale groundcover for sandy sites. It is best in coastal gardens and for erosion control on sandy slopes. The plant will survive burial in shifting sand by producing new shoots from the internodes.

European beach grass prefers sandy soil in full sun or light shade. Plants resent heavy wet clay. Plants withstand wind and are salt-tolerant.

CULTURE AND PROPAGATION: Division is best, as seeds are often sterile. Divide plants in spring or fall. Make large divisions, with 1 to 2 feet of rhizome, and plant them deep in the sand.

PESTS AND PROBLEMS: The only problem you may have with European beach grass is if mail-order plants dehydrate during shipping. Plants are often shipped bareroot, since sand won't stay on the roots. Keep divisions cool and moist and do not let them dry out until plants are established.

ANDROPOGON
BLUESTEM, BEARDGRASS, ANDROPOGON

The *Andropogon* genus contains over 200 species that are found all over the world. In North America, bluestem comprised a large part of what used to be extensive tall- and shortgrass prairies, found naturally in almost every state in the continental United States. Bluestems are now greatly reduced in their native habitats. Their common names refer to their reddish purple to silvery blue flower stems and their fluffy, beardlike blooms.

Most bluestems tolerate dry conditions, though many species prefer moist or boggy soil. They vary in height from 1-foot-tall compact miniatures to giants approaching 10 feet tall. It has been written that a man would have to stand on his horse to see over the top of mature stands of big bluestem. Early descriptions of the prairie often evoked images of oceans or seas. Bluestems quite literally were the original amber waves seen by the first European settlers on the prairie.

Botanists recently split the genus *Andropogon* into two groups, *Andropogon* and *Schizachyrium*. Many older grass references do not contain this recent division. Therefore, the two genera are often confused and substituted correctly or incorrectly for one another. Many andropogons also

have incredibly large areas of distribution. This translates into numerous forms and variations that have yet to be accurately described. To add to the confusion, plants grow differently in different climates. For example, big bluestem, which can easily reach 8 feet or more in the East, is rarely 5 feet tall in New Mexico and may not reach 3 feet in Southern California.

As a group, the bluestems are at their best in large drifts or masses. Many are excellent as a large-scale groundcover for parks, highways, medians, and slopes. Most are easy to propagate from seed and division. Seed from locally collected populations is usually preferred as it should be best adapted to local conditions.

Overlooked by early European grass enthusiasts, the bluestems are enjoying new attention as many new species are making their way into the American nursery trade. The native plant movement has done much to popularize these stunning native grasses. Named cultivars selected for height, and for intensive fall colors from red to purple and orange, will soon be introduced into nurseries and garden centers.

BOTANICAL NAME	***Andropogon gerardii***
PRONUNCIATION	an-droh-POH-gon jer-AR-dee-eye
COMMON NAME	Big bluestem, turkey foot
USDA HARDINESS ZONE	4 to 10
ORIGIN	North America from Oklahoma to Canada
PREFERRED SITES	Dry soils, open prairie

DESCRIPTION: Big bluestem was the primary grass of the tallgrass prairies that once extended from Ohio to Colorado and from Oklahoma to Canada. Today, very little pure prairie remains. Often growing taller than 6 feet, this

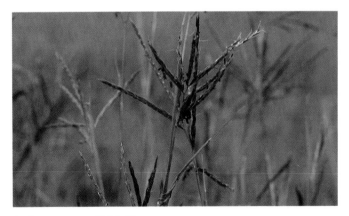

Andropogon gerardii, big bluestem.

inland sea of grass was the original sod that the first farmers plowed under, destroying forever the rich tapestry of flora and fauna associated with it.

A deciduous, clumping, warm-season grass, big bluestem ranges in color from shades of blue-green to silvery blue. The foliage grows in clumps from 4 to 7 feet tall and can reach 10 feet tall with optimum conditions. The purplish flower spikes, ¼ to ½ inch wide, emerge in August and September. Also distinctive is its three-branched seed head, which suggested one of its common names, turkey foot.

LANDSCAPE USES: Big bluestem is useful as a tall background plant or screen. At home in mass plantings or naturalized areas, it excels along highways and is a good plant to use for erosion control. In perennial borders, a single specimen can be very dramatic. Big bluestem has good fall color in varying bronze tones, and the color persists into winter. Use cut flowers in fresh or dried arrangements.

CULTURE AND PROPAGATION: Big bluestem grows best in full sun in moist, well-drained soil. It tolerates considerable drought but will be shorter and more compact. In its original habitat, it receives considerable summer moisture; in arid southwest climates, it will benefit from water in summer. Not shy of heat, big bluestem can be effective in hot spots in the garden, against a south wall, or near paving.

Propagate by seed, or by division in early spring.

PESTS AND PROBLEMS: Big bluestem has no known pests or problems.

SOME *Andropogon gerardii* CULTIVARS ARE:

'Champ' ('Champ' big blue-stem): grows 5 to 6 feet tall with good fall color; best in sandy soils.

'Roundtree' ('Roundtree' big bluestem): upright; reaches 6 to 7 feet; early-blooming.

'Kaw' ('Kaw' big bluestem): southerly selection that is later-flowering.

'Pawnee' ('Pawnee' big blue-stem): somewhat weeping 5- to 6-foot foliage; subject to rust in high-rainfall areas.

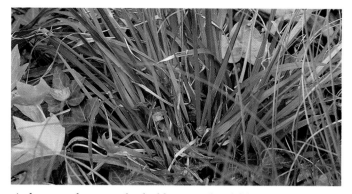

Andropogon glomeratus, bushy bluestem—basal foliage in winter color.

BOTANICAL NAME	***Andropogon glomeratus***
PRONUNCIATION	an-DROH-poh-gon gloh-mer-AH-tus
COMMON NAME	Bushy bluestem
USDA HARDINESS ZONE	5 to 10
ORIGIN	Eastern and southern United States
PREFERRED SITES	Widespread, generally moist locations, water margins

DESCRIPTION: Clumping, deciduous bushy bluestem is distinguished by its dense, fluffy clusters of cottony flowers. Bright, glossy green leaves, ¼ to ½ inch wide and 10 to 18 inches long, form a tight, handsome clump of foliage 1 to 2 feet tall and as wide. The flowers emerge from August through September and rise 2 to 3 feet above the foliage. The flowers mature to fluffy plumes that form whisklike clusters at the tops of the stems. These cottony plumes are effective at catching light. In the fall the flower spikes turn a warm orange and the leaves turn reddish purple.

LANDSCAPE USES: Bushy bluestem is at its best near water, along streams, and in bogs or tubs. Plant it against a dark background or where early morning and late afternoon sunlight can backlight the flowers. Bushy bluestem makes a good accent planted alone or massed in drifts or groups. The flowers are stunning in fresh arrangements.

CULTURE AND PROPAGATION: Bushy bluestem grows best in moist, fertile loam in full sun. It tolerates light shade but does not do well in too much shade. It tolerates hot climates and coastal conditions as long as constant moisture is present. Bushy bluestem will readily naturalize in moist areas. Under ideal conditions it can become invasive.

Propagate by seed or division.

PESTS AND PROBLEMS: Bushy bluestem has no known pests or problems.

BOTANICAL NAME	***Andropogon saccharoides*** **(also known as *Bothriochloa saccharoides*)**
PRONUNCIATION	an-DROH-poh-gon sak-uh-ROY-deez
COMMON NAME	Silver beardgrass, silver bluestem
USDA HARDINESS ZONE	5 to 9
ORIGIN	Southwestern United States
PREFERRED SITES	Prairies, openings in woods, rocky slopes, sandy banks

DESCRIPTION: Silver beardgrass is a clumping, deciduous grass that is somewhat similar to split beard bluestem (*Andropogon ternarius*). Silver beardgrass is admired for the silky flower puffs that clothe its vertical stems, and it is better suited to dry climates than split beard bluestem. Silver beardgrass forms dense tufts of glossy green foliage 12 to 18 inches tall and as wide. Erect vertical flower spikes grow 2 to 3 feet above the foliage. They appear from May through September and mature to display showy, fluffy white seed heads. As fall progresses, the leaves begin to turn from red to purple or burnt orange. The contrast of the leaves with the fluffy panicles creates a breathtaking effect in the fall and early winter. Like most other bluestems, this grass holds its fall color deep into winter.

LANDSCAPE USES: Silver beardgrass is an effective flowering accent planted alone or in groups. It makes a good large-scale groundcover on rocky slopes or sandy banks and makes a spectacular winter accent. Its flowers are stunning in fresh arrangements.

CULTURE AND PROPAGATION: Silver beardgrass prefers well-drained, fertile soil in full sun. Good drainage is essential

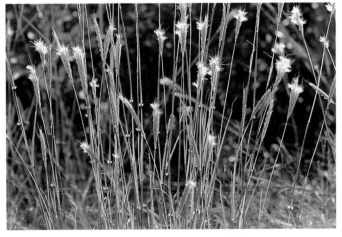

Andropogon saccharoides, silver beardgrass, in fall glory.

for good growth. It tolerates light shade but will flop over in too much shade.

Propagate by division or seed.

PESTS AND PROBLEMS: Silver beardgrass has no known pests or problems.

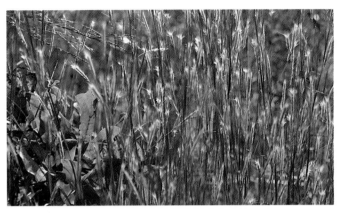

Andropogon ternarius, split beard bluestem, in fall color.

BOTANICAL NAME	***Andropogon ternarius***
PRONUNCIATION	an-DROH-poh-gon ter-NAIR-ee-us
COMMON NAME	Split beard bluestem
USDA HARDINESS ZONE	6 to 9
ORIGIN	Widespread from eastern United States to Kansas and from Florida to Texas
PREFERRED SITES	Dry sandy soils, openings in woods

DESCRIPTION: Split beard bluestem is distinguished by its erect, vertical columns of fluffy, cottony plumes. The plant forms a tight clump of deciduous foliage that varies in color from glossy green to green with purplish tints. There are only a few small leaves; the bulk of the plant is composed of flower spikes. Plants form clumps of leaves 1 to 1½ feet tall and as wide. The flower spikes reach 4 to 5 feet tall. Pairs of cottony racemes, silvery to creamy or grayish, are found along the vertical flower stems. When properly situated, this grass evokes images of shooting fireworks.

LANDSCAPE USES: Split beard bluestem is an effective flowering accent planted alone or in mass. It is a good erosion control and slope planting in poor or sandy soils and is a strong performer in coastal gardens. It is stunning in fresh flower arrangements.

CULTURE AND PROPAGATION: Split beard bluestem grows best in well-drained, fertile soil in full sun. It tolerates a wide variety of soil conditions and exposures, including light shade and coastal conditions. This species reseeds readily and can be invasive; it is not invasive in dry western climates.

Propagate by seed or division; it is easier to propagate by seed.

PESTS AND PROBLEMS: Split beard bluestem has no known pests or problems.

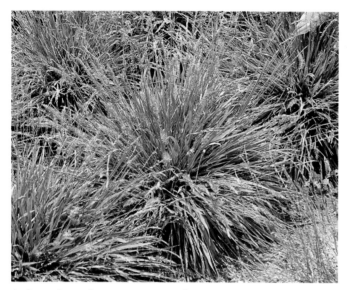

Anthoxanthum odoratum, sweet vernal grass.

BOTANICAL NAME	***Anthoxanthum odoratum***
PRONUNCIATION	an-thoh-ZAN-thum oh-dor-AH-tum
COMMON NAME	Sweet vernal grass
USDA HARDINESS ZONE	5 to 10
ORIGIN	Eurasia; now naturalized from Newfoundland to Louisiana and Michigan; Pacific Coast from British Columbia to central California
PREFERRED SITES	Open pastures, meadows

DESCRIPTION: Sweet vernal grass is a clumping, evergreen, cool-season grass. Its soft, medium green leaves grow ¼ to ½ inch wide and 6 to 8 inches tall. The foliage has a high coumarin content and is fragrant when crushed or brushed against. The flowers emerge a silky green with showy yellow stamens on slender, cylindrical, spikelike panicles that grow 12 to 16 inches above the foliage in May through June; they dry to golden yellow in early summer. The flowers are showy on the plant from spring to late fall.

LANDSCAPE USES: Use sweet vernal grass as a border or edging along pathways, where its pleasant scent can be enjoyed. It will tolerate considerable foot traffic; in fact, if plants are placed close together they can be an occasionally mowed lawn. Sweet vernal grass makes an excellent meadow or mass planting and is effective along median strips and parkways. Its cut leaves remain fragrant for days.

CULTURE AND PROPAGATION: Sweet vernal grass grows best in full sun, but tolerates light shade. In hot, arid climates, light shade or half-day sun is best. Sweet vernal grass grows in just about any soil, but fertile acid loam is best. It takes damp or dry conditions, but in dry conditions it will not be as lush.

Propagate by seed, or by division in spring or fall.

PESTS AND PROBLEMS: Sweet vernal grass has no known pests or problems.

BOTANICAL NAME	***Aristida purpurea***
PRONUNCIATION	a-ris-TIH-dah pur-pur-EE-ah
COMMON NAME	Purple three awn
USDA HARDINESS ZONE	6 to 9
ORIGIN	Southwestern North America, from Arkansas to California; northern Mexico and throughout Texas
PREFERRED SITES	Dry hills, plains

DESCRIPTION: This semi-evergreen, clumping grass is the drought-tolerant grass of the shortgrass prairie. Fine-textured, sage green foliage forms dense tufts ¹/₃₂ to ¹/₁₆

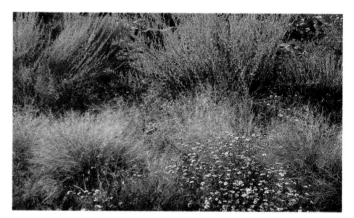

Aristida purpurea, purple three awn.

inch wide and 6 to 12 inches long. The flowers emerge on erect spikes 1½ to 2½ feet tall, and delicate, nodding panicles emerge a silky greenish purple, becoming more purple as the seed matures. The three segmented awns are needlelike and are very effective at catching the light. At maturity, the purple bleaches to a whitish golden-brown. The flowers are showy and persist on the plant.

LANDSCAPE USES: Purple three awn is good planted in groups and masses and is an excellent groundcover in hot, dry situations. A striking flowering accent for southwestern gardens, it is extremely drought-tolerant and heat-resistant. The flowers are beautiful in fresh or dried arrangements.

CULTURE AND PROPAGATION: Purple three awn grows best in well-drained soil in full sun. It resents moist or boggy conditions.

Propagate by seed, or by division in spring.

PESTS AND PROBLEMS: Purple three awn naturalizes in favorable conditions and can even become somewhat weedy. Depending on where it is planted, it can be a problem, since the dried seed heads adhere to clothing and pets.

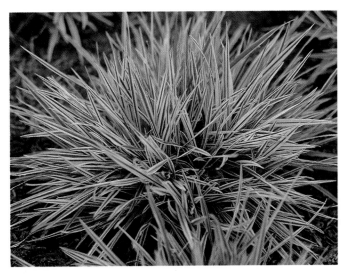

Arrhenatherum elatius var. *bulbosum* 'Variegatum', bulbous oat grass.

CULTURE AND PROPAGATION: Bulbous oat grass grows best in moist, well-drained, acid soil. Plant it in full sun in cool climates, and in partial shade in hot climates. It is not a good grass for sunny, hot climates, and it can look shabby in the summer. It may languish in heavy wet clays.

Propagate by division in spring or fall.

PESTS AND PROBLEMS: Bulbous oat grass is particularly susceptible to rust and can be quite unattractive when infected. Treat with an appropriate organic fungicide (see page 23) or cut back foliage and fertilize if the plants become unsightly.

BOTANICAL NAME	***Arrhenatherum elatius var. bulbosum* 'Variegatum'**
PRONUNCIATION	ah-ren-AH-ther-um el-AH-tee-us bul-BOH-sum var-ee-uh-GAH-tum
COMMON NAME	Bulbous oat grass
USDA HARDINESS ZONE	4 to 9
ORIGIN	Horticultural selection
PREFERRED SITES	Moist, well-drained areas

DESCRIPTION: Bulbous oat grass is a clumping, cool-season grass noted for its white-striped foliage. It is called bulbous oat grass because of the peculiar bulbous nodes found below the foliage at the base of the stem. The nodes resemble a rattlesnake tail and may be seen only by pulling away the foliage or cutting back the plant. It is prized for its showy white foliage, ⅛ to ¼ inch wide and 6 to 12 inches tall. A small, erect, oatlike spike emerges from May through June and is showy throughout the summer.

LANDSCAPE USES: Clumps of bulbous oat grass are effective as specimens in rock gardens or perennial borders. New spring growth is striking when planted with silver- and gray-foliaged plants. It is a good accent for both its flowers and its foliage.

BOTANICAL NAME	***Arundo donax***
PRONUNCIATION	ah-RUN-doh DOH-nax
COMMON NAME	Giant reed
USDA HARDINESS ZONE	6 to 10
ORIGIN	Southern Europe
PREFERRED SITES	Streamsides in canyons near moisture

DESCRIPTION: Giant reed is perhaps the best example of the definition of a weed as "a plant out of place." Originally brought to the New World by Spanish colonizers, it is now labeled a noxious weed in California and several southern states. Yet its grace and utility in cold climates make it a treasured perennial and a much sought-after specimen. This tall grass was the bamboo of the New World. Fast-growing and tolerant of sun, heat, and drought, it was a most utilitarian plant for early settlers. Its stout canes could be used in all manner of construction, as fences, animal pens, cages, and roof thatching, and in innumerable other

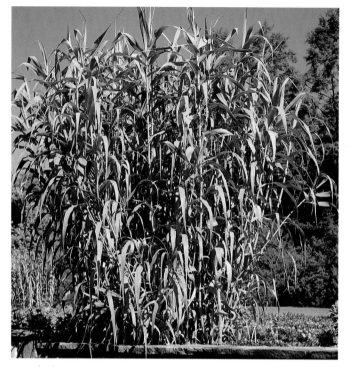

Arundo donax, giant reed.

crafts. Giant reed canes are still the source of reeds for woodwind instruments. In California, the Spanish mission fathers introduced giant reed and planted it up and down the state. In addition to its construction value, it provided shade and an effective windbreak. Today, giant reed has invaded natural habitats. Though maligned and misunderstood, it is still a valuable ornamental in its proper place.

Giant reed has vigorous, upright, arching canes that can reach 10 to 25 feet tall. Its blue-green foliage grows 2 to 3 inches wide and 18 to 24 inches long. The foliage clasps the hollow canelike stem. These canes sprout from dense, woody rhizomes. Flowers are fluffy panicles 18 to 30 inches tall and 6 to 10 inches wide. They emerge in September and persist on the plant into winter. In mild climates, the foliage is evergreen, and second-year canes may branch in warmer climates. Giant reed turns beige with the first frost and remains a giant dormant skeleton of its former self, making an attractive winter display.

LANDSCAPE USES: Giant reed is an outstanding tall screen and windbreak. It is stunning planted alone or in groups. When backlit or silhouetted against walls or buildings, this plant has a dramatic architectural quality. Its form is also attractive at or near the water's edge, where its canes can arch over the bank and be reflected in the water. Cut flowers are striking in arrangements. Giant reed tolerates sand or alkaline conditions and is a superior choice for seacoast gardens, where it serves as a windbreak and sand stabilizer.

CULTURE AND PROPAGATION: Giant reed grows best in fertile, moist, well-drained soil, but with a little moisture it will grow just about anywhere, in any soil. It will tolerate heat and seacoast conditions with equal vigor. Clumps may eventually get too large and require thinning. Even in mild climates, in a garden situation, giant reed is best cut to the ground in February or March to keep the plant neat and attractive. By midsummer, mature plants can reach 20 feet from clumps cut to the ground in March. Control plant size and spread in arid climates by adding or withholding water. In cold climates at the edge of its hardiness range, plants may not flower before the onset of winter.

Propagate by division, or by cuttings of basal stems in the spring.

PESTS AND PROBLEMS: In moist situations, plants can colonize quite rapidly and could become invasive; however, this rarely happens in cold climates.

BOTANICAL NAME	***Arundo donax* 'Variegata'**
PRONUNCIATION	ah-RUN-doh doh-nax var-ee-uh-GAH-tah
COMMON NAME	Striped giant reed

DESCRIPTION: Similar in most respects to the species, *Arundo donax*, striped giant reed is distinguished by creamy yellow-white variegated leaves. Not as tall as the species, it usually reaches a height of 6 to 12 feet, and even higher in hot climates, depending on moisture and location. The stripes are most pronounced in the spring and tend to fade by late summer, when the yellow color is found only at the tips. Like the species, it turns beige with the first frost, and goes completely dormant in cold climates.

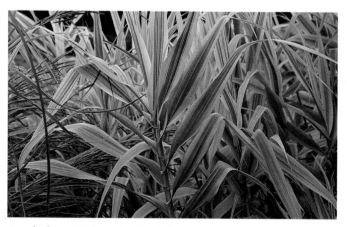

Arundo donax 'Variegata', striped giant reed.

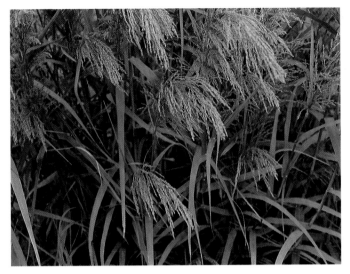

Arundo pliniana, arrow reed.

BOTANICAL NAME	*Arundo pliniana*
PRONUNCIATION	ah-RUN-doh plih-nee-AH-nah
COMMON NAME	Arrow reed
USDA HARDINESS ZONE	6 to 10
ORIGIN	Eurasia
PREFERRED SITES	Moist places, streamsides

DESCRIPTION: The sharp, stiff leaves and slender upright canes of this odd reed make it mostly a collector's item. The bluish leaves are stiff and attach to the culm at almost a right angle. The leaves, ¾ to 1 inch wide and 3 to 5 inches long, are sharply pointed and rather sparse along the culms, which are 1 to 1½ inches wide and grow 6 to 10 feet tall in odd, almost animated clumps. The flowers, long fluffy panicles, bloom in fall and are persistent on the plant. Becoming dormant with a hard freeze, arrow reed's curious skeleton makes an interesting winter sculpture.

LANDSCAPE USES: Arrow reed is a unique specimen or accent plant in the garden. It is a fine pot or tub plant. It makes a good verticle accent for smaller gardens. It will also thrive in coastal and water gardens.

CULTURE AND PROPAGATION: Arrow reed prefers fertile, moist soil in full sun. It tolerates a wide range of extremes, including wet and boggy conditions. It will grow in shallow water 1 to 2 inches deep and in deeper water with age. It tolerates wind and salt spray.
Propagate by division or seed.

PESTS AND PROBLEMS: Arrow reed is extremely sharp, so take care when working near the plant to avoid serious eye injury and painful pricks.

BOTANICAL NAME	***Bothriochloa barbinoides* (also known as *Andropogon barbinoides*)**
PRONUNCIATION	boh-three-OH-kloh-ah bar-bih-NOY-deez
COMMON NAME	Cane bluestem
USDA HARDINESS ZONE	7 to 9
ORIGIN	Southwestern United States
PREFERRED SITES	Mesas, rocky slopes, coastal chaparral

DESCRIPTION: A close relative of the *Andropogon* bluestems, clump-forming cane bluestem is deciduous in cold climates and semideciduous in coastal Mediterranean climates. The plant grows 3 to 4 feet tall and as wide. It has sprawling, somewhat floppy foliage and flower spikes. Its hairy leaves, ⅛ to ¼ inch wide and 3 to 8 inches long, are held on wiry stems. Silky flowers emerge cream-colored from May through October, becoming silvery at maturity. In the fall, the foliage blushes orange, red, even peach. In cold climates the foliage becomes completely dormant in the winter.

LANDSCAPE USES: Cane bluestem is best used for naturalizing as a groundcover. It is good for informal meadow plantings and in coastal gardens in California. A somewhat coarse grass, it is best planted in groups or drifts.

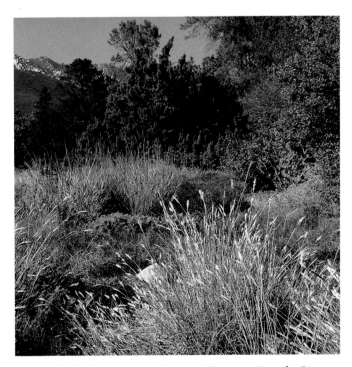

Bothriochloa barbinoides, cane bluestem (foreground), at the Santa Barbara Botanic Garden.

CULTURE AND PROPAGATION: Cane bluestem grows best in moist, well-drained soil. It will tolerate extreme conditions, from heavy soil to sandy, rocky, calcareous soil, but it grows poorly in shady sites. It is tolerant of coastal conditions and is drought-tolerant in coastal gardens. It prefers some summer water in hot inland climates.

Propagate by seed or division; it is easier to propagate by seed.

PESTS AND PROBLEMS: Cane bluestem has no known pests or problems.

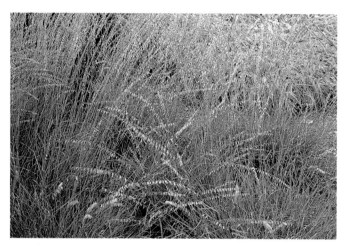

Bouteloua curtipendula, side oats gramma.

BOTANICAL NAME	***Bouteloua curtipendula***
PRONUNCIATION	boo-tuh-LOO-ah kur-tih-PEN-dyoo-lah
COMMON NAME	Side oats gramma
USDA HARDINESS ZONE	4 to 9
ORIGIN	North America, from Canada to the Gulf of Mexico and from the Eastern Seaboard to the California desert
PREFERRED SITES	Plains, prairies, rocky hills

DESCRIPTION: Side oats gramma is a clumping, warm-season grass. It is drought-tolerant and adapts to a wide range of habitats and garden conditions. Its common name derives from the one-sided arrangement of the spikelets along the stem, rather like a banner in the wind. The gray-green, fine-textured leaves are ⅛ to ¼ inch wide and grow 1 to 2 feet tall and almost as wide. The purple-tinted, erect flowers emerge in June and grow 5 to 15 inches tall. They mature to a golden color that bleaches white as cold weather approaches; it blushes purple again with the first frost, and finally dries to a straw color in winter.

LANDSCAPE USES: Side oats gramma makes a very showy groundcover and can be used in meadow and mass plantings, and to help control erosion on dry slopes and roadsides. The flowers are stunning in fresh or dried arrangements.

CULTURE AND PROPAGATION: Side oats gramma grows best in well-drained, fertile soil in full sun, although it tolerates heavy or sandy soils and poor fertility. Once established, plants withstand heat, drought, occasional mowing, and light foot traffic. It is a tough plant for harsh climates.

Propagation is easy by seed, or by division in the spring.

PESTS AND PROBLEMS: Side oats gramma has no known pests or problems.

BOTANICAL NAME	***Bouteloua gracilis***
PRONUNCIATION	boo-tuh-LOO-ah grah-SIL-is
COMMON NAME	Blue gramma, mosquito grass
USDA HARDINESS ZONE	3 to 10
ORIGIN	North America, from Canada to Texas, and from the Ohio River valley to the California desert
PREFERRED SITES	Plains

DESCRIPTION: Blue gramma is another important grass of the original North American shortgrass prairie. Fine-textured and warm-season-growing, with light green-gray foliage, it makes an ideal lawn grass, mowed or unmowed. Unmowed foliage clumps grow 8 to 24 inches tall; they can be mowed to an attractive turf 1 to 1½ inches tall. The leaves, ⅛ to ¼ inch wide, tolerate considerable foot traffic. Flowers on unmowed plants reach 12 inches above the foliage. Attached to the stem at a right angle, they resemble

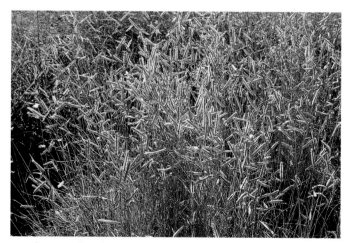

Bouteloua gracilis, blue gramma.

tiny combs or mosquito larvae, giving rise to this species' other common name, mosquito grass. Emerging silvery white, these delicate seed heads turn purplish with maturity. The entire plant turns purple with the first frost and bleaches to a straw color by winter.

LANDSCAPE USES: Blue gramma is particularly useful as a mowed or unmowed turf in the southwestern and prairie states. It is unsuitable as a lawn in the Midwest, and is largely untested as a lawn in the Northeast. Tolerant of drought and poor soils, it makes an excellent choice for unmowed meadows. When cultivated for a mowed lawn, it is often mixed with buffalo grass (*Buchloe dactyloides*) in a ratio of 40 percent blue gramma to 60 percent buffalo grass. Stunning planted in masses or groups, it also looks lovely in rock gardens as a single specimen. The flowers are attractive in fresh and dried arrangements.

CULTURE AND PROPAGATION: Easy to establish and basically pest- and disease-free, blue gramma thrives in loamy or sandy soils in full sun. Mowing promotes thick sod development. Tolerant of extreme cold and heat, blue gramma is one of the best grasses for the arid West.

Propagation is easy by seed, or by division in the spring.

PESTS AND PROBLEMS: Blue gramma has no known pests or problems.

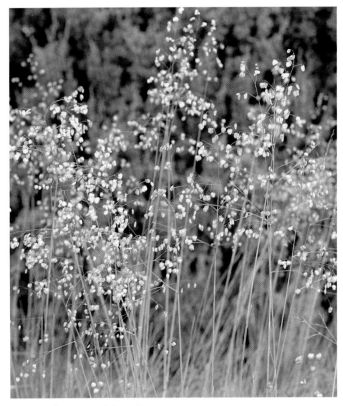

Briza media, perennial quaking grass.

BOTANICAL NAME	*Briza media*
PRONUNCIATION	BREYE-zah MEE-dee-ah
COMMON NAME	Perennial quaking grass, rattlesnake grass
USDA HARDINESS ZONE	4 to 10
ORIGIN	Mediterranean region
PREFERRED SITES	Moist meadows, prairies

DESCRIPTION: Perennial quaking grass is a small, clumping, cool-season-growing, evergreen grass with showy flowers. It is adaptable to many climates and is one of the easiest and most dependable ornamental grasses to grow. Its medium green leaves, ¼ to ½ inch wide and 12 to 18 inches tall, are soft to the touch and form dense clumps. The small, heart-shaped florets resemble tiny rattlesnake tail segments and emerge an iridescent green from April through June, turning golden with maturity. The flowers rise 12 to 18 inches above the foliage and quiver or shake in the breeze, hence the common name perennial quaking grass. The flowers persist on the plant well into summer before becoming tattered and shattering to the ground.

LANDSCAPE USES: Perennial quaking grass is an excellent all-purpose grass, both used as a single specimen and massed in groups. It makes a fine groundcover for large areas. It accents other spring-blooming perennials such as iris and campanula. A consistent performer in perennial borders, the delicate flowers of perennial quaking grass make it a beautiful, unusual accent in the foreground and mid-ground of the border and as an edging plant. The intriguing flowers can be added to fresh or dried flower arrangements at all stages of maturity. It is reported in A. J. Oakes's *Ornamental Grasses* that "cutting the flower heads when they are light green in the spring or in the summer after they are mature and grayish white results in dried flower heads of different colors."

CULTURE AND PROPAGATION: Perennial quaking grass grows best in rich, fertile soil in full sun. While it prefers moist loam, it tolerates a wide range of soils. In light shade it may not bloom well. It tolerates hot, dry climates but must have regular water. Old flower spikes should be removed in the summer if they become unsightly. Cutting back tired or worn foliage several inches from the crown will encourage new, fresh growth.

Propagate by division in spring or fall in cold climates, or year-round in mild climates.

PESTS AND PROBLEMS: Perennial quaking grass has no known pests or problems.

BOTANICAL NAME	***Buchloe dactyloides***
PRONUNCIATION	boo-KLOH-ee dak-til-LOY-deez
COMMON NAME	Buffalo grass
USDA HARDINESS ZONE	3 to 9
ORIGIN	North America, Canada to Texas, plains to Rocky Mountains
PREFERRED SITES	Dry plains

DESCRIPTION: Gray-green, fine-textured, warm-season-growing buffalo grass is a major component of the short-grass prairie. Slowly spreading from rhizomes, it grows only 4 to 6 inches tall with flowers that barely reach over the foliage. It can be mowed or left as is. The non-showy flowers resemble those of blue gramma (*Bouteloua gracilis*), except they are shorter and not as profuse. The gray-green foliage takes on a purplish cast with the first frost, then turns beige, remaining so throughout the winter.

LANDSCAPE USES: Buffalo grass makes a wonderful lawn or meadow. Tolerant of heat, cold, and varying soils, it is one of the finest grasses for arid regions, where it provides erosion control and soil stabilization.

CULTURE AND PROPAGATION: Buffalo grass grows best with good drainage in full sun. This hardy grass can grow in any soil, but prefers slightly clayey soil. It resents overwatering and fertilization. Runners bind the soil as they grow but do not spread invasively. Cultivars are available in nurseries and garden centers, and new ones, developed for improved vigor, color, and compactness, should be available in the near future.

Propagate by seed, or by division in early spring after the danger of a hard freeze has passed.

PESTS AND PROBLEMS: If buffalo grass has a fault, it is that it is slow to establish and spread.

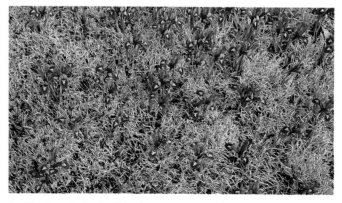

Buchloe dactyloides, buffalo grass, in winter color with *Iris reticulata.*

SOME ***Buchloe dactyloides*** CULTIVARS ARE:	
'D. D. B-1' ('D. D. B-1' buffalo grass): soon to be released; most compact growth of all, with a maximum height of 2 to 3 inches.	**'609'** ('609' buffalo grass): fine texture; low growth habit. Bluer green than prairie buffalo grass; produces no pollen or seed.
'Prairie' ('Prairie' buffalo grass): fine texture and low growth; produces no pollen or seed.	**'Texoka'** ('Texoka' buffalo grass): improved forage for cattle; useful for meadows and pastures. Can be planted from seed.

BOTANICAL NAME	***Calamagrostis acutiflora* 'Stricta'**
PRONUNCIATION	kal-ah-mah-GROS-tis ah-KYOO-tih-flor-ah STRIK-tah
COMMON NAME	Feather reed grass
USDA HARDINESS ZONE	5 to 9
ORIGIN	Eurasia
PREFERRED SITES	Moist meadows, open woods

DESCRIPTION: Feather reed grass is one of the showiest flowering ornamental grasses grown today. Its appearance can vary widely, depending on the climate zone it is grown in. A somewhat cool-season grass, it may go completely deciduous in cold climates, yet remain mostly evergreen in mild climates. A hard frost may turn the foliage orange-yellow in mild climates, but almost always some green remains. The stiff-edged leaves, ¼ to ½ inch wide, grow in an upright, arching clump 18 to 24 inches tall. In dry or mild climates the foliage usually reaches 2 to 3 feet. In optimum colder climates and moist, rich soils it can reach 3 to 4 feet. Although the medium green foliage is handsome and architectural in habit, it is the flowers that really distinguish the plant. In May to June, depending on climate zone, tall, upright flower spikes emerge greenish with red-bronze tones. These slender spikes rise 3 to 4 feet above the foliage and dry to a golden color, bleaching to buff by late fall. The flower spikes persist into the winter. Feather reed grass may bloom sporadically if at all in mild climates.

LANDSCAPE USES: Feather reed grass has many garden uses. Used as a specimen, it makes a stunning vertical accent. In groups, it creates a horizontal band of golden flowers that bend and sway in the wind. It is an effective addition planted at the rear of a border. Its narrow, erect panicles,

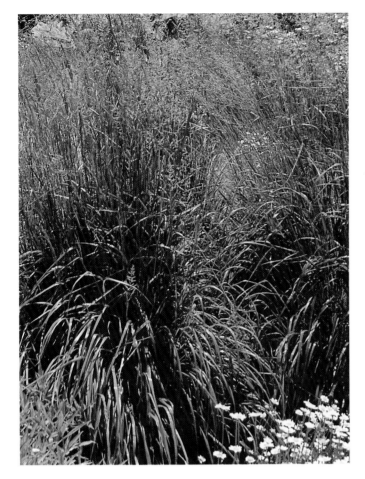

Calamagrostis acutiflora 'Stricta', feather reed grass, with newly emerging flowers.

BOTANICAL NAME	***Calamagrostis arundinacea* var. *brachytricha***
PRONUNCIATION	kal-ah-mah-GROS-tis ah-run-din-AH-see-ah BRAK-ee-trik-ah
COMMON NAME	Fall-blooming reed grass
USDA HARDINESS ZONE	5 to 9
ORIGIN	Eurasia
PREFERRED SITES	Meadows, open woods

DESCRIPTION: Fall-blooming reed grass is a clumping, warm-season grass graced with rich green foliage and showy flowers. The leaves, ¼ to ⅜ inch wide, reach 1½ to 2½ feet tall. New spring growth is a rich green color that adds beauty to the garden. The foliage turns bright yellow with the approach of fall and goes completely dormant even in mild climates. Flower spikes emerge from late summer to early fall, arching up and out, 1½ to 2 feet above the foliage. The flowers emerge green blushed with pink and mature to a wheat color in early fall. The flowers of fall-blooming reed grass are fatter and fluffier than those of other feather reed varieties.

LANDSCAPE USES: Fall-blooming reed grass is prized for its flowering accent and fall color. Since it will bloom in considerable shade, it can be an asset to lightly shaded borders, woodland plantings, and areas too shady for fountain grass (*Pennisetum* spp.). It appears equally beautiful alone or in masses.

CULTURE AND PROPAGATION: Fall-blooming reed grass grows best in moist, fertile soil in full sun. Tolerant of a variety of soil conditions, it does not like to be too dry, and it performs well in light shade. Water weekly in hot climates, and provide light or afternoon shade.

Propagate by division in spring or fall.

PESTS AND PROBLEMS: Fall-blooming reed grass has no known pests or problems.

borne on long, stiff stems, make feather reed grass a good cut flower.

CULTURE AND PROPAGATION: Feather reed grass prefers moist, rich soil in full sun. It tolerates heavy soils and withstands heat if plenty of moisture is present. In light shade it will not bloom well and the flowers may flop over.

Propagate by division in the fall or spring, though spring planting gives better results in cold climates.

PESTS AND PROBLEMS: Feather reed grass has no known pests or problems.

ANOTHER CULTIVAR OF ***Calamagrostis acutiflora*** IS:

'Overdam' ('Overdam' feather reed grass): white variegated foliage; requires partial shade in hot climates.

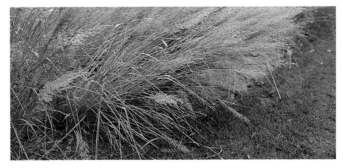

Calamagrostis arundinacea var. *brachytricha*, fall-blooming reed grass.

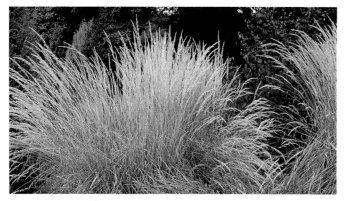

Calamagrostis arundinacea 'Karl Foerster', Foerster's feather reed grass.

BOTANICAL NAME	***Calamagrostis arundinacea* 'Karl Foerster'**
PRONUNCIATION	kal-ah-mah-GROS-tis ah-run-din-AH-see-ah
COMMON NAME	Foerster's feather reed grass
USDA HARDINESS ZONE	5 to 9
ORIGIN	Eurasia
PREFERRED SITES	Meadows, open woods

DESCRIPTION: In mild climates Foerster's feather reed grass is almost identical to feather reed grass (*Calamagrostis acutiflora* 'Stricta'). In colder climates, Foerster's grows slightly more compact and blooms 2 to 3 weeks earlier. In hotter climates, the difference between these two grasses is invisible. This grass is virtually indistinguishable from *C. arundinacea* 'Stricta', with differences determined by local growing conditions.

LANDSCAPE USES: Foerster's feather reed grass is preferred by gardeners in the colder reaches of its hardiness range, where it is quicker to bloom. In warmer climates, this attribute may be of little consequence, but in short growing seasons it can prove desirable. Otherwise, it can be treated the same as feather reed grass.

CULTURE AND PROPAGATION: Foerster's feather reed grass prefers moist, rich soil with full-day sun. It tolerates heavy soils and will take the heat if plenty of moisture is present. In light shade it will not bloom as well and its flowers may flop over.
  Propagate by division in fall or spring.

PESTS AND PROBLEMS: Foerster's feather reed grass has been constantly confused with *C. acutiflora* 'Stricta' throughout the United States. Even reputable nurseries may not be growing true *C. arundinacea* 'Karl Foerster'.

BOTANICAL NAME	***Calamagrostis nutkaensis***
PRONUNCIATION	kal-ah-mah-GROS-tis noot-kay-EN-sis
COMMON NAME	Pacific reed grass
USDA HARDINESS ZONE	8 to 9
ORIGIN	Pacific coast, from Alaska to Point Concepcion, California
PREFERRED SITES	Coastal slopes, meadows, boggy areas

DESCRIPTION: Pacific reed grass is a rather coarse, clumping, cool-season grass. It has medium green glossy blades ½ to ¾ inch wide and 2 to 3 feet tall. The flowers rise 1 to 2 feet above the foliage, emerging purplish from April through May and maturing to a wheat color.

LANDSCAPE USES: Pacific reed grass is an excellent choice for coastal meadows, mass plantings, and erosion control on steep coastal banks. Its ability to tolerate wind and salt spray makes it a good choice for beach plantings.

CULTURE AND PROPAGATION: Pacific reed grass prefers moist, rich soil in full sun. However, it tolerates considerable summer drought and a wide range of soils, from heavy clay to rocky serpentine. It requires more moisture in sandy soils. It tolerates moderate shade and grows better inland if planted in some shade.
  It propagates easily by division in the fall or spring, and may also be raised from seed.

PESTS AND PROBLEMS: Pacific reed grass may be affected by rust during wet periods of weather conducive to rust; treat accordingly with an appropriate organic fungicide (see page 23). Infestations are rarely severe, and rust generally disappears with the onset of new growth.

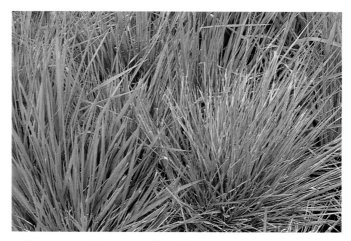

Calamagrostis nutkaensis, Pacific reed grass.

CAREX
SEDGES

There are over 2,000 species of *Carex,* commonly called sedges, found in many habitats, from sandy beaches to alpine scree. Their foliage can be red, orange, copper, silver, brown, and every shade of green. They come in many shapes and sizes, some becoming dense tussocks forming black trunks 2 to 3 feet tall and topped with flowing hairlike foliage. New Zealand hair sedge (*C. comans*) grows streamside with 6-foot-long leaves coursing down the water's edge. Still others, like miniature variegated sedge (*C. conica* 'Marginata'), are delightful miniatures for rock and dish gardens.

Although most commonly associated with moist habitats, some sedges have a wide tolerance that allows them to adapt to drought and heat. Many grow in water or tolerate moist, boggy soils. Sedges are generally at home in or around pond and stream gardens and many excel as groundcovers at the water's edge. Many tolerate seasonal submersion along a pond or streamside.

Sedges often grow in shady habitats and, therefore, are indispensable for shade gardens. Sedges make good fillers and groundcovers and many combine well with ferns, hostas, and other traditional shade-loving plants. Their varied foliage colors can accent dark areas.

Some species have showy flowers and/or seed heads. Their interesting shapes range from the long, pendulous, catkinlike flowers of drooping sedge (*C. pendula*) to the clusters of bright red-orange seeds of crimson seed sedge (*C. baccans*). Gray's sedge (*C. grayi*) has greenish seed pods that are reminiscent of spiked clubs. Flower and seed spikes like these are stunning in fresh and dried flower arrangements.

Some sedges form clumps, while others spread from underground runners. Clumps can range from slow-growing, delicate miniatures to fast-growing, dense tufts. Running or creeping types can be invasive in some situations, so take care when planting these. However, colonizing traits can be desirable for large areas or erosion control. Most *Carex* cultivars and varieties are mild mannered and well-behaved in the garden.

Some sedges are used as meadows or lawns. A few currently undergoing testing are being considered for closely mowed turf. Perhaps the drought-tolerant, no-mowing-needed dwarf lawn grass of the future won't be a grass at all, but a sedge!

The sedges are too numerous to be completely covered in this encyclopedia. Instead, those currently being offered in nurseries or garden centers, or soon to be offered, are mentioned here. More are sure to come from this huge family of plants.

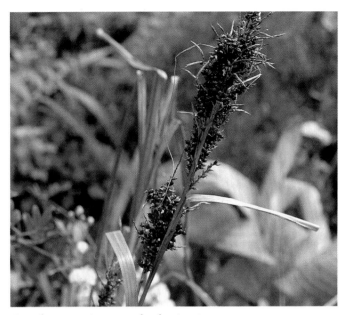

Carex baccans, crimson seed sedge, in winter.

BOTANICAL NAME	***Carex baccans***
PRONUNCIATION	KAIR-ex bah-KANZ
COMMON NAME	Crimson seed sedge
USDA HARDINESS ZONE	8(?) to 9 (hardiness untested; may grow in Zone 8)
ORIGIN	India
PREFERRED SITES	Moist areas

DESCRIPTION: Clumping, evergreen crimson seed sedge produces dark green leaves ½ to ¾ inch wide and 2 to 3 feet long. Its flower spike arches up and out from the clump and is graced by greenish flowers that grow 2 to 3 inches wide and 6 to 12 inches long. The flowers form small green clusters of seeds that change to bright red-orange at maturity. Though the seeds are only the size of sand grains, the spike bends under their weight.

LANDSCAPE USES: Crimson seed sedge makes a good accent plant in areas with full and partial shade. Use it as an accent draped over the water's edge, where its seed heads can dangle. It makes an excellent cut flower.

CULTURE AND PROPAGATION: Crimson seed sedge grows best in moist, fertile loam in full or partial shade. Like most sedges, it tolerates a wide range of conditions, though this sedge does not like to be dry. Crimson seed sedge is not known to naturalize.

Propagation is difficult by seed but easy by division.

PESTS AND PROBLEMS: Crimson seed sedge has no known pests or problems.

BOTANICAL NAME	***Carex buchananii***
PRONUNCIATION	KAIR-ex byoo-kah-NAN-ee-eye
COMMON NAME	Leather leaf sedge
USDA HARDINESS ZONE	7 to 9
ORIGIN	New Zealand
PREFERRED SITES	Moist areas, streamsides

DESCRIPTION: The evergreen, or ever-brown, leather leaf sedge is a clumping perennial with showy, coppery, red-brown leaves. The fine-textured leaves grow $1/16$ inch wide and 1 to 2 feet tall; they may reach 3 feet under optimum conditions. Vertical when young, leaves tend to spread with age. The leaf tips appear almost cylindrical and may curl. The inconspicuous flowers nestle among the foliage.

LANDSCAPE USES: The copper-colored foliage of leather leaf sedge provides marvelous contrast to silver, blue, and dark green foliage. Attractive in groups, leather leaf sedge can be used in rock and water gardens and will grow in peat beds. It also makes an interesting container subject.

CULTURE AND PROPAGATION: Leather leaf sedge grows best in constantly moist, fast-draining, rocky soil. In its native habitat, it tolerates a wide range of soil conditions and exposures. In hot climates, it grows best in partial shade. In coastal climates, it grows best in full sun. Moisture is necessary, but established plants can tolerate some drought. This sedge may be hardy north of Zone 7 if given protection.

Propagate by seed, or by division in the spring.

PESTS AND PROBLEMS: Leather leaf sedge, like many New Zealand sedges, may be short-lived, usually lasting two to three years in the garden. Therefore, it is risky in mass plantings of desired permanence. Dense clumps can get aphids and mealybugs in hot climates. A cool root run and constant moisture with excellent drainage is the best preventive (see also page 23).

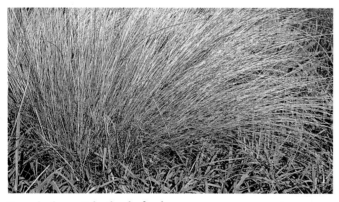

Carex buchananii, leather leaf sedge.

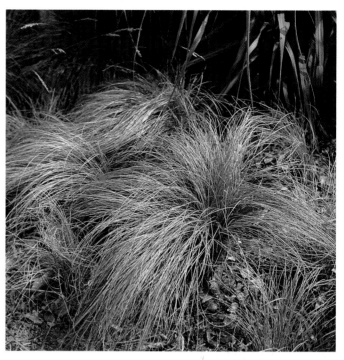

Carex comans, New Zealand hair sedge.

BOTANICAL NAME	***Carex comans* (also known as *C. comans* 'Stricta', *C. albula, C. albula* 'Frosty Curls', and *C. vilmorinii*)**
PRONUNCIATION	KAIR-ex KOH-manz
COMMON NAME	New Zealand hair sedge
USDA HARDINESS ZONE	7 to 9
ORIGIN	New Zealand
PREFERRED SITES	Moist places, streamsides

DESCRIPTION: This extremely variable plant is a source of considerable confusion. True New Zealand hair sedge has many forms that have been distributed under several names and varieties. Many seedling variations may exist.

The fine-textured, clumping, evergreen sedge grows hair-like leaves $1/16$ inch wide that form dense tufts. Iridescent, light green, and almost cylindrical, the leaves usually grow 1 foot tall but can reach 3 to 6 feet under ideal growing conditions. In its natural habitat the foliage grows along streamsides, the leaves spilling down into the water. The inconspicuous flowers appear among the foliage from June through August.

LANDSCAPE USES: Allow the fine, weeping foliage of New Zealand hair sedge to spill over rocky slopes or walls. A mass planting on a slope gives the wonderful illusion of falling water. Enjoy single specimens in pots or tubs, especially when the leaves reach their mature length.

CULTURE AND PROPAGATION: New Zealand hair sedge grows best in moist, fast-draining soil. It does equally well in full sun or partial shade, though some shade is best in hot climates. It often naturalizes, although not invasively. When cutting back, leave 3 to 4 inches above the crown, as plants dislike a close shearing.

Propagate by seed, or by division in the spring.

PESTS AND PROBLEMS: New Zealand hair sedge may be short-lived, often dying out after three or four years. Old, dense clumps may get mealybugs and aphids and should be treated accordingly (see page 23).

BOTANICAL NAME	***Carex comans* 'Bronze' (also known as *C. comans* 'Bronce' and *C. comans* 'Bronze Form')**
PRONUNCIATION	KAIR-ex KOH-manz
COMMON NAME	'Bronze' New Zealand hair sedge

DESCRIPTION: 'Bronze' New Zealand hair sedge resembles the species but has fine brownish white foliage. The plant appears dead all the time, which makes it a curious conversation piece for the garden. The brown foliage can be effective in rock and dish gardens. This plant also makes an interesting pot or tub subject.

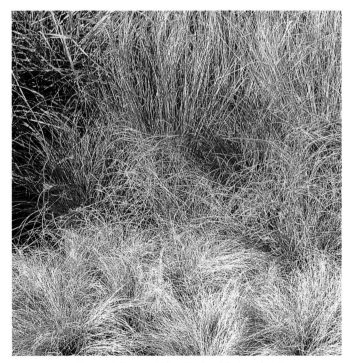

Carex comans 'Bronze', 'Bronze' New Zealand hair sedge, bottom.

BOTANICAL NAME	***Carex comans* 'Frosty Curls'**
PRONUNCIATION	KAIR-ex KOH-manz
COMMON NAME	'Frosty Curls' New Zealand hair sedge

DESCRIPTION: 'Frosty Curls' New Zealand hair sedge, similar to New Zealand hair sedge, is more compact and has leaves that form curly pigtails at the tips. Leaves are $1/6$ inch wide, and the tips appear iridescent and almost white. The clumps grow ½ to 1 foot tall, then flop over.

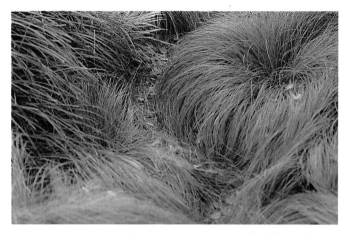

Carex comans 'Frosty Curls', 'Frosty Curls' New Zealand hair sedge.

BOTANICAL NAME	***Carex conica* 'Marginata' (also known as *C. conica* 'Variegata' and *C. conica* 'Himekansuge')**
PRONUNCIATION	KAIR-ex KON-ih-kah mar-jih-NAH-tah
COMMON NAME	Miniature variegated sedge
USDA HARDINESS ZONE	5 to 9
ORIGIN	Southern Korea and Japan
PREFERRED SITES	Open woods, forests

DESCRIPTION: Small, clumping, evergreen miniature variegated sedge is noted for its silvery white variegation. The dark green leaves grow ⅛ to ⅜ inch wide and rarely reach higher than 6 inches. The flowers are inconspicuously borne on the foliage from May through July.

LANDSCAPE USES: One of the most popular sedges for rock and dish gardens, miniature variegated sedge is also effective between stepping stones or as a low groundcover. It prefers shady, or partly shady, moist areas of the garden.

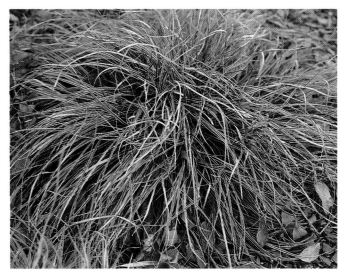

Carex conica 'Marginata', miniature variegated sedge.

CULTURE AND PROPAGATION: Miniature variegated sedge grows best in moist, fertile soil in partial shade. It must have regular moisture and light to moderate shade in hot, dry climates. Slow to moderate growth makes this miniature sedge an agreeable border plant.

Propagate by division in the spring.

PESTS AND PROBLEMS: Old foliage may develop dead tips. The foliage can be cut back in early spring, 2 to 3 inches above the crown.

BOTANICAL NAME	***Carex elata* 'Bowles Golden' (also known as *C. acuta*, *C. flava*, *C. flava* 'Bowles Golden', and *C. stricta* 'Bowles Golden')**
PRONUNCIATION	KAIR-ex eh-LAH-tah
COMMON NAME	'Bowles Golden' sedge, golden variegated sedge, yellow sedge
USDA HARDINESS ZONE	5 to 9
ORIGIN	Species originated in Eastern Europe
PREFERRED SITES	Moist streamsides, marshes

DESCRIPTION: Although confusing from a nomenclature standpoint, 'Bowles Golden' sedge has a beauty that is unmistakable. Bright yellow foliage with green edges distinguishes this clumping semi-evergreen sedge. The leaves are ⅛ to ½ inch wide, and a clump usually grows 2 feet tall and 2 feet wide; under optimum conditions it can reach 3 to 5 feet wide. Bright yellow new spring growth is particularly

striking, but the yellow color fades by late summer. Emerging May through June, the flowers are brownish in color and arch up and out from the foliage. They are noticeable but not particularly showy.

LANDSCAPE USES: This moisture-loving sedge looks its best in or near water. Its golden foliage casts a beautiful reflection on ponds, streams, and water gardens and will lighten a moist, shady area. Single specimens are dramatic; masses or groups are almost overwhelming.

CULTURE AND PROPAGATION: 'Bowles Golden' sedge must be constantly wet to thrive. It prefers acid soil and half-day sun to look its best. It will grow in shallow water, 2 to 3 inches deep; new plants should be planted in water no deeper than 4 inches. Plants languish in too much shade. It usually does not grow taller than 1 foot in hot, dry climates, where humidity, moisture, and light shade are lacking. 'Bowles Golden' sedge does not like to be dry or exposed to hot, dry winds.

Propagate by division in the spring.

PESTS AND PROBLEMS: 'Bowles Golden' sedge has no known pests or problems.

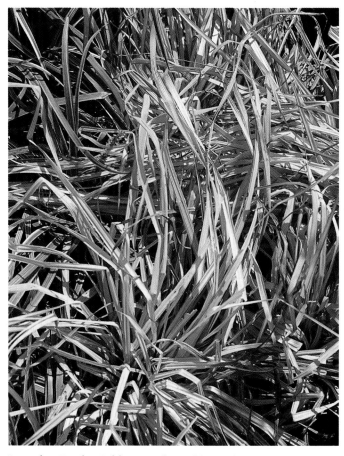

Carex elata 'Bowles Golden', 'Bowles Golden' sedge.

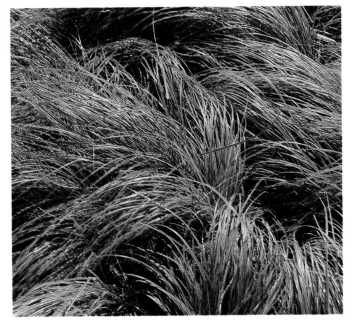

Carex elegantissima 'Variegata', golden-edged sedge.

BOTANICAL NAME	*Carex flagelifera*
PRONUNCIATION	KAIR-ex flah-jel-IH-fer-ah
COMMON NAME	Weeping brown New Zealand sedge
USDA HARDINESS ZONE	7 to 9
ORIGIN	New Zealand
PREFERRED SITES	Moist streamsides

DESCRIPTION: This evergreen, or rather ever-brown, sedge has iridescent, coppery brown foliage that is both unusual and attractive. Its fine-textured leaves, $^1/_{16}$ inch wide, emerge from a clump that arches upward 1½ to 2 feet before spilling back to the ground. The leaves may eventually reach 6 feet long. The flowers are borne along the stems as they lie on the ground.

LANDSCAPE USES: Weeping brown New Zealand sedge is very versatile in the garden. Its distinctive foliage makes a stunning accent planted alone or in masses. It grows well in rock gardens and lightly shaded areas. An excellent filler and spiller, it tumbles down slopes and over rocks.

CULTURE AND PROPAGATION: Weeping brown New Zealand sedge grows best in moist, well-drained, fertile soil in light shade. In coastal climates, it will tolerate drier soils and full sun.

Propagation is easy by seed, or by division in the spring.

PESTS AND PROBLEMS: Weeping brown New Zealand sedge may live only three to five years. Older plants accumulate dead leaves that bleach gray and can look quite unattractive. Shear these 4 to 5 inches above the crown, if necessary. Plants may be slow to return from a severe "haircut." This sedge is occasionally subject to mealybugs and aphids, which should be properly treated (see page 23).

BOTANICAL NAME	*Carex elegantissima* 'Variegata'
PRONUNCIATION	KAIR-ex el-eh-gan-TISS-ih-mah var-ee-uh-GAH-tah
COMMON NAME	Golden-edged sedge
USDA HARDINESS ZONE	8 to 9
ORIGIN	Uncertain; probably Asia
PREFERRED SITES	Most likely moist places

DESCRIPTION: Fine-textured, clumping, evergreen golden-edged sedge lives up to its name with gilt edges that catch the light in a most enchanting way. Its olive-green leaves, ⅛ inch wide, are graced by golden yellow edges. The dense clump grows 18 to 24 inches tall in an upward arch. The flowers bloom on wiry stems that arch out 6 to 12 inches from the foliage.

LANDSCAPE USES: Grow golden-edged sedge as an accent or specimen in a shady garden. Plant it where sunlight can play on its gilt-edged margins.

CULTURE AND PROPAGATION: Golden-edged sedge grows best in moist, well-drained, fertile soil in light shade. Plants resent hot, dry soil. They tolerate more sun in coastal gardens, but the foliage may burn in full sun in hot climates.

Propagate by division in fall or spring.

PESTS AND PROBLEMS: Aphids can attack in hot-summer climates and should be treated appropriately (see page 23).

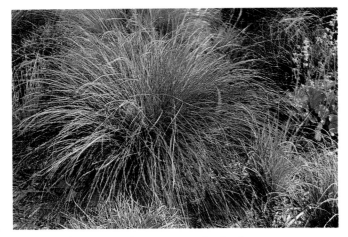

Carex flagelifera, weeping brown New Zealand sedge.

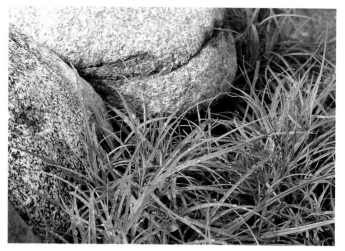

Carex glauca, blue sedge.

BOTANICAL NAME	**Carex glauca (also known as C. flacca)**
PRONUNCIATION	KAIR-ex GLOU-kah
COMMON NAME	Blue sedge
USDA HARDINESS ZONE	5 to 9
ORIGIN	Europe
PREFERRED SITES	Wet to dry fields

DESCRIPTION: The slowly creeping, rhizomatous blue sedge has handsome blue-gray foliage. It is semideciduous in all but the mildest climates. Its medium- to fine-textured leaves are ⅛ to ¼ inch wide and 6 to 12 inches long. The plant rarely exceeds 6 inches tall, forming a creeping mat. The inconspicuous flowers bloom in June and July.

LANDSCAPE USES: Blue sedge makes an excellent ground-cover and filler. Slowly creeping and not invasive by habit, it is not difficult to control if it spreads where it is unwanted. It makes an interesting blue-gray lawn that tolerates light traffic and light shade.

CULTURE AND PROPAGATION: Blue sedge grows best in moist, fertile loam in full sun, but it tolerates far worse conditions. It has shown some drought-tolerance once it is established, tolerates light to medium shade, and will grow in competition with tree roots. It is not particular as to soil type and looks best with regular watering. Unkempt foliage can be cut back to 2 to 3 inches above the crown to force new, fresh growth.

Propagate by seed or division; division is easiest in the spring or fall.

PESTS AND PROBLEMS: Blue sedge has no known pests or problems.

BOTANICAL NAME	**Carex grayi**
PRONUNCIATION	KAIR-ex GRAY-eye
COMMON NAME	Gray's sedge, morning star sedge
USDA HARDINESS ZONE	5 to 9
ORIGIN	North America
PREFERRED SITES	Meadows, wet in spring, dry in summer

DESCRIPTION: Clumping and semi-evergreen, Gray's sedge bears light green leaves ¼ to ½ inch wide and 2 to 3 feet tall. The plant is distinguished by clustered, 1-inch fruits that resemble spiked clubs. The fruit emerges greenish yellow and persists on the plant, drying to brown.

LANDSCAPE USES: Gray's sedge is lovely planted alone or in groups. It thrives at or near water in pools, ponds, and puddles. Its attractive fruit makes the plant an interesting accent and pot subject. The fruit is stunning in fresh or dried arrangements.

CULTURE AND PROPAGATION: Gray's sedge grows best in moist, fertile soil in full sun, though it tolerates some shade. Because it resents drying out, it suffers in dry soils and hot climates. Even with light shade and continual moisture, in hot climates it will not reach 2 feet.

Propagate by seed, or by division in the spring.

PESTS AND PROBLEMS: Gray's sedge has no known pests or problems.

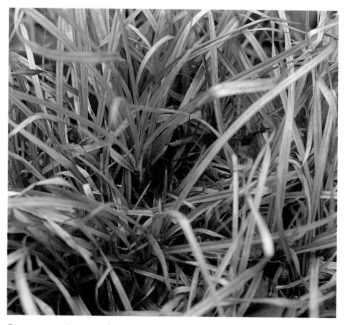

Carex grayi, Gray's sedge, in winter color.

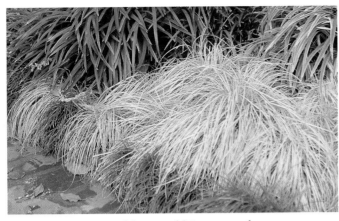

Carex hachioensis 'Evergold', 'Evergold' Japanese sedge.

BOTANICAL NAME	***Carex hachioensis*** ***'Evergold' (also known as*** ***C. morrowii aureo*** ***variegata 'Old Gold' and C.*** ***morrowii aureo variegata*** ***'Everbrite')***
PRONUNCIATION	KAIR-ex hah-chee-oh-EN-sis
COMMON NAME	'Evergold' Japanese sedge, variegated Japanese sedge
USDA HARDINESS ZONE	7 to 9
ORIGIN	Japan
PREFERRED SITES	Volcanic soils, moist areas

DESCRIPTION: The clumping, evergreen 'Evergold' Japanese sedge, called by various botanical names in the last decade or so, is distinguished by bright creamy yellow, center-striped leaves and lush, arching foliage. Even with green-margined leaves, this plant appears golden yellow in the garden. The leaves, ¼ to ⅜ inch wide and 12 to 16 inches tall, gracefully arch back to the ground, where the plant can reach 18 to 24 inches long. The lustrous leaves usually hide the nondescript, brownish flower spikes.

LANDSCAPE USES: 'Evergold' Japanese sedge is an effective accent plant whether planted alone or massed as a groundcover. It is a good plant for rock gardens and for spilling over rocky slopes. It will grow indoors with constant moisture, good drainage, and strong light.

CULTURE AND PROPAGATION: 'Evergold' Japanese sedge grows best in moist, gravelly soil in light shade or half-day sun. It tolerates full sun in coastal climates but needs some shade in hot interior climates. This plant resents drying out and will languish in too much shade. 'Evergold' Japanese sedge has been known to revert back occasionally to its green form. Tissue-cultured plants may be even more unstable.

The variegated portion may be protected by removing reversions when they appear. However, the glossy green reversion is also attractive and worthy of garden attention. Known to be short-lived, in some garden situations this sedge may live only two to three years. Cutting back, if required, should be to 4 to 5 inches above the crown.

Propagate by division, ideally in spring.

PESTS AND PROBLEMS: 'Evergold' Japanese sedge has no known pests or problems.

BOTANICAL NAME	***Carex morrowii*** ***'Goldband'***
PRONUNCIATION	KAIR-ex mor-ROH-ee-eye
COMMON NAME	'Goldband' Japanese sedge, golden variegated Japanese sedge
USDA HARDINESS ZONE	7 to 9
ORIGIN	Japan
PREFERRED SITES	Moist places

DESCRIPTION: Evergreen 'Goldband' Japanese sedge grows lustrous green leaves edged with golden yellow bands. It is similar to silver variegated Japanese sedge (*Carex morrowii* 'Variegata') in form and habit, but its gold margins give it a distinct golden yellow cast. Its leaves, ¼ to ½ inch wide, stiffly ascend to 1 foot and then arch outward and gracefully spill back to the ground. The flowers are inconspicuous brownish spikes.

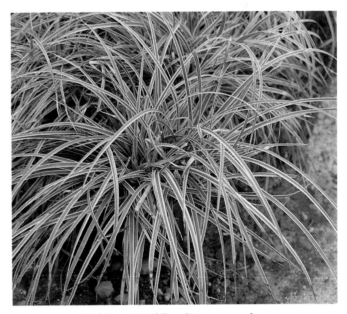

Carex morrowii 'Goldband', 'Goldband' Japanese sedge.

LANDSCAPE USES: 'Goldband' Japanese sedge makes an attractive accent planted alone or in masses. It is stunning when early morning or late-afternoon sun backlights its handsome, gold-edged foliage. It grows well near water, in moist borders, and alongside shade perennials, such as hostas, forget-me-nots (*Myosotis* spp.), and bellflowers (*Campanula* spp.). It can be grown indoors if given good drainage, constant moisture, and strong light.

CULTURE AND PROPAGATION: 'Goldband' Japanese sedge grows best in well-drained, fertile loam with constant moisture and light shade. The color of the plant is far richer viewed in shade than in full sun. Avoid reflected heat and light in hot climates, and do not let the plant dry out.
   Propagate by division in the spring.

PESTS AND PROBLEMS: 'Goldband' Japanese sedge has no known pests or problems.

LANDSCAPE USES: Silver variegated Japanese sedge is a good plant for groundcovers and mass plantings. It makes a good underplanting for trees and in shady borders with other shade-loving perennials, such as heuchera, hellebore, and cimicifuga.

CULTURE AND PROPAGATION: To look its best, silver variegated Japanese sedge should be grown in moist, rich loam in partial shade. It tolerates considerable shade but will also grow in full sun in all but hot climates, where light to moderate shade is a must. Do not plant it against reflective surfaces such as concrete walls. In full, hot sun, the plant may bleach to an unattractive yellow.
   Propagate by division in the spring.

PESTS AND PROBLEMS: Silver variegated Japanese sedge has no known pests or problems.

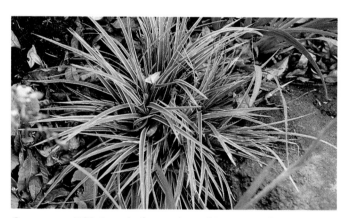

Carex morrowii 'Variegata', silver variegated Japanese sedge.

BOTANICAL NAME	*Carex morrowii* 'Variegata'
PRONUNCIATION	KAIR-ex mor-ROH-ee-eye var-ee-uh-GAH-tah
COMMON NAME	Silver variegated Japanese sedge
USDA HARDINESS ZONE	5 to 9
ORIGIN	Japan
PREFERRED SITES	Moist places, wet meadows

DESCRIPTION: Silver variegated Japanese sedge is a clumping evergreen sedge, distinguished by faint silver margins on its lustrous, delicately variegated foliage. The hint of silver is enough to make the slightly sharp leaf edges glisten. The stiff leaves, ¼ to ½ inch wide, generally reach 1 foot tall, although the arching foliage can grow to 18 to 24 inches long. The flowers, noticeable but not showy, are typical of the species—elongated brownish spikes.

BOTANICAL NAME	*Carex muskingumensis*
PRONUNCIATION	KAIR-ex mus-kin-goo-MEN-sis
COMMON NAME	Palm sedge
USDA HARDINESS ZONE	4 to 9
ORIGIN	The Great Lakes region of the United States and Canada
PREFERRED SITES	Marshes and streamsides

DESCRIPTION: This slowly creeping, semideciduous sedge has attractive foliage that resembles palm fronds. Its arching culms, 2 to 3 feet long, have leaves ¼ inch wide and 4 to 8 inches long. The leaves radiate from the culm in three distinct planes, giving the plant a unique, somewhat tropical appearance. Noticeable but not showy flowers top the light green foliage in May and June. The plant tends to flop, spill, and then slowly creep. The first hard frost turns it yellow.

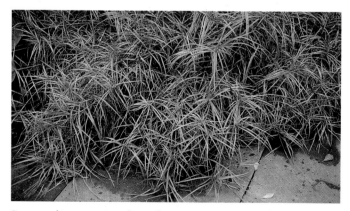

Carex muskingumensis, palm sedge.

LANDSCAPE USES: Palm sedge is an excellent groundcover and mass planting for moist, lightly shaded areas. It can be used as a tall lawn substitute under trees and near ponds or streams and provides good erosion control for moist banks. It is a showy plant for pots, tubs, and water gardens.

CULTURE AND PROPAGATION: Palm sedge prefers moist loam and is equally happy in sun or shade, provided moisture is ample; plants resent drying out. In hot climates, plant palm sedge in light shade. The foliage becomes more noticeably yellowish green in full sun. Palm sedge will grow in shallow water, 3 to 4 inches deep, and will grow in deeper water as it ages.

Propagate by seed, or by division in spring or fall.

PESTS AND PROBLEMS: Palm sedge will flop in too much shade.

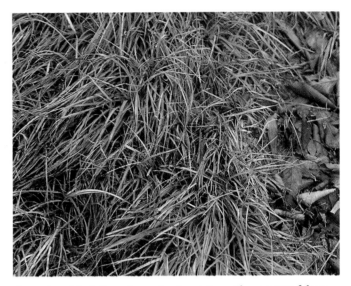

Carex nigra, black-flowering sedge, in winter, with emerging foliage.

ONE CULTIVAR OF **Carex muskingumensis** IS:

'Wachtposten' (Sentry tower palm sedge): new upright cultivar with uniform dark green foliage.

BOTANICAL NAME	*Carex nigra*
PRONUNCIATION	KAIR-ex NIH-grah
COMMON NAME	Black-flowering sedge
USDA HARDINESS ZONE	4 to 8
ORIGIN	Eurasia
PREFERRED SITES	Wet soils

DESCRIPTION: Black-flowering sedge is nearly identical to, and often interchanged with, blue sedge (*Carex glauca*), although it is somewhat taller growing and more coarse in texture. The soft, blue-gray foliage with a powdery white underside is mostly evergreen in all but the coldest climates. The leaves are ⅛ to ¼ inch wide, curling 6 to 9 inches tall, and slowly creeping. Blackish flowers, appearing mostly in the spring, usually bloom close to the foliage. The flowers are noticeable but not really showy. (For more showy black flowers, see California black-flowering sedge [*C. nudata*].)

LANDSCAPE USES: Black-flowering sedge is a good groundcover. Its blue-gray foliage can accent green plants or blend with other blue-gray plants, such as columbine, iris, and lamium. A fine pot and tub subject, it is also good for water gardens. Although spreading in habit, it is not invasive.

CULTURE AND PROPAGATION: Black-flowering sedge grows best in moist, fertile soil in light shade. In hot climates, it needs constant moisture and resents drying out. It will grow in shallow water, 3 to 4 inches deep, and can grow in deeper water as it ages.

Propagate by seed, or by division in the spring.

PESTS AND PROBLEMS: Black-flowering sedge has no known pests or problems.

BOTANICAL NAME	*Carex nudata*
PRONUNCIATION	KAIR-ex noo-DAH-tah
COMMON NAME	California black-flowering sedge
USDA HARDINESS ZONE	7 to 9
ORIGIN	Northern California, coastal ranges
PREFERRED SITES	Streamsides

DESCRIPTION: This clumping, deciduous sedge is distinguished by showy black flowers that emerge on upright spikes 18 to 24 inches tall over the foliage. The gray-green leaves, ⅛ to ¼ inch wide and 1½ to 2½ feet long, form a dense mound. The foliage turns bright yellow and orange with the first frost. The winter foliage is a tawny brown and persists on the plant. The unusual, almost animated, flowers emerge in late winter and early spring.

LANDSCAPE USES: California black-flowering sedge is an excellent groundcover for moist stream banks or at the water's edge, where its delicate spikes can nod gently in a breeze. It is equally effective planted alone or in groups. It grows in shallow water and can be used in pots or tubs. It also makes an effective fall and winter accent. It is stunning in fresh or dried flower arrangements.

CULTURE AND PROPAGATION: California black-flowering sedge grows best in moist, fertile soil in full sun or light shade. It tolerates a variety of soil types and deeper shade, and it will grow in shallow water, 3 to 4 inches deep, and deeper with age. Some people prefer to cut the foliage back after the fall color display so that next year's flowers can emerge from the clump before the new foliage. Others prefer the look of old, dormant foliage with the black flowers above.

Propagate by seed, or by division in spring.

PESTS AND PROBLEMS: California black-flowering sedge has no known pests or problems.

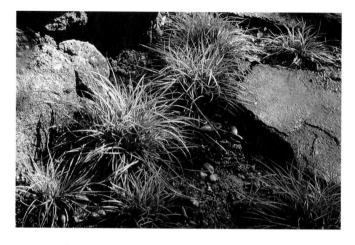

Carex ornithipoda 'Variegata', variegated bird's foot sedge, emerging from winter dormancy.

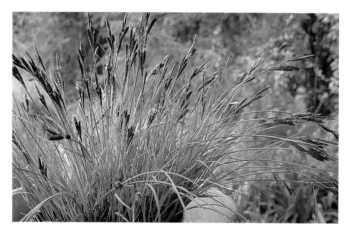

Carex nudata, California black-flowering sedge.

blooming flower that resembles a clawlike bird's foot. The green leaves, ⅛ to ⅜ inch wide, have a creamy white center stripe. The small clumps usually grow 4 to 6 inches tall with soft, recurving foliage. The plant rarely flowers in the upper ranges of its hardiness zone.

LANDSCAPE USES: Variegated bird's foot sedge is a treasure in rock and dish gardens. Its soft white foliage makes a delicate groundcover and accent plant in light shade.

CULTURE AND PROPAGATION: Variegated bird's foot sedge grows best in loose, humus-rich soil with constant moisture and good drainage. It grows best in light shade. It burns in full sun and performs poorly in dense shade.

Propagate by division only.

PESTS AND PROBLEMS: Variegated bird's foot sedge is a difficult plant to grow in interior hot climates but is worth the challenge. It does not grow strong unless conditions are absolutely perfect.

BOTANICAL NAME	***Carex ornithipoda*** **'Variegata'**
PRONUNCIATION	KAIR-ex or-nih-thih-POH-dah var-ee-uh-GAH-tah
COMMON NAME	Variegated bird's foot sedge
USDA HARDINESS ZONE	7 to 9
ORIGIN	Eastern Europe
PREFERRED SITES	Pine and oak forests on calcareous, loose, humus-rich soil

BOTANICAL NAME	***Carex pansa***
PRONUNCIATION	KAIR-ex PAN-sah
COMMON NAME	California meadow sedge
USDA HARDINESS ZONE	8 to 10
ORIGIN	California to Washington
PREFERRED SITES	Sand dunes, coastal plains

DESCRIPTION: Variegated bird's foot sedge is a diminutive evergreen sedge noted for its charming white, longitudinally variegated leaves. Its name is derived from its spring-

DESCRIPTION: Creeping California meadow sedge makes a fine lawn substitute or unmowed meadow. Growing no taller than 3 to 4 inches, its dark green color and smooth glossy foliage make it a good groundcover for southern and western gardens. The rich lustrous green leaves, 1/16 to ⅛ inch wide and 4 to 8 inches long, spread from rhizomes to form dense colonies of curling foliage. The fuzzy, cream-colored flower spikes are held on slender stems just above the foliage. The flowers appear in early spring and are noticeable but not particularly showy. The foliage is evergreen in mild climates, with little winter discoloration.

LANDSCAPE USES: California meadow sedge makes a durable, lawnlike surface that can grow in shade and with tree roots. It tolerates occasional mowing but also does well as an unmowed lawn. Its rhizomatous nature makes it good for dog runs and children's play areas. It tolerates moderate traffic and grows equally well in sun or shade. Reasonably drought-tolerant by the coast, it needs regular water to stay green in hot inland climates.

CULTURE AND PROPAGATION: California meadow sedge prefers moist, well-drained soil in full sun or partial shade. It tolerates a wide variety of conditions and exposures, including coastal conditions, wind, salt spray, and heavy soils. It tolerates some summer drought, but goes dormant if no summer water is applied.

Propagation is easy from division; it is possible to propagate from seed.

PESTS AND PROBLEMS: California meadow sedge's spreading nature may prove invasive in some situations.

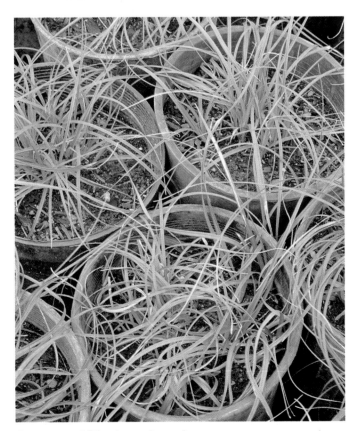

Carex pansa, California meadow sedge.

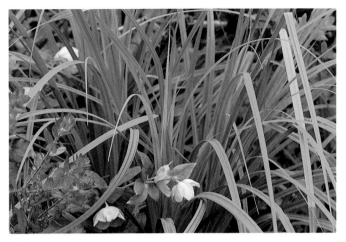

Carex pendula, drooping sedge.

BOTANICAL NAME	***Carex pendula***
PRONUNCIATION	KAIR-ex PEN-dyoo-lah
COMMON NAME	Drooping sedge
USDA HARDINESS ZONE	5 to 9
ORIGIN	Great Britain; eastern, western, southern Europe; North Africa; Asia Minor; Caucasus Mountains
PREFERRED SITES	Moist places, streamsides

DESCRIPTION: Drooping sedge is noted for its long, arching flower spikes and vertically hanging flowers and fruit. The dark evergreen leaves, ½ to ¾ inch wide, emerge from a dense clump 3 to 4 feet tall. The flower spikes rise up and out from the foliage 1 to 2½ feet. The brownish, drooping, 3- to 5-inch catkinlike flowers appear from July through August and persist on the plant into winter.

LANDSCAPE USES: Drooping sedge is an effective accent plant along the water's edge, where the flowers and foliage can be reflected, or along a path or walk, where one can touch the drooping seed heads. It is also attractive in groups and as a background planting. It grows in shallow water and in pots, tubs, and pools. The flowers are stunning in fresh and dried arrangements.

CULTURE AND PROPAGATION: Drooping sedge grows best in moist, rich soil in light shade. It tolerates full sun if it has constant moisture, but suffers in dry conditions. Since drooping sedge is a slow grower, its size can be underestimated; remember to leave plenty of room for its future growth when planting it.

Propagate by seed, or by division in the spring.

PESTS AND PROBLEMS: Drooping sedge has no known pests or problems.

BOTANICAL NAME	***Carex petrei***
PRONUNCIATION	KAIR-ex PEE-tree-eye
COMMON NAME	Dwarf brown sedge
USDA HARDINESS ZONE	7(?) to 9 (hardiness untested; may grow above Zone 7)
ORIGIN	North and south island mountains of New Zealand
PREFERRED SITES	Moist volcanic soils, to 5,000 feet in elevation; streamsides

DESCRIPTION: Dwarf brown sedge is a handsome, clumping sedge with distinctive copper-brown, curly-tipped leaves. The fine-textured leaves are $1/32$ to $1/16$ inch wide and 4 to 6 inches long. Because of its brown color, it often appears dead. The flowers, held down in the foliage, are quite inconspicuous. This plant resembles a miniature version of leather leaf sedge (*Carex buchananii*).

LANDSCAPE USES: Dwarf brown sedge is an excellent rock garden subject. Its compact habit makes it a good choice for pot or tub gardens. The copper-brown foliage makes a striking accent when played off of silver- and blue-foliaged plants. Dwarf brown sedge is also a good filler plant.

CULTURE AND PROPAGATION: Dwarf brown sedge has some-what exacting requirements, as it must stay constantly moist and have good drainage. If these two conditions are met, it tolerates both full sun and heavy shade. Dwarf brown sedge does not like to dry out, nor does it like boggy, oxygenless conditions.

Propagation is easier by seed, but plants can be divided in the spring.

PESTS AND PROBLEMS: Like many other New Zealand sedges, it is short-lived in hot climates, dying out in its third or fourth year in the garden. Should aphids and mealybugs appear, treat appropriately (see page 23).

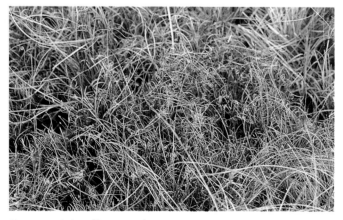

Carex petrei, dwarf brown sedge.

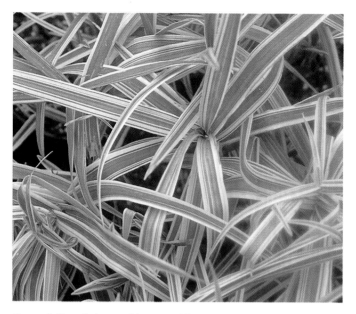

Carex phyllocephala 'Sparkler', 'Sparkler' sedge.

BOTANICAL NAME	***Carex phyllocephala* 'Sparkler'**
PRONUNCIATION	KAIR-ex fih-low-SEF-ah-lah
COMMON NAME	'Sparkler' sedge
USDA HARDINESS ZONE	8 to 10
ORIGIN	Japan and China
PREFERRED SITES	Moist areas, streamsides

DESCRIPTION: 'Sparkler' sedge is a handsome sedge distin-guished by bright yellow-white variegation and an interest-ing upright form. The upright culms, pencil thick, have a red-purple coloring. The lustrous leaves, green with white edges and occasional white streaks, are 8 to 12 inches long and $1/2$ to $3/4$ inch wide, tapering to a fine point. The flowers are a showy terminal cluster of 8 to 10 brownish spikes 3 to 4 inches long. The coloring and growth habit of this plant make its common name a most appropriate descrip-tion. This sedge goes dormant in all but mild climates.

LANDSCAPE USES: 'Sparkler' sedge makes a fine accent or specimen plant that is good in pots and tubs, along the water's edge near pools and ponds, and in shade gardens and rockeries.

CULTURE AND PROPAGATION: 'Sparkler' sedge prefers fertile, moist soil in full sun or partial shade. It grows best in half-day sun or partial shade in hot inland climates. It does not like to dry out and resents hot, drying winds.

Propagate by division.

PESTS AND PROBLEMS: 'Sparkler' sedge has no known pests or problems.

BOTANICAL NAME	***Carex plantaginea***
PRONUNCIATION	KAIR-ex plan-ta-jin-EE-ah
COMMON NAME	Plantain-leaved sedge
USDA HARDINESS ZONE	4 to 9
ORIGIN	Eastern forests of North America
PREFERRED SITES	Shady woods

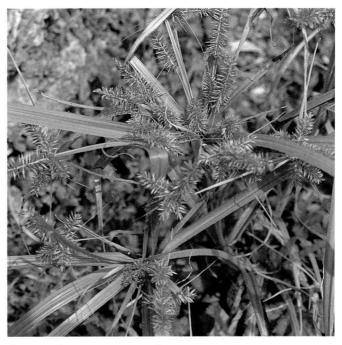

Carex pseudocyperus, cyperus sedge.

DESCRIPTION: An eastern United States native, plantain-leaved sedge is a delightful, clumping, evergreen sedge best suited for shady woodland settings. Its broad, flat leaves make a striking accent. They are bright green with many veins, ¾ to 1 inch wide, and form a clump 1 to 1½ feet in height and width. The flowers are somewhat showy and generally emerge before the foliage in early spring. They resemble many other sedge spikes, brownish black in color, arching 6 to 12 inches above the crown of newly emerging leaves.

LANDSCAPE USES: Plantain-leaved sedge makes a good foliage accent planted either alone or in masses. It makes an excellent companion planting for other shade-loving perennials, woodland plants, ferns, and spring-blooming bulbs. It is a good sedge to grow near ponds, pools, and water gardens, especially shaded ones. The flowers are stunning in fresh or dried arrangements.

CULTURE AND PROPAGATION: Plaintain-leaved sedge grows best in moist, fertile soil in light shade. In the northeastern United States, it tolerates dry, shady conditions. In hot and dry climates, it must have moisture and shade to perform well. Although tolerant of drier conditions in its native range, plantain-leaved sedge must have shade and moisture in hot southern and western areas or the leaves will show burnt edges and poor growth.

Propagate by seed or division.

PESTS AND PROBLEMS: Plantain-leaved sedge has no known pests or problems.

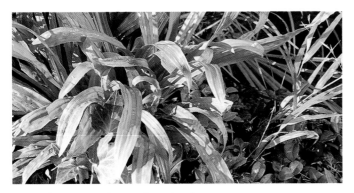

Carex plantaginea, plantain-leaved sedge.

BOTANICAL NAME	***Carex pseudocyperus***
PRONUNCIATION	KAIR-ex soo-doh-SEYE-per-us
COMMON NAME	Cyperus sedge
USDA HARDINESS ZONE	5 to 9
ORIGIN	A circumpolar plant found in temperate zones of North America, Europe, and eastern Asia
PREFERRED SITES	Wet areas, swampy sites

DESCRIPTION: Clumping, deciduous cyperus sedge is distinguished by nodding flower spikes that resemble cypress plants. The yellow-green leaves are ¼ to ⅜ inch wide. The 1- to 2-foot-tall flowers emerge in spring on sturdy 2- to 3-foot-tall attractive, persistent spikes. The brownish, mature flowers contrast strikingly against the yellow-green foliage.

LANDSCAPE USES: Cyperus sedge is an interesting flowering accent in moist, boggy areas or along the water's edge. It is attractive in shallow water in pots, tubs, and ponds. The flowers are stunning in fresh and dried arrangements.

CULTURE AND PROPAGATION: Cyperus sedge grows best in moist, rich soils in full sun or half shade. It tolerates moderate shade and prefers shade in hot, arid climates. Moisture is the key to successful growth.

Propagate by seed, or by division in the spring.

PESTS AND PROBLEMS: Cyperus sedge has no known pests or problems.

BOTANICAL NAME	***Carex siderostica***
	'Variegata'
PRONUNCIATION	KAIR-ex sih-der-OH-stih-kah
	var-ee-uh-GAH-tah
COMMON NAME	Creeping variegated
	broad-leaved sedge
USDA HARDINESS ZONE	7 to 9
ORIGIN	Eastern China to Manchuria,
	Japan
PREFERRED SITES	Moist woodlands

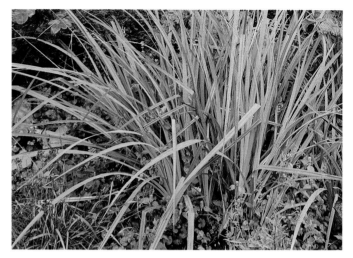

Carex spissa, San Diego sedge.

DESCRIPTION: This striking Asian sedge has broad leaves similar to plantain-leaved sedge's (*Carex plantaginea*), but differs in coloring and growth habit. It is also deciduous. Its leaves, ½ to ¾ inch wide and 12 to 18 inches long, are medium to dark green with creamy white margins and white-streaked centers. Slowly spreading from underground stems, the plant forms stunning, noninvasive colonies of handsome foliage. The foliage is tawny in winter. New spring growth emerges a showy pink. Typical sedge brownish black flowers, 6 to 12 inches long on thin wiry spikes, are noticeable but not showy.

LANDSCAPE USES: Creeping variegated broad-leaved sedge makes an attractive groundcover for shady woodland gardens, especially when dappled sunlight can play on the variegated leaves. It grows well in moist, shady areas near ponds or streams. It is effective planted alone or in masses.

CULTURE AND PROPAGATION: Creeping variegated broad-leaved sedge grows best in rich soil with humus, constant moisture, and light shade.
   Propagate by division only.

PESTS AND PROBLEMS: Creeping variegated broad-leaved sedge needs protection from the sun and drought in hot, arid climates.

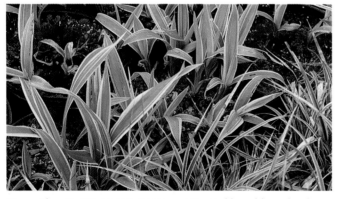

Carex siderostica 'Variegata', creeping variegated broad-leaved sedge.

BOTANICAL NAME	***Carex spissa***
PRONUNCIATION	KAIR-ex SPEE-sah
COMMON NAME	San Diego sedge
USDA HARDINESS ZONE	8 to 9
ORIGIN	Southern California from Baja
	to San Luis Obispo and into
	Arizona
PREFERRED SITES	Stream banks, marshy ground

DESCRIPTION: Silver-gray, evergreen San Diego sedge has richly colored foliage and a handsome clumping habit. Of considerable stature, the foliage can easily reach 4 to 5 feet under optimum conditions. In most garden conditions, the ¾- to 1-inch-wide powdery gray leaves grow 3 to 4 feet tall. The typical sedge brownish black flower spikes, noticeable but not particularly showy, arch up and out from the foliage 12 to 18 inches. They emerge golden in early spring and become tan with age.

LANDSCAPE USES: Its large clumping habit makes San Diego sedge a good background plant, effective in or near water, planted alone or in groups. It grows well in pots and tubs.

CULTURE AND PROPAGATION: San Diego sedge grows best in moist, loamy soil in full sun or partial shade. It tolerates a wide range of conditions and will endure summer drought once established. Plants are slow to moderate growers, needing at least a year to come into their own. The foliage color is richer in light shade or half-day sun.
   Propagate by seed or division.

PESTS AND PROBLEMS: Although tolerant of heat and drought, San Diego sedge will show stress unless given constant moisture.

BOTANICAL NAME	***Carex sylvatica***
PRONUNCIATION	KAIR-ex sil-VAH-tee-kah
COMMON NAME	Forest sedge, sylvan sedge
USDA HARDINESS ZONE	7 to 9
ORIGIN	Eurasia
PREFERRED SITES	Moist forest floors

DESCRIPTION: Clumping, semi-evergreen forest sedge has medium green foliage and slender, arching flower spikes. The leaves, ⅛ to ¼ inch wide, form dense tufts 18 to 24 inches long. The foliage turns yellowish with the first frost. Long, fine-textured flowers bloom in mid-spring on wiry stems and produce narrow, drooping fruits. The flowers are quite prolific, rising up and out from the clump 2 to 3 feet. While noticeable, they are not particularly showy.

LANDSCAPE USES: Forest sedge is an attractive groundcover when planted in groups and masses, especially along streamsides or at water's edge. It is a good understory plant beneath trees, on wooded slopes, and in other shady areas.

CULTURE AND PROPAGATION: Forest sedge likes rich, fertile soil and constant moisture in light shade. It tolerates full sun if moisture is constant. It stays more compact in arid climates, rarely reaching 18 inches in height and width.
   Propagate by seed, or by division in the spring.

PESTS AND PROBLEMS: Forest sedge must have some protection from the sun in hot southern and western climates or the foliage will burn.

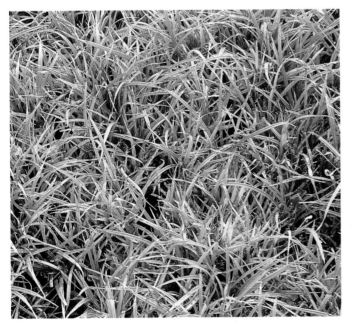

Carex sylvatica, forest sedge.

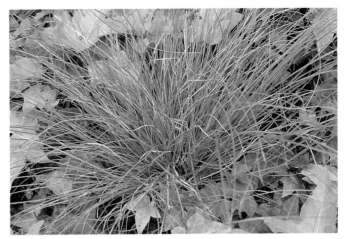

Carex testacea, orange-colored sedge.

BOTANICAL NAME	***Carex testacea***
PRONUNCIATION	KAIR-ex tes-TAY-see-ah
COMMON NAME	Orange-colored sedge
USDA HARDINESS ZONE	8 to 9
ORIGIN	New Zealand
PREFERRED SITES	Moist streamsides

DESCRIPTION: The clumping, fine-textured evergreen glossy foliage of orange-colored sedge is truly unique. The foliage, ¹⁄₃₂ to ¹⁄₁₆ inch wide and 1 to 1½ feet tall, gracefully arches over. It may reach 8 feet in length under optimum conditions. The iridescent foliage emerges olive green, turning intense orange as it ages. Mature foliage is more coppery in color. The flowers are insignificant and are held in the long flowing strands of hairlike foliage.

LANDSCAPE USES: Orange-colored sedge is a unique accent plant, spilling down rocky slopes or over walls and in rock gardens. Its long, fine-textured leaves are also beautiful cascading out of pots or tubs.

CULTURE AND PROPAGATION: Orange-colored sedge likes moist, well-drained, rocky soil. It grows in sun or shade but thrives on moist, gravelly soil. It tolerates full sun in all but the hottest climates. It may be a weak grower in too much shade. It resents being completely dry and will display brown, dead foliage tips if subjected to too much drought stress. It also may lose its orange coloring if it is in too much shade. For best coloring, it needs strong light for half of the day.
   Propagation is easy by seed, or by division in the fall or spring.

PESTS AND PROBLEMS: Like other New Zealand sedges, orange-colored sedge may be short-lived in hot climates.

BOTANICAL NAME	*Carex texensis*
PRONUNCIATION	KAIR-ex tex-EN-sis
COMMON NAME	Catlin sedge, Texas sedge
USDA HARDINESS ZONE	7 to 10
ORIGIN	Southwestern United States; naturalized in Southern California, San Gabriel Mountains
PREFERRED SITES	Streamsides

DESCRIPTION: Catlin sedge takes its name from the famous Southern California horticulturist and artist, Jack Catlin, who grew the plant as a groundcover for his fabulous bonsai collection. This low, clumping, evergreen sedge has shown great promise as a candidate for the dwarf lawn of the future.

Its medium green, lustrous leaves, 1/16 inch wide, usually grow no taller than 3 to 4 inches. Early spring-blooming flowers are held on long, leaflike stems that lie flat on the leaves. The flowers are inconspicuous.

LANDSCAPE USES: Catlin sedge makes a handsome lawn, either mowed or unmowed. It makes an excellent groundcover in both sun and shade, perfect for displaying flowering spring bulbs. Its dwarf habit makes it a good choice between stepping stones or as a garden path, where one might typically plant a lawn. Tough and durable, it is a strong performer where traffic is heavy, including children's play areas. Interplanting with dwarf grassy sweet flag (*Acorus gramineus* 'Pusillus') creates a fragrant lawn. Enjoy individual specimens in small pots and tubs.

CULTURE AND PROPAGATION: Sun- and shade-tolerant and capable of enduring heavy traffic and drought, this dwarf sedge needs only occasional mowing to make an attractive

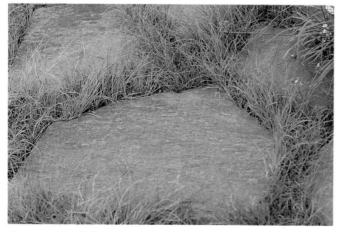

Carex texensis, Catlin sedge.

lawn. It is currently being tested as a "never-needs-to-be-mowed" lawn. Currently of limited availability, it should be readily and abundantly available in the coming years.

Catlin sedge grows best in moist, fertile soil in light or partial shade. It tolerates a wide range of conditions, including sun or shade, low moisture, and shallow water, 1 to 2 inches deep. It will grow in all but the deepest shade and grows more compactly in dry situations. This sedge may sunburn or appear yellowish in hot, arid climates unless planted in light or partial shade. For lawn applications, the closer the spacing, the more comfortable it is to walk on. Plugs should be set out no less than 6 inches apart. For meadows, space plants 12 to 16 inches apart.

Propagate by seed or division.

PESTS AND PROBLEMS: Catlin sedge has no known pests or problems.

BOTANICAL NAME	*Carex tumulicola*
PRONUNCIATION	KAIR-ex toom-yoo-lih-KOH-lah
COMMON NAME	Berkeley sedge
USDA HARDINESS ZONE	8 to 10
ORIGIN	Northern California
PREFERRED SITES	Moist streamsides

DESCRIPTION: The clumping, evergreen Berkeley sedge is one of the best for creating lush meadowlike effects along the west coast of California. It can reach 18 to 24 inches tall and as wide, although it usually forms a clump 8 to 12 inches tall. Its lustrous, dark green leaves, 1/8 inch wide and 12 to 18 inches long, arch out gracefully from the clump. The inconspicuous, brownish, spring-blooming flowers are held on long, wiry, floppy stems.

LANDSCAPE USES: Berkeley sedge makes an attractive groundcover for large areas and is good for creating evergreen meadows. It is also useful as a single specimen or in small groupings in shade plantings. It makes a good groundcover under trees, since it tolerates tree root competition. Plant it in combination with ferns and other shade- and moisture-loving plants. It tolerates traffic and, once established (usually after one season), will take considerable abuse; thus it is a good choice for dog yards.

CULTURE AND PROPAGATION: Berkeley sedge tolerates a wide variety of soils and grows in sun or shade. Although somewhat drought-tolerant once established, it looks best with regular watering. It tolerates wet or boggy areas and

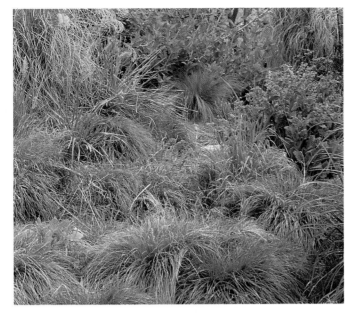

Carex tumuicola, Berkeley sedge.

can survive in the shallow water of ponds or tubs. Berkeley sedge is a moderately fast grower, quick to establish in one season. Though it does not require mowing, cutting it back once or twice a year will keep it looking fresh and tidy. It may go semideciduous in cold climates on the edge of Zone 8.

Propagation is easy by seed, or by division in fall or spring.

PESTS AND PROBLEMS: Berkeley sedge has no known pests or problems.

BOTANICAL NAME	***Carex*** × **'The Beatles'**
PRONUNCIATION	KAIR-ex
COMMON NAME	'The Beatles' sedge, mop-headed sedge
USDA HARDINESS ZONE	7 to 9
ORIGIN	Horticultural: a presumed hybrid between *C. digitata* and *C. ornithipoda*
PREFERRED SITES	Rich, moist soils

DESCRIPTION: Regardless of its questionable parentage, 'The Beatles' sedge is one of the best low evergreen sedges. Its slow-creeping habit and fine-textured leaves make it a useful plant in almost any garden. Its soft, dark green leaves, 1/16 to 1/8 inch wide, usually grow 3 to 4 inches tall. The soft foliage makes a cool place on which to lie. The inconspicuous flowers are held down in the foliage.

LANDSCAPE USES: 'The Beatles' sedge is one of the best sedges to plant as a low groundcover between stepping stones and for lining paths. It is a good filler between other plantings and is useful in rock gardens and pots. It tolerates light foot traffic as a lawn substitute or low meadow. Its foliage makes a nice background for bulbs, especially miniatures.

CULTURE AND PROPAGATION: 'The Beatles' sedge grows best in moist, rich soil in light shade. It tolerates less than perfect conditions, but in hot climates it must have light shade and constant moisture.

Propagate by division only.

PESTS AND PROBLEMS: 'The Beatles' sedge has no known pests or problems.

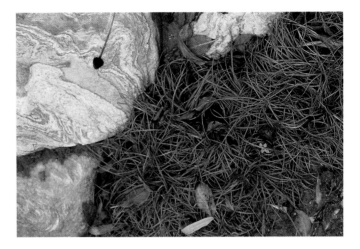

Carex × 'The Beatles', 'The Beatles' sedge.

OTHER SEDGE SPECIES ARE:

Carex aurea (Golden-fruited sedge): beautiful, deciduous dwarf sedge; grows 4 to 6 inches tall; showy golden yellow fruits; excellent in rock gardens.

Carex digitata (Finger sedge): a fine, deciduous sedge growing 4 to 6 inches tall; best in cool climates.

Carex flacca (Creeping forest sedge): an invasive, deciduous, creeping sedge growing 1 to 2 feet tall; good as a large-scale groundcover.

Carex speciosa 'Velebit Humilis' (Grassy forest sedge, velebit sedge): semi-evergreen clumping sedge with fine-textured grasslike leaves growing 6 to 8 inches tall. Good for low meadow effects.

BOTANICAL NAME	***Chasmanthium latifolium***
PRONUNCIATION	kas-MAN-thee-um
	lat-ih-FOL-ee-um
COMMON NAME	Northern sea oats, wild oats
USDA HARDINESS ZONE	5 to 9
ORIGIN	Southern, central, and eastern
	North America
PREFERRED SITES	Rich woodlands, shaded
	streamsides

DESCRIPTION: Northern sea oats is a clumping, deciduous grass treasured for its showy, drooping flowers and rich, bamboolike foliage. Its sturdy stems, 2 to 3 feet tall, are clothed with light green leaves, ½ to ¾ inch wide and 4 to 6 inches long. The attractive foliage changes from green in spring to copper in fall to brown in winter. It is particularly arresting when contrasted against a mantle of snow. Though vertical in youth, the weight of the mature flower spikes causes the stems to droop. The flat flower spikes are ¾ to 1 inch long. Like the foliage, the flowers are green in the summer, maturing to copper. They are persistent on the plant well into winter, when they appear a celadon gray. A warm-season grass, northern sea oats makes a most attractive winter skeleton.

LANDSCAPE USES: Northern sea oats is a versatile performer in the garden, noted for both its foliage and flower. It is effective planted in masses in tubs and containers. It is a good flowering accent in shady and damp situations, and its drooping habit is beautifully displayed along the water's edge. Its salt tolerance makes it a dependable choice for

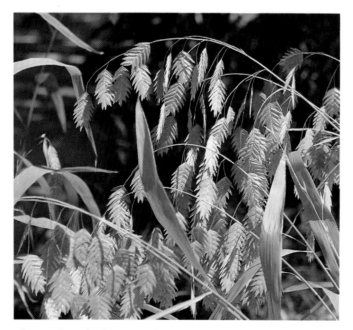

Chasmanthium latifolium, northern sea oats.

coastal gardens, and its bamboolike foliage creates a lovely tropical effect. Since its flowers are beautiful at all stages of maturity, this grass is good in fresh and dried arrangements.

CULTURE AND PROPAGATION: Northern sea oats grows best in deep, rich soil in partial shade with plenty of moisture, although it will grow in less than ideal conditions. In shade, the foliage appears darker green. In full sun, the leaves bleach to a light yellow-green. In hot inland climates, partial shade is best or plants will sunburn. Northern sea oats tolerates a variety of soil conditions, including full sun and dry soil, as long as it has constant moisture; however, the foliage tips and leaves may burn if the plants dry out completely.

Propagation is easy by seed, or by division in spring. The grass does reseed itself but usually not invasively so.

PESTS AND PROBLEMS: Northern sea oats has no known pests or problems.

BOTANICAL NAME	***Chloris virgata***
PRONUNCIATION	KLOR-is ver-GAH-tah
COMMON NAME	Finger grass, feather finger grass
USDA HARDINESS ZONE	8 to 10
ORIGIN	Tropical and subtropical areas
PREFERRED SITES	Open, sunny meadows and
	coastal areas

DESCRIPTION: Subtropical, evergreen finger grass has glossy green leaves that blush reddish purple with the first frost. They are slow-spreading and clumping, ½ to ¾ inch wide and 4 to 6 inches long. The foliage grows 6 to 18 inches tall, depending on the availability of moisture. The delicate flower spikes grow 12 to 18 inches above the foliage; immature spikes are silky and droop from the top of the spikelike silk tassels. Once mature, they fluff up and become upright like a feather duster. They are showy and persistent on the plant. Finger grass also has an attractive fall color.

LANDSCAPE USES: Finger grass is effective alone as a flowering accent or in masses, and is a good choice for dry gardens since it tolerates hot, dry climates. It grows well in pots and tubs. The flowers are stunning in fresh or dried arrangements.

CULTURE AND PROPAGATION: Finger grass grows best in moist, well-drained soil in full sun. It tolerates a wide variety of soil conditions, from sand to clay, and from moist to dry to

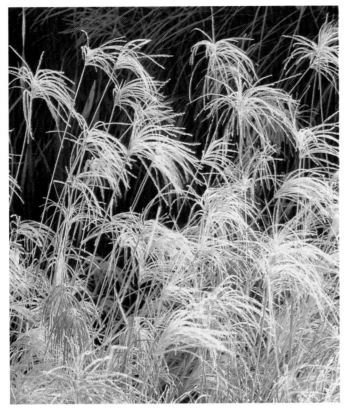

Chloris virgata, finger grass.

seacoast conditions. Full sun is best for flower production; flowers can become floppy in too much shade. In cold climates, plants can be overwintered in greenhouses.

Propagation is easy by seed; plants can also be divided in the spring.

PESTS AND PROBLEMS: Finger grass reseeds readily and can become invasive in some situations. Removing flower spikes prior to maturity requires diligence, as they mature throughout the season.

BOTANICAL NAME	***Coix lacryma-jobi***
PRONUNCIATION	COY LAK-ree-mah-JOH-bee
COMMON NAME	Job's tears, Christ's tears, tear grass
USDA HARDINESS ZONE	9 to 10
ORIGIN	Subtropical Asia
PREFERRED SITES	Wet areas

DESCRIPTION: Tender, evergreen Job's tears is believed to be one of the first grasses cultivated by humans for purely ornamental purposes. The hard seeds were prized for use in bead necklaces, dresses, and rosaries. In some parts of Asia, the seeds were ground to make food.

Job's tears is an upright, clumping grass with shiny, light green, tropical-looking leaves. Its stiff, erect, much-branched stems are clothed by leaves 3 to 12 inches long and ½ to 1½ inches wide. The plant grows from 3 to 6 feet tall in an upright, fountaining form. The flowers emerge in midsummer and continue through the fall. They are short, grayish white, drooping tassels on which hard, beadlike seeds form. The ¼-inch tear-shaped seeds begin a shiny light green and mature into whitish, bluish gray, or black seeds. The seeds drop at maturity.

LANDSCAPE USES: Job's tears is grown mostly as a curiosity and for its beadlike seeds. It is used in western and tropical climates for background foliage and as an accent. In warm climates, it is an effective screen or hedge. In colder climates, it is grown as an annual.

CULTURE AND PROPAGATION: Job's tears grows best in moist, rich soil in full sun. The plants tolerate a variety of soils but resent drying out. They languish and flop over in too much shade.

Propagate by seed, or by division in spring.

PESTS AND PROBLEMS: When grown on the edge of Zone 9, Job's tears freezes to the ground. It has survived short periods of 15°F but will not tolerate sustained cold, wet conditions.

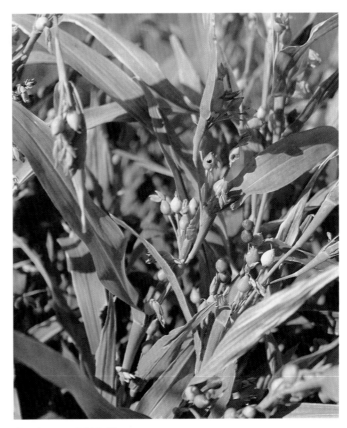

Coix lacryma-jobi, Job's tears.

CORTADERIA
PAMPAS GRASS

Most of the 24 species of pampas grass are native to South America and New Zealand. This genus is often considered the royalty of the ornamental grasses. The South American pampas grasses are native to the great Argentine grasslands known as the pampas, giving them their common name. Their stunning flowers and architectural form have made them popular in gardens since Victorian times. Although many named species and cultivars exist, most of these superior forms are just now becoming available in nurseries and garden centers.

Much confusion exists about pampas grass, as careless seed dealers have often sold plants not true to type and, in some cases, substituted one species for another. The resulting confusion has given all members of the genus a bad name, especially in California, where several weedy species have become naturalized and have invaded the native chaparral vegetation. However, not all cultivars are weedy and aggressive, and some are considerably hardier than others. Dwarf and compact forms have great potential in today's gardens. Some pampas grasses are either male or female plants; others have both male and female parts on the same plant. Female plants tend to have showier flowers than male plants and are preferred for garden cultivation. Plants can be quite variable from seed, so asexual propagation is preferred and is required for cultivars with superior traits. As a cut flower accent or as a specimen in the garden, pampas grass has a majesty few grasses can equal.

BOTANICAL NAME	***Cortaderia jubata***
PRONUNCIATION	kor-tah-DEER-ee-ah joo-BAH-tah
COMMON NAME	Purple pampas grass, pink pampas grass
USDA HARDINESS ZONE	8 to 10
ORIGIN	Western South America, Argentina
PREFERRED SITES	Grasslands

DESCRIPTION: Purple pampas grass is similar to pampas grass (*Cortaderia selloana*), differing mainly in its greener foliage and loose, pinkish flowers. This plant has been known to reach 15 feet on moist coastal California slopes but usually grows 9 to 12 feet in dense, mounding clumps. Razor-sharp edges on green leaves, ½ to 1 inch wide, are formidable. The flower spikes are borne on stems 6 to 9

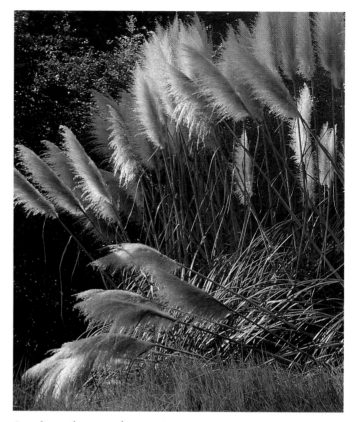
Cortaderia jubata, purple pampas grass.

feet above the foliage as fluffy, loose plumes 1½ to 2 feet tall from September to October. Their color varies from pink, red, and purple, to even yellowish. This plant is often inadvertently offered as pampas grass.

LANDSCAPE USES: The foliage and flower of purple pampas grass make a large and beautiful accent. Grown in a mass, the grass forms an impenetrable hedge and windbreak.

CULTURE AND PROPAGATION: Purple pampas grass grows best in moist, rich loam with regular water. Under ideal conditions, a small nursery plant can reach 8 feet in one season. Because of its eventual large size, care must be taken in placement of this grass. It tolerates less than ideal conditions, including wet soil, drought, wind, and aridity, with measured but steady persistence, although in cold climates it grows more slowly and will not reach such immense proportions.

Selected color forms must be propagated by division, as seedling-grown plants can be highly variable. Named varieties should be propagated by division only, which is best done in late spring.

PESTS AND PROBLEMS: Purple pampas grass has some serious faults, not the least of which is its aggressive, weedy reseeding in mild climates. In California, native plant enthusiasts sadly watched it invade the chaparral and coastal forests, choking out the native vegetation and forming dense, impenetrable thickets. In addition to its weediness, the flower spikes of purple pampas grass are prone to breakage in high winds, and the plant is considerably less hardy than even most pampas grass clones. In most situations, named cultivars of *C. selloana* are far superior to this plant.

BOTANICAL NAME	***Cortaderia selloana***
PRONUNCIATION	kor-tah-DEER-ee-ah sell-oh-AN-ah
COMMON NAME	Pampas grass
USDA HARDINESS ZONE	8 to 10
ORIGIN	South America, from Argentina to Brazil
PREFERRED SITES	grasslands

DESCRIPTION: This is the true pampas grass of horticultural fame and is probably the most popular ornamental grass. There are a considerable number of types of pampas grass, varying in size and flowering characteristics. Even the typical species, if grown from seed, varies in size, vigor, and hardiness, and its flower may vary in size and form. There are quite a few cultivars of pampas grass now in nurseries and garden centers and perhaps many more to follow.

This evergreen grass forms a dense clump of sharp-edged grayish to greenish foliage. Its leaves, ½ to 1 inch wide, can grow into a clump 8 to 12 inches tall and as wide. The 6- to 12-inch-wide flowers are held on sturdy stalks ½ to 1 inch in diameter. Showy panicles grow above the foliage. The plumes are silky at first, becoming fluffy with maturity. In the typical species, 2- to 4-inch-long flower spikes rise erectly from the well-foliaged clump. Flower color varies from silvery white to creamy white to pinkish tones. Flowers bloom mostly from late July through August and are persistent and showy on the plant into early winter.

LANDSCAPE USES: Pampas grass is planted mainly for its dramatic flowering accent. In mild climates, its evergreen foliage is graceful and durable. It can be planted alone as an accent or massed in groups. Taller varieties are effective as screens or windbreaks. It makes a useful plant for coastal gardens, dry slopes, or the water's edge, or as a lawn or grouped near a lawn. Try to place plants where a dark background will make the flowers stand out. It is dramatic when placed where both morning and evening light can shine through the foliage and flower. Pampas grass makes

an excellent cut flower, in fresh or dried arrangements. Flowers should be cut when they are fresh and newly open; flowers picked later in the day have a tendency to shatter. Flowers are often dyed for arrangements. Because of its eventual size and its razor-sharp edges, pampas grass can quickly become a formidable presence in the garden. If poorly situated, such as planted too close to a walkway, it can become a nuisance, requiring considerable effort to remove.

CULTURE AND PROPAGATION: Pampas grass prefers fertile, well-drained soil with adequate moisture. It will tolerate a wide range of conditions, but will be slower-growing in drier, poorer soils. Although it will tolerate wet soil for short periods of time, it does not like to be in cold, soggy, constantly wet soil. The plant prefers full sun, but will tolerate light shade, especially in hot, inland climates. In cold climates and areas of marginal hardiness, foliage may go partially or wholly deciduous. Shield clumps planted in wet climates from overwatering by placing them in a well-drained, protected site. In cold-winter areas, pampas grass needs a winter protection of mulch and/or its dormant foliage. Cut back in the spring.

Propagate by seed, or by divisions from seed. Since seed is viable for only a short period of time, division is the best

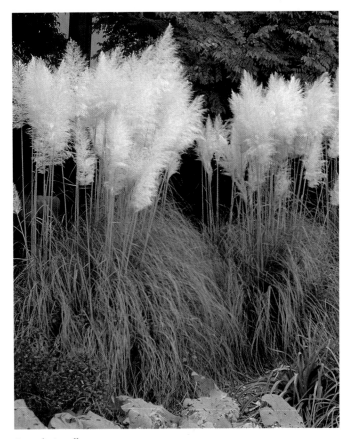

Cortaderia selloana, pampas grass.

method of propagation, and the only way to ensure that clonal characteristics are continued. Division is best in early spring, although fall divisions, if protected in the winter, may also be successful.

PESTS AND PROBLEMS: Caution and forethought should be given to the placement of pampas grass in the garden because of its enormous size. Avoid placing it too close to walks or swimming pools, where its sharp-edged foliage can be a hazard.

Cutting back, thinning, or removing old clumps can be quite a chore, requiring gloves, a long-sleeved shirt, goggles, and boots. A fiendishly sharp axe or mattock is needed. The best way to cut back foliage is with a weed eater fitted with a blade attachment. Cutting and thinning every one to two years will keep the task from becoming too monumental.

The compact clump is slow-growing, reaching 4 to 6 feet tall and as wide. Its flower, a stately vertical spike, tends to be more erect than the other yellow variegated pampas variety, *Cortaderia selloana* 'Sun Stripe'. It is also more compact than *C. selloana* 'Sun Stripe'. Plants will grow in shady conditions, but may not bloom as well. Its creamy white flowers usually appear from late August through September. The flowers bloom sporadically and seldom bloom the first year.

BOTANICAL NAME	*Cortaderia selloana* 'Pumila'
PRONUNCIATION	kor-tah-DEER-ee-ah sell-OH-ana pyoo-MILL-ah
COMMON NAME	Dwarf pampas grass

DESCRIPTION: Dwarf pampas grass is similar to the species, but has a delightful miniature size and a prolific blooming habit. Its compact foliage, gray-green in color, forms dense evergreen clumps 4 to 6 feet tall, depending on the type of soil and moisture availability. Its narrow leaves, ½ to ¾ inch wide, are sharp, like those of the species. Creamy

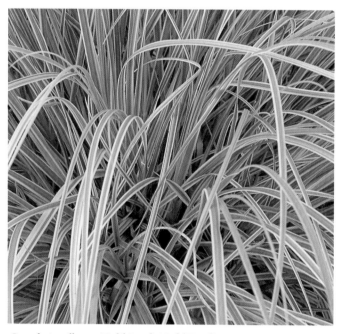

Cortaderia selloana 'Gold Band', 'Gold Band' pampas grass.

BOTANICAL NAME	*Cortaderia selloana* 'Gold Band'
PRONUNCIATION	kor-tah-DEER-ee-ah sell-oh-AN-ah
COMMON NAME	'Gold Band' pampas grass

DESCRIPTION: Similar to pampas grass in flower and habit, this golden variegated dwarf pampas grass is distinguished by golden foliage and a compact habit. Yellow-green leaves, ½ to ¾ inch wide, are edged with golden yellow stripes.

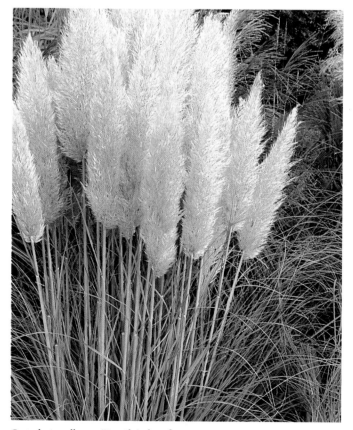

Cortaderia selloana 'Pumila', dwarf pampas grass.

white silky flowers emerge as spikes 3 to 4 feet tall and 6 to 8 inches wide in August and are showy into the winter. A mature plant can have 50 to 100 blossoms at a time, while a small specimen planted in the spring may have 3 to 5 flower spikes by August. It does not reseed itself and is an excellent choice for gardens with limited space.

If you want pampas grass, this is the cultivar to plant. Its smaller size makes it more suitable for the majority of home gardens.

Propagate by division only, since all plants are female and usually do not set seed. Division in late winter and early spring is best. Fall divisions can be successful if protected in winter.

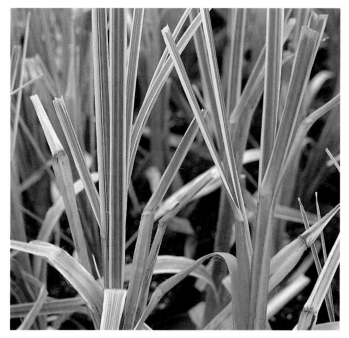

Cortaderia selloana 'Silver Stripe', 'Silver Stripe' pampas grass.

BOTANICAL NAME	*Cortaderia selloana* **'Silver Stripe' (also known as *C. selloana* 'Albo-Lioneata')**
PRONUNCIATION	kor-tah-DEER-ee-ah sell-oh-AN-ah
COMMON NAME	'Silver Stripe' pampas grass

DESCRIPTION: This beautiful female clone is graced by pure white, linear, variegated leaves. 'Silver Stripe' is a compact grower and is slow to achieve its eventual size. Its dense clumping foliage reaches 4 to 5 feet tall and as wide. It has creamy white flowers, but blooms sporadically and may not flower at all the first or second year. 'Silver Stripe'

pampas grass makes a beautiful foliage accent whether planted alone or in groups. Although slow-growing, it is stunning in the garden and makes an excellent accent in gray and silver borders. It is a good choice for hot climates or drought-tolerant plantings where variegated Japanese silver grass (*Miscanthus sinensis* 'Variegatus') would be inappropriate.

Propagate by division only, in late winter or early spring. Fall division is possible with winter protection.

BOTANICAL NAME	*Cortaderia selloana* **'Sun Stripe'**
PRONUNCIATION	kor-tah-DEER-ee-ah sell-oh-ana
COMMON NAME	'Sun Stripe' pampas grass

DESCRIPTION: This bright yellow cultivar was discovered in Monrovia Nursery in Azuza, California. The typical pampas leaves have bright yellow centers and yellow-green margins. 'Sun Stripe' grows 4 to 6 feet tall. The plant is almost too yellow to blend easily with other plants: Its bright yellow color is sure to be noticed. Its flowers are topped by fluffy white plumes in late summer. A dependable bloomer, it blooms well from the second year on, though flower spikes tend to flop over.

Propagate by division in late winter and early spring.

This plant is protected by a plant patent; thus, vegetative propagation is licensed only from Monrovia Nursery.

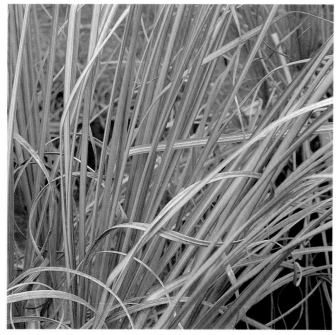

Cortaderia selloana 'Sun Stripe', 'Sun Stripe' pampas grass.

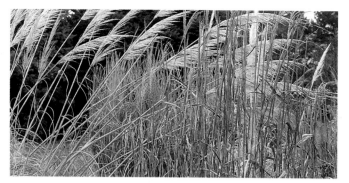

Cortaderia selloana 'Sunningdale Silver', 'Sunningdale Silver' pampas grass, at left, in late winter.

BOTANICAL NAME	***Cortaderia selloana 'Sunningdale Silver'***
PRONUNCIATION	kor-tah-DEER-ee-ah sell-oh-AN-ah
COMMON NAME	'Sunningdale Silver' pampas grass

DESCRIPTION: While similar to pampas grass in most respects, this cultivar has a distinctive flower and form. This hardy female clone is distinguished by large, robust clumps 6 to 10 feet tall and as wide, topped by symmetrical, large, white flowers held well above the foliage. The flowers can reach 6 to 9 feet tall and are large fluffy plumes. There is a distinct separation between foliage and flower that enhances its glorious flowering display. Be sure to give it enough room, as the plant is vigorous and can get quite large in a short period of time. *Cortaderia selloana* 'Sunningdale Silver' may be hard to find.

ANOTHER CULTIVAR OF *Cortaderia selloana* IS:

'Carminea Rendatleri' (Pink pampas grass): plants 6 to 12 feet tall and as wide; pink flowers 3 to 6 feet above the foliage.

OTHER PAMPAS GRASS SPECIES ARE:

Cortaderia fulvida (Kakaho, tussock grass, toe toe): a showy, flowering New Zealand native growing 4 to 6 feet tall; evergreen; not invasive.

Cortaderia richardii (Plumed toe toe, black pampas grass, plumed tussock): an evergreen New Zealand native with showy flowers growing 6 to 8 feet tall; clumping.

BOTANICAL NAME	***Cymbopogon citratus***
PRONUNCIATION	sim-boh-POH-gon cih-TRAH-tus
COMMON NAME	Lemon grass
USDA HARDINESS ZONE	9 to 10
ORIGIN	Old World tropics; widely cultivated in India and Sri Lanka
PREFERRED SITES	Some tropical grasslands, widely cultivated in tropical regions

DESCRIPTION: The fragrant citrus aroma of the leaves of this plant are used in soup, as medicinal herbs, and as perfume. It has just recently come to be appreciated as a garden plant in American gardens. This plant has been cultivated for a thousand years or more.

This subtropical clumping grass is a tender evergreen that requires protection in all but the most tropical gardens of Zone 10. The bright yellow-green foliage grows 3 to 4 feet tall and as wide. The new and old growth of its soft, translucent leaves, 2 to 3 feet long and 1 to 1½ inches wide, is often a bluish, purplish red. Flowers, rare in cultivation and not particularly showy, are a fluffy panicle of small spikelets that bloom sporadically if at all. Flowering usually occurs from August through September.

LANDSCAPE USES: The attractive, fast-growing foliage of lemon grass is best displayed where morning and evening light causes the leaves to look like they are glowing. It is effective planted along walkways, where it emits its pleasant lemon fragrance when crushed or brushed against. It is a good plant for hot locations, and in fact thrives under these conditions. It is also a good grass to grow in pots, in

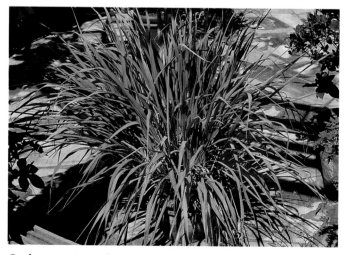

Cymbopogon citratus, lemon grass.

tubs, in windows, and in herb and culinary gardens as long as strong light is provided.

CULTURE AND PROPAGATION: Lemon grass prefers moist, fertile, well-drained loam in full sun. However, it tolerates a wide range of soils and exposures, and light shade. It will perform slowly in damp, dark conditions. In arid western climates, it prefers some additional summer watering. Though drought-tolerant when established, it resents drying out completely.

Propagate by seed, division, or cuttings. Division is best in late spring or early summer; otherwise, a hothouse is required. Cuttings can be rooted under mist with high heat and humidity as long as the stem contains a piece of rhizome.

PESTS AND PROBLEMS: In cold climates, treat lemon grass as an annual. The plant is best planted in spring well after the threat of frost has passed.

CYPERUS
UMBRELLA SEDGES

This large group of plants, members of the Cyperaceae family, has over 600 species and is found primarily in tropical and subtropical habitats, with some temperate-climate members. The umbrella sedges are generally moisture-loving plants, many growing in or near water. They range from 1-foot-tall miniatures to giant reedlike plants reaching 10 to 12 feet tall, forming a huge thicket over wide areas. The leaves of many umbrella sedges are very small, with three-sided culms making up the bulk of the plant's "foliage." Culms are usually topped by a flat cluster of flowerlike bracts that may be compound or simple. The true flowers are usually small or inconspicuous, set atop the bracts.

Umbrella sedges make excellent pot and tub plants and are great companion plants for water lilies and other aquatic plantings. Most need the protection of a greenhouse to overwinter in cold climates, and subtropical and tropical varieties need protection from wind, especially hot, dry winds. Most umbrella sedges look their best in high humidity. Many will grow indoors with high light and high humidity.

Although umbrella sedges have been cultivated for centuries, there has not been a comprehensive botanical treatment agreed upon by both botanists and horticulturists. More often than not, this leads to serious confusion. The following names are the most commonly used in the nursery trade among water plant growers.

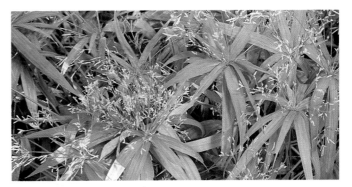

Cyperus albostriatus, broadleaf umbrella plant.

BOTANICAL NAME	***Cyperus albostriatus* (also known as *C. diffusus, C. elegans,* and *C. flabelliformis*)**
PRONUNCIATION	SEYE-per-us al-boh-stree-AH-tus
COMMON NAME	Broadleaf umbrella plant
USDA HARDINESS ZONE	9 to 10
ORIGIN	South Africa
PREFERRED SITES	Damp, shady places near openings of woods

DESCRIPTION: Known by many names, broadleaf umbrella plant is a fine garden plant. It is distinctly different from its close cousin, umbrella plant (*Cyperus alternifolius*), by virtue of its broader, softer, more opaque leaflike bracts and its compact, more refined habit. The bright green leaflike terminal bracts are ½ to ¾ inch wide, narrowing to a soft point 4 to 6 inches long. The flowers, 2 to 6 inches long, are held along wiry stems and form a delicate greenish haze. These spikelets mature to a light brown and are showy and persistent on the plant. The overall height of the plant is generally 1½ to 2 feet tall and as wide. It forms a slowly spreading clump. Broadleaf umbrella plant has several cultivars, all of which have great charm and appeal.

LANDSCAPE USES: Broadleaf umbrella plant is a fine addition to any lightly shaded border or garden; it is a nice filler in shady gardens with ferns and other shade-loving perennials. It makes a nice accent planted alone or in mass. It is an excellent potted subject and will also grow in shallow water or bog gardens.

CULTURE AND PROPAGATION: Broadleaf umbrella plant grows best in moist, fertile soil in light shade or half-day sun. Constant moisture, high humidity, and strong indirect light are keys to good-looking foliage. It resents strong light and drying winds, yet suffers in too much shade. When growing in water, place it close to the surface or slightly above. This species is more difficult to grow indoors than other *Cyperus* species. It is quite well behaved, is never invasive like umbrella plant, and does not seed itself in the garden. It is also more frost-tender.

Propagate by division in late spring.

PESTS AND PROBLEMS: Broadleaf umbrella plant has no known pests or problems.

BOTANICAL NAME	*Cyperus albostriatus* **'Nanus'**
PRONUNCIATION	SEYE-per-us al-boh-stree-AH-tus
COMMON NAME	Dwarf broadleaf umbrella plant

DESCRIPTION: Dwarf broadleaf umbrella plant is similar to the species, differing in that it grows no taller than 12 to 16 inches. Its leaves, stems, and flowers are similar to those of the species, but are longer, narrower, and finer-textured, giving the entire plant a more refined look.

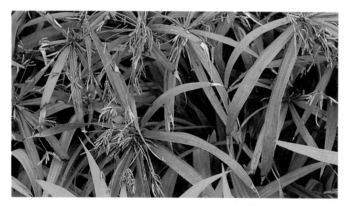

Cyperus albostriatus 'Nanus', dwarf broadleaf umbrella plant.

BOTANICAL NAME	*Cyperus albostriatus* **'Variegatus'**
PRONUNCIATION	SEYE-per-us al-boh-stree-AH-tus var-ee-uh-GAH-tus
COMMON NAME	Variegated broadleaf umbrella plant

DESCRIPTION: Variegated broadleaf umbrella plant is similar to the species, differing in its rich, creamy, white-streaked foliage. The variegation is quite subtle, appearing

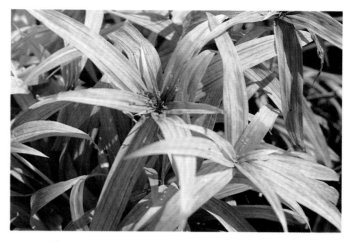

Cyperus albostriatus 'Variegatus', variegated broadleaf umbrella plant.

as if delicately airbrushed onto the foliage. Occasionally, stems and leaf rosettes appear pure white. The coloring is most pronounced on the new growth and tends to fade somewhat by fall. The flowers are similar to those of the species, except that the wiry stems holding the flowers are closer to the leafy rosettes and are not as showy. Variegated broadleaf umbrella plants are compact, generally growing 1 to 1½ feet tall and as wide.

ANOTHER CULTIVAR OF *Cyperus albostriatus* IS:
'Nanus Variegatus' (Dwarf variegated broadleaf umbrella plant): similar to dwarf broadleaf umbrella plant with white, linear stripes on the leaflike terminal bracts; grows 1 to 1½ feet tall; creeping.

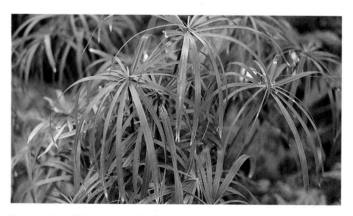

Cyperus alternifolius, umbrella plant.

BOTANICAL NAME	**_Cyperus alternifolius_**
PRONUNCIATION	SEYE-per-us
	ahl-TERN-ih-FOH-lee-us
COMMON NAME	Umbrella plant, umbrella palm
USDA HARDINESS ZONE	9 to 10
ORIGIN	Madagascar; widely naturalized in tropical and subtropical marshes worldwide
PREFERRED SITES	Wet, marshy areas

DESCRIPTION: The umbrella plant has been cultivated in pots and water gardens for over 200 years, and it remains a favorite today. Although it can be killed by temperatures below 15°F and damaged at 32°F, it can still be found in water gardens throughout the world. Its dark green foliage grows 3 to 5 feet wide in dense clumps. The foliage actually consists of three-sided or round culms topped by leaflike bracts that resemble the ribs of an umbrella. These bracts, ⅛ to ⅝ inch wide and 4 to 12 inches long, are topped by flat clusters of greenish flowers that turn brown at maturity. The flowers are showy and persistent on the plant.

LANDSCAPE USES: The umbrella plant is at its best by pools or ponds, in pots and tubs, and in water. It will grow indoors as a houseplant or greenhouse specimen. It is an excellent plant for tropical and subtropical effects and exhibits striking silhouettes when casting a shadow. The plants are indispensable in fresh flower arrangements.

CULTURE AND PROPAGATION: Umbrella plant grows best in constantly moist, fertile soil in sun or partial shade. In hot inland climates, plants need at least half-day shade or they tend to sunburn. Plants will tolerate extreme heat as long as moisture is present. In hot climates, avoid placing umbrella plant against a hot wall in full sun. To keep plants looking good, protect from drying winds and hot, direct sun. They will grow in shallow water 2 to 3 inches deep. Inside the house, umbrella plant does best in an area with high light and high humidity.

Propagate by division of culms or by seed. Plantlets will also form on detached flower heads placed upside down and floated on water, though it may be difficult to propagate some of the dwarf and variegated cultivars by this method.

PESTS AND PROBLEMS: Watch for spider mites indoors. If they prove troublesome wash them off with a steady spray of water. In mild climates this plant seeds itself readily and can easily overtake a small garden. It is best to remove flower heads before they shatter or keep copious seedlings pulled. In a small pool, keep the plant in a container to confine its growth.

BOTANICAL NAME	**_Cyperus alternifolius_ 'Variegatus'**
PRONUNCIATION	SEYE-per-us
	ahl-TERN-ih-FOH-lee-us
	var-ee-uh-GAH-tus
COMMON NAME	Variegated umbrella plant

DESCRIPTION: Similar in most respects to umbrella plant (*Cyperus alternifolius*), variegated umbrella plant has creamy, white-streaked culms, with some bracts growing completely white. The variegation is usually unstable, and plants have a tendency to revert to nonvariegated forms. It is not as vigorous or invasive as umbrella plant, growing only 2 to 3 feet tall. The white variegation is streaked horizontally on the stems and bracts.

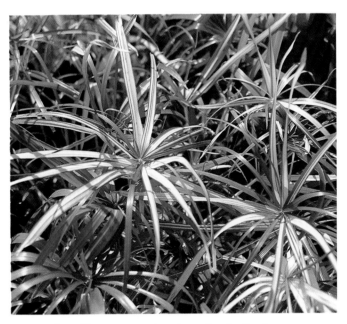

Cyperus alternifolius 'Variegatus', variegated umbrella plant.

ANOTHER CULTIVAR OF *Cyperus alternifolius* IS:

'Gracilis' (Miniature papyrus): a compact cultivar similar to the species with fine-textured foliage; grows 1 to 1½ feet tall.

BOTANICAL NAME	**_Cyperus isocladus_ (also known as _C. haspans_ and _C. papyrus_ 'Nanus')**
PRONUNCIATION	SEYE-per-us eye-soh-CLA-dus
COMMON NAME	Dwarf papyrus, miniature papyrus
USDA HARDINESS ZONE	9 to 10
ORIGIN	Zanzibar, South Africa, western Africa
PREFERRED SITES	Marshes, swampy places

DESCRIPTION: This small aquatic sedge resembles its giant cousin, Egyptian papyrus (*Cyperus papyrus*), but reaches only 2 to 3 feet tall. Its fine-textured terminal bracts have a threadlike appearance. The glossy green umbels grow 3 to 4 inches in diameter. The flowers are borne in noticeable brown spikes that are persistent on the plant. Unlike many other papyrus species, its heads tend to look messy as they mature.

LANDSCAPE USES: Dwarf papyrus is an effective accent in small pools, ponds, pots, and tubs. The plants are stunning in fresh or dried arrangements.

CULTURE AND PROPAGATION: Dwarf papyrus prefers constantly moist, fertile soil in light shade or half-day sun. It grows best in strong indirect light and high humidity. Plants resent drying out, and in arid climates the umbels may be reduced in size. Dead seed heads should be constantly removed to keep plants attractive.

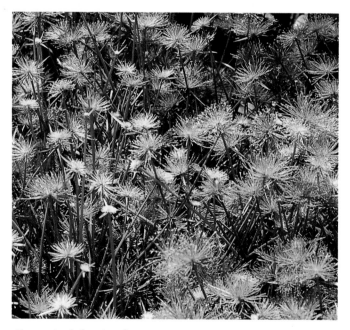

Cyperus isocladus, dwarf papyrus.

Propagate by seed, division, or cuttings of terminal bracts. Place the flower heads upside down on the surface of the water and new plantlets will emerge from the axils of the bracts.

PESTS AND PROBLEMS: Dwarf papyrus has no known pests or problems.

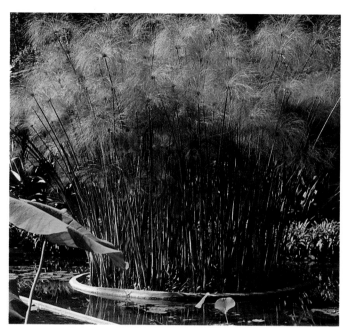

Cyperus papyrus, Egyptian papyrus.

BOTANICAL NAME	**_Cyperus papyrus_**
PRONUNCIATION	SEYE-per-us pah-PEYE-rus
COMMON NAME	Egyptian papyrus, papyrus, paper plant
USDA HARDINESS ZONE	9 to 10
ORIGIN	North Africa, tropical Africa
PREFERRED SITES	Banks and shores of slowly flowing water

DESCRIPTION: This is the plant from which the Egyptians first made paper, making it one of the most historically important grasses. Along the banks of the Nile River, this giant sedge can reach over 15 feet tall. In gardens, its thick, triangular stems grow 1 to 2 inches wide and 4 to 10 feet tall or more. The terminal bracts are threadlike and numerous, sometimes over 100 to a cluster. They can reach 18 inches long, and form graceful nodding flower heads. The flowers are small, greenish spikelets that become brown at maturity, and are noticeable and persistent on the plant. The plants flower from June through September.

LANDSCAPE USES: Egyptian papyrus makes a bold, dramatic statement in the garden. Its use as a tall accent or tall background planting can be stunning. Plants are at their best in or near water, as they would be found in nature, and make good container subjects. It can be grown as a house-plant but requires humid warmth and high light. Its foliage is attractive in fresh arrangements.

CULTURE AND PROPAGATION: Egyptian papyrus prefers constantly moist, fertile soil in full sun or partial shade. It tolerates a wide variety of soil conditions as long as constant moisture is present. Plants look their best protected from hot, drying winds, which will break or damage the heads. Egyptian papyrus is a tender tropical plant that needs winter protection in all but the mildest of climates. In cold climates, lift plants from the garden before the first hard frost and protect in a greenhouse.

Propagate by division or seed. Cut flower heads floated upside down on water will sprout new plants.

PESTS AND PROBLEMS: Egyptian papyrus has no known pests or problems.

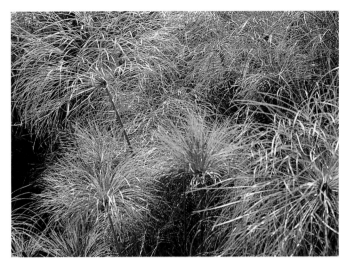

Cyperus papyrus 'Mexico', 'Mexico' papyrus.

near water and in pots and tubs. The tall, arching stems and seed heads nod under the weight of the umbels, swaying in the slightest breeze. It is quite dramatic in fresh and dried flower arrangements.

CULTURE AND PROPAGATION: 'Mexico' papyrus prefers constantly moist, fertile soil in full sun or partial shade. It grows in shallow water 2 to 4 inches deep and can grow in deeper water when mature. Protect plants from hot, drying winds.

Propagate by seed or division.

PESTS AND PROBLEMS: 'Mexico' papyrus has no known pests or problems.

BOTANICAL NAME	***Cyperus papyrus* 'Mexico'**
PRONUNCIATION	SEYE-per-us
COMMON NAME	'Mexico' papyrus
USDA HARDINESS ZONE	9 to 10
ORIGIN	Tabasco, Mexico
PREFERRED SITES	Swampy marshes

DESCRIPTION: This recently introduced, undescribed cultivar of *papyrus* was brought to the nursery trade by famed California plantsman Gary Hammer. Identical in most aspects to the well-known Egyptian papyrus (*Cyperus papyrus*), this selection has twice-divided heads, giving the plant a lush, wispy look. It has quickly caught the attention of the western nursery trade.

Its tall, stout, triangular stems can reach 8 to 10 feet tall. The terminal bracts, threadlike with over 100 to a cluster, arch out gracefully 8 to 12 inches and then divide into two more threads that may reach an additional 6 to 8 inches long. The overall cluster approaches 1½ to 2 feet in diameter. The flowers are borne at the ends of the terminal bracts and are noticeable, showy, and persistent on the plant. A recent introduction, 'Mexico' papyrus may be hard to find in nurseries and garden centers.

LANDSCAPE USES: 'Mexico' papyrus is best used as a tall accent or background plant. It is spectacular planted in or

BOTANICAL NAME	***Cyperus testacea***
PRONUNCIATION	SEYE-per-us tes-TAY-see-ah
COMMON NAME	Slender papyrus
USDA HARDINESS ZONE	9 to 10
ORIGIN	South Africa
PREFERRED SITES	Wet, marshy areas

DESCRIPTION: This species was introduced by Gary Hammer of Sunland, California. Clumping, evergreen slender papyrus resembles a refined, elegant, dark green version of the well-known umbrella plant (*Cyperus alternifolius*). Slender papyrus's thin, strong stems, ¼ to ½ inch thick, grow 5 to 7 feet tall. The stiff rosette of terminal bracts bends at a distinct 45° angle from the stem. The terminal bracts are sparse, with only 10 to 15 per cluster, and are only ¼ to ½ inch wide and 4 to 6 inches long. Slender papyrus has attractive greenish flowers and often forms plantlets in the

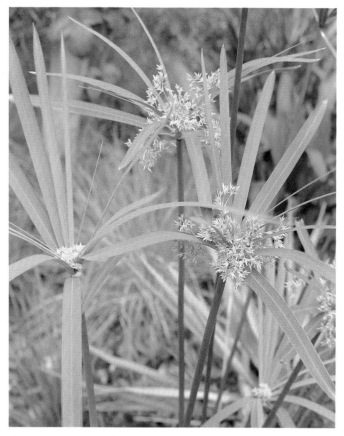

Cyperus testacea, slender papyrus.

BOTANICAL NAME	***Dactylis glomerata 'Variegata'***
PRONUNCIATION	DAK-til-is glom-er-AY-tah var-ee-uh-GAH-tah
COMMON NAME	Variegated orchard grass, variegated cocksfoot grass
USDA HARDINESS ZONE	4 to 9
ORIGIN	Horticultural selection from a species common in Eurasia, where it escaped from cultivation
PREFERRED SITES	Woods and meadows

DESCRIPTION: Orchard grass, often grown as a pasture grass in continental Europe and England, is a common weed-grass along roadsides and fields in the United States. Variegated orchard grass has soft, grayish green leaves with white linear variegation growing in sprawling dense clumps of semi-evergreen foliage 1 to 2 feet tall. The leaves are medium-textured, ⅛ to ⅜ inch wide, and 3 to 5 inches long. The clumps spread moderately fast, forming dense colonies. The flowers are open, white, fluffy spikelets that dance above the foliage. Its 6- to 12-inch-tall flowers are sometimes absent in cultivation.

LANDSCAPE USES: Variegated orchard grass makes an excellent accent planted in small masses and groups. Although somewhat vigorous, it can add interest to rock gardens. It makes an effective groundcover for small areas.

CULTURE AND PROPAGATION: Variegated orchard grass prefers moist, well-drained, fertile soil in light shade or part-day sun. It tolerates full sun in all but the hottest inland

axils of the terminal bracts. The heads nod under the weight of the plantlets. Slender papyrus is the darkest green of all the papyrus species.

LANDSCAPE USES: Slender papyrus makes a fine specimen or accent in small ponds and pools since it is at its best in or near water; it also grows well in tubs or containers. Its noninvasive nature makes it a fine substitute for umbrella plant (*C. alternifolius*). The foliage is stunning in fresh or dried arrangements.

CULTURE AND PROPAGATION: Slender papyrus grows best in moist, fertile soil in light shade or half-day sun. It resents drying out and looks best with constant moisture. It grows in water 2 to 3 inches deep and will grow in deeper water with age. Slender papyrus is perhaps the hardiest of all the papyrus species, tolerating temperatures as low as 24°F with no damage to the foliage. Its ultimate hardiness is untested, but slender papyrus's great beauty is sure to encourage further tests.

Propagate by division or from plantlets formed in the foliage.

PESTS AND PROBLEMS: Slender papyrus has no known pests or problems.

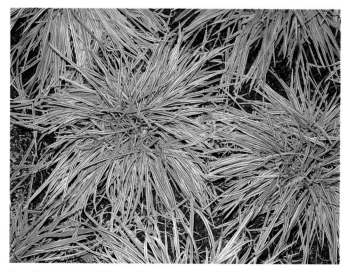

Dactylis glomerata 'Variegata', variegated orchard grass.

climates, but looks better with some shade. Although tolerant of heavy soil, it may perform poorly in heavy, wet clay. This grass is basically a cool-season grass and can look shabby throughout the summer; cut back to 3 to 4 inches above the crown if plants appear too ragged. Plants will be slow to recover in midsummer and may also revert to the green form. Green plants should be removed, as they are more vigorous than the variegated form.

Propagate by division in spring or fall.

PESTS AND PROBLEMS: Variegated orchard grass has no known pests or problems.

DESCHAMPSIA
HAIRGRASS

Deschampsia, named after the French botanist Deschamps, comprises over 50 cultivars and varieties of annuals and perennials. Most grow naturally in moist places, but some are quite drought-tolerant. Hitchcock's *Manual of Grasses of the United States* says that tufted hairgrass grows naturally from Alaska to Southern California and from Greenland to Virginia. The great bulk of hairgrasses currently offered in nursery and garden centers are reputed to be of continental European heritage. Below is a description of the most popular cultivars and varieties available today. Readers should be aware that native hairgrasses may outperform imported clones. Note that hairgrasses are a favored treat of rabbits.

BOTANICAL NAME	**Deschampsia caespitosa**
PRONUNCIATION	deh-SHAMP-see-ah ses-pih-TOH-sah
COMMON NAME	Tufted hairgrass, fairy wand grass
USDA HARDINESS ZONE	4 to 9
ORIGIN	Found throughout the Northern Hemisphere on all continents
PREFERRED SITES	Usually in meadows, wet areas, woods

DESCRIPTION: Tufted hairgrass is a cool-season, mostly evergreen grass that forms dense tufts of dark green foliage 1 to 3 feet tall and as wide. Its leaves are ⅛ to ½ inch wide. The handsomely pleated foliage gives a neat, clean look.

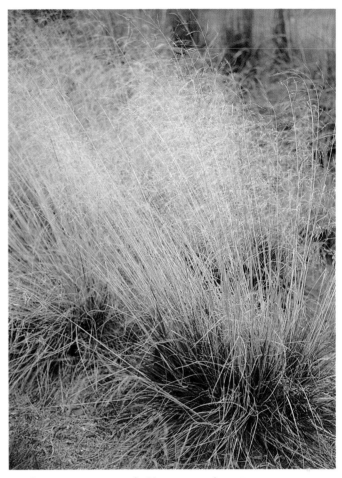

Deschampsia caespitosa, tufted hairgrass, in late winter.

While it remains evergreen in Zones 8 and 9, in colder climates it may freeze back, causing exposed foliage to go dormant. In mild climates, a hard freeze will turn foliage tips yellowish orange. Most cultivars are noted for their flowers, which emerge silky green in late May, and, depending upon the stage of maturation, range from yellow to gold and shades of bronze to almost purple. Plants grown from seed may exhibit mixed flower color and form. The flowers generally appear in loose, airy panicles that occur in such profusion that they totally obscure the foliage. The flowers generally arch upward and out from the plant, 2 to 3 feet above the foliage. They are showy well into summer.

LANDSCAPE USES: Tufted hairgrass tolerates a fair amount of shade, making it a practical companion for ferns, hostas, and other shade- and moisture-loving plants. It is effective planted alone or in masses and is an excellent groundcover for lightly shaded, moist slopes and along the water's edge. As a spring-flowering accent, tufted hairgrass is indispensable, since it is one of the earliest grasses to bloom. Its flowers are particulary showy when backlit by early morning or late evening light, or on sites where the loose, drooping panicles can be viewed from below.

CULTURE AND PROPAGATION: Tufted hairgrass grows best in moist, rich soil in light shade. Plants do not like to dry out and resent hot, dry situations. Full, hot sun will often discolor the foliage, especially in hot climates. Plants are not as particular about sun in cool summer areas, and while they grow in deep shade, they may fail to bloom effectively.

Propagate by seed or division. Plants are quite variable from seed. Propagate cultivars by division only, in the fall and spring.

PESTS AND PROBLEMS: Tufted hairgrass of European origin seems to do poorly in hot or mild climates. Its performance varies in the Deep South and mild-winter areas of California. In California, less showy native clones may outperform European ones in flowering and drought tolerance.

BOTANICAL NAME	***Deschampsia caespitosa*** **'Bronzeschleier'**
PRONUNCIATION	deh-SHAMP-see-ah ses-pih-TOH-sah bron-zah-SCHLEYE-er
COMMON NAME	Bronze veil tufted hairgrass

DESCRIPTION: Bronze veil tufted hairgrass grows 2½ to 3 feet to the top of the bronze-yellow flowers. It is one of the better bloomers for mild climates.

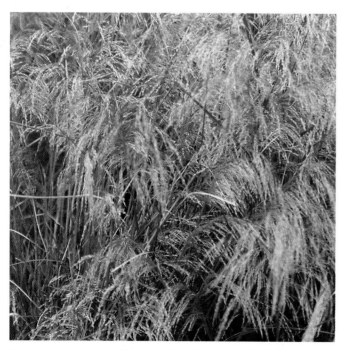

Deschampsia caespitosa 'Bronzeschleier', bronze veil tufted hairgrass.

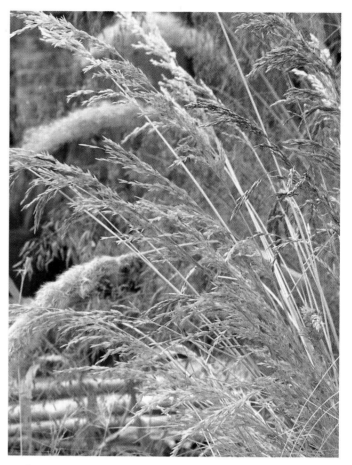

Deschampsia caespitosa 'Holciformis', Pacific hairgrass, in dried arrangement with cottony plumes of *Imperata brevifolia*, satintail.

BOTANICAL NAME	***Deschampsia caespitosa*** **'Holciformis'**
PRONUNCIATION	deh-SHAMP-see-ah ses-pih-TOH-sah hol-sih-FOR-mis
COMMON NAME	Pacific hairgrass

DESCRIPTION: Evergreen, cool-season Pacific hairgrass is quite different from the fairy wand grasses of European origin. Its bright green foliage and dense narrow panicles are completely unlike its Euroepan cousins. Not nearly as showy as its kin, Pacific hairgrass is a fine groundcover in hotter Mediterranean climates where European *Deschampsia* species flower poorly.

Pacific hairgrass grows in dense tufts 1½ to 2 feet tall and as wide, with fine-textured leaves ¹⁄₁₆ to ⅛ inch wide and 1 to 1½ feet long, tapering to a fine point. The flowers, erect, narrow panicles that rise 1½ to 3 feet above the foliage, emerge greenish in late spring and become golden. Showy at first, they bleach to a grayish color at maturity and can look ragged late in the season.

OTHER ***Deschampsia caespitosa*** CULTIVARS ARE:

'Bronze Veil' ('Bronze Veil' tufted hairgrass): English version; weeping bronze flowers.

'Fairy's Joke' ('Fairy's Joke' tufted hairgrass): forms tiny plantlets on the flower spikes; foliage 1½ to 2 feet with flower spikes 1 to 1½ feet above foliage.

'Goldgehaenge' (Gold pendant tufted hairgrass): blooms dependably in mild climates; nodding golden yellow flowers reach 2 to 3 feet.

'Goldschleier' (Gold veil tufted hairgrass): late-blooming, golden yellow flowers reach 1 to 2 feet above foliage.

'Schottland' (Scotland tufted hairgrass): robust flower spikes reach 1½ to 2½ feet above 2- to 3-foot dark green foliage.

'Tardiflora' (Late-blooming tufted hairgrass): late-blooming cultivar reaching 2 to 3 feet tall.

'Tautraeger' (Dew-bearer tufted hairgrass): compact late-blooming form with dark, almost bluish panicles that become golden at maturity.

'Waldschatt' (Forest shade tufted hairgrass): dark brown panicles reach 2 to 3 feet tall.

BOTANICAL NAME	***Deschampsia flexuosa* (also known as *Aira flexuosa* and *Avenella flexuosa*)**
PRONUNCIATION	deh-SHAMP-see-ah flex-yoo-OH-sah
COMMON NAME	Crinkled hairgrass, wavy hairgrass
USDA HARDINESS ZONE	4 to 8 (9) (hardiness untested; may grow into Zone 9)
ORIGIN	Northern Hemisphere: Eurasia; North America, Greenland to Alaska, south to Georgia
PREFERRED SITES	Moist meadows, rocky wet spots

DESCRIPTION: Crinkled hairgrass is a tufted, cool-season, evergreen grass with shiny green foliage and delicate, airy flowers. Its leaves form a tight clump of smooth, almost oily-looking foliage 1 to 2 feet tall and as wide. The leaves are narrow and wiry, 1/16 to 1/8 inch wide and 6 to 12 inches long. The glossy, nodding, sometimes purple-tinged panicles emerge in June and July, maturing to yellowish brown. Twisted or bent awns give this grass its common name.

LANDSCAPE USES: This showy, fine-textured, small, flowering grass makes an excellent accent in lightly shaded borders. It can be planted alone or in groups to create dramatic displays. Crinkled hairgrass is a good groundcover to naturalize in lightly shaded areas. It is also a good rock garden plant. The small flowers are often used in fresh and dried arrangements.

CULTURE AND PROPAGATION: Crinkled hairgrass prefers cool summers and moist, acid soil with humus to look its best. In cooler climates, full sun is fine if the grass is given sufficient moisture. Crinkled hairgrass grows poorly in hot-summer areas.

Propagate by seed or division. Cultivars should be propagated by division only.

PESTS AND PROBLEMS: Crinkled hairgrass has no known pests or problems.

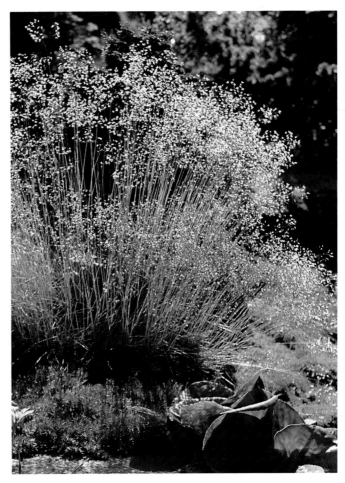

Deschampsia flexuosa, crinkled hairgrass.

BOTANICAL NAME	***Dichromena latifolia***
PRONUNCIATION	dye-KROH-men-ah lah-tih-FOH-lee-ah
COMMON NAME	Star sedge, white-bracted sedge
USDA HARDINESS ZONE	9 to 10
ORIGIN	Caribbean, Gulf Coast of the United States to North Carolina
PREFERRED SITES	Sandy margins of moist areas, open grassy meadows

DESCRIPTION: A protected plant in some Gulf states, star sedge is distinguished by its showy white bracts, which appear below the true flowers. Bright, glossy, yellow-green foliage grows 6 to 12 inches tall and as wide. This slowly spreading plant is rarely invasive. The chartreuse-colored leaves are ⅛ to ¼ inch wide and 4 to 7 inches long.

The flowers appear on erect, wiry stalks 6 to 12 inches above the foliage in early summer. In ideal conditions, the flowers can reach 3 feet tall, though the plant, including flowers, is usually no taller than 1½ feet. The star-shaped bracts below the inconspicuous flowers can range from pure white to white with green tips.

LANDSCAPE USES: This attractive sedge is excellent for naturalizing in sandy, southern meadows and coastal gardens. It makes a fine accent plant in light shade and is at home in or near ponds and pools. It will grow in shallow water 1 to 2 inches deep and makes a good tub or pot plant. Star sedge can be used as a houseplant if it has high light and high humidity. The flowers are good in fresh arrangements.

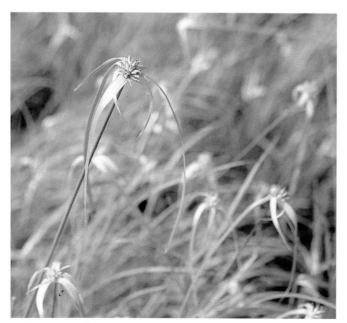

Dichromena latifolia, star sedge.

CULTURE AND PROPAGATION: Star sedge grows best in fertile soil with high humidity. It tends to grow slowly and less vigorously in hot, arid climates, where it rarely reaches 1 foot tall. In hot, dry climates, filtered shade is best, since plants tend to sunburn in full, hot sun. Star sedge resents drying out.

Propagate by division or seed.

PESTS AND PROBLEMS: Subtropical cultivars may be killed at temperatures below 28°F.

This plant may be protected in your community, so check with native plant associations before digging existing populations.

ELYMUS, LEYMUS
WILD RYE, LYME GRASS, DUNE GRASS

There are over 50 species of rye, growing mostly in temperate climates around the world. The most famous ornamental, blue Lyme grass (*Elymus arenarius* 'Glaucus'), has been used in gardens for over 100 years. It is known incorrectly as *Elymus glaucus,* and it may take some time to right this nomenclatural confusion. The true *Elymus glaucus* is native to California and is fast becoming widely used in that state.

To add to the confusion, *Elymus* is soon to be split by botanists into two genera, *Elymus* and *Leymus*. Be careful when ordering plants; many nurseries are not aware of the proper names.

BOTANICAL NAME	***Elymus arenarius* 'Glaucus' (also known as *Leymus arenarius* 'Glaucus'; often mislabeled *Elymus glaucus*)**
PRONUNCIATION	EL-lee-mus ayr-eh-NAYR-ee-us GLOU-kus
COMMON NAME	Blue Lyme grass, European blue dune grass
USDA HARDINESS ZONE	4 to 10
ORIGIN	Eurasia; this cultivar is a horticultural selection
PREFERRED SITES	Sand dunes

DESCRIPTION: Almost metallic blue foliage graces this deciduous, spreading grass, known extensively, and incorrectly, as *Elymus glaucus.* It has grown in gardens since 1900 and was a favorite plant of famous English gardener

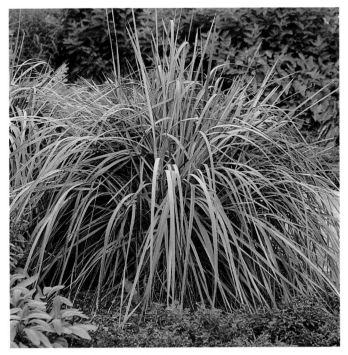

Elymus arenarius 'Glaucus', blue Lyme grass.

Gertrude Jekyll. Its leaves, ¼ to ½ inch wide, are 12 to 18 inches long on stout, thick rhizomes. The plant grows 1 to 3 feet tall but stoops over, giving an effective height of 1 to 2 feet. Flowers bloom sporadically from June through August and are not particularly showy. They emerge bluish gray, turning wheat color with age.

LANDSCAPE USES: Plant blue Lyme grass wherever its blue foliage can be enjoyed. To control its invasive, rhizomatous habit in perennial borders, plant it in a drainage tile or concrete barrier. In dune plantings, its colonizing habit may be used to advantage as a dune stabilizer and for erosion control on coastal bluffs. It will tolerate both salt spray and ocean winds. Its foliage is striking against a dark background or combined with vibrant flower colors. Along the water's edge, its blue foliage is reflected dramatically. It is a good drought-tolerant grass for dry coastal sites.

CULTURE AND PROPAGATION: Blue Lyme grass grows in just about any soil type, in full sun or light shade. It is less invasive in heavy clays and dry soils. In mild climates, it may never go completely dormant. Mowing or cutting it back will stimulate new growth and keep the foliage fresh and blue. In cold climates, a brief yellowish fall color precedes dormant winter foliage.

To perpetuate its blue foliage, propagate by division, since it produces different shades of blue from seed.

PESTS AND PROBLEMS: Blue Lyme grass has no known pests or problems.

ANOTHER CULTIVAR OF *Elymus arenarius* IS:

'Findhorn' ('Findhorn' wild rye): compact cultivar.

BOTANICAL NAME	***Elymus canadensis***
PRONUNCIATION	EL-lee-mus kan-ah-DEN-sis
COMMON NAME	Canada wild rye
USDA HARDINESS ZONE	3 to 8
ORIGIN	North America
PREFERRED SITES	Mostly dry soils

DESCRIPTION: A member of the tallgrass prairie that once stretched from Massachusetts to Montana and south to Texas, Canada wild rye is a deciduous, clumping, cool-season grass that is a fast grower and can adapt to a wide range of soil types and climates. It is primarily used as a cover crop since plants are generally short-lived; by the third or fourth year they tend to yield to other grasses and prairie plants. Blue-green foliage of medium texture grows 2 to 5 feet tall and generally reaches maturity from early

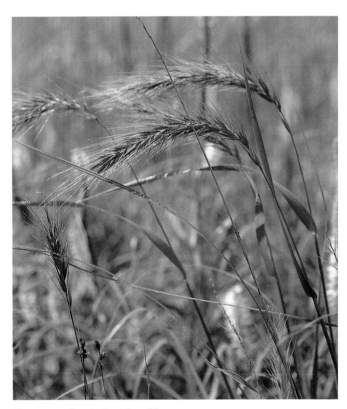

Elymus canadensis, Canada wild rye.

April to early June. Greenish panicles, 6 to 9 inches long, droop under their own weight.

LANDSCAPE USES: Canada wild rye is useful for naturalizing and prairie plantings. It grows quickly in the cool season and offers an effective, quick groundcover and means of erosion control. It is attractive in borders, where its blue-green foliage contrasts with flowering perennials and other dark-foliaged plants. Its seeds provide a winter food source for birds, and were once used as a food source by Native Americans. This plant is valuable for establishing prairies in midwestern climates. The flowers are stunning in fresh or dried arrangements.

CULTURE AND PROPAGATION: Canada wild rye grows best in moist, fertile soil in full sun. It prefers regular moisture during the growing season to look its best; lack of regular moisture will result in early summer dormancy. It tolerates a wide latitude of soils and exposures and is extremely cold-hardy.

Propagate by seed or division. It is easiest to grow from seed but can be quite variable. Division is best in spring, and is the recommended means to retain good blue-green color.

PESTS AND PROBLEMS: Canada wild rye has no known pests or problems.

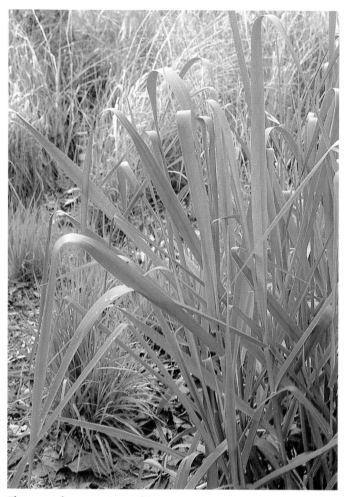

Elymus condensatus, giant wild rye.

BOTANICAL NAME	***Elymus condensatus***
PRONUNCIATION	EL-lee-mus kon-DEN-sah-tus
COMMON NAME	Giant wild rye
USDA HARDINESS ZONE	8 to 10
ORIGIN	Mostly coastal ranges from Baja California to Northern California
PREFERRED SITES	Rocky or sandy soils

DESCRIPTION: Robust, semi-evergreen giant wild rye has green to gray-green foliage that grows 3 to 6 feet tall in a slowly spreading clump. The glossy leaves, ½ to 1 inch wide and 12 to 18 inches long, grow on stout stems. The flowers are borne on erect stems that reach 2 to 4 feet above the foliage. Bluish green flowers emerge 10 to 16 inches long and ½ to 1 inch wide, drying to an attractive wheat color. In inland situations and cold canyons, giant wild rye turns brilliant yellow-orange with the first hard frost. The plant usually goes summer dormant in dry-summer climates.

LANDSCAPE USES: Giant wild rye is an effective soil stabilizer and windbreak in sandy soils and is a great drought-tolerant grass. The plants remain dormant until late winter rains; warming soil temperatures stimulate new growth. Giant wild rye will grow in dune sand in windy coastal conditions. It is an excellent plant for erosion control and for bank and streamside plantings. It tolerates considerable shade and can be effective as a tall mass planting under a canopy of deciduous trees. The flowers are stunning in fresh or dried arrangements.

CULTURE AND PROPAGATION: Giant wild rye prefers sandy loam in full sun. It tolerates extremes in soil conditions, from heavy, wet clay to dry, rocky slopes. It can be kept somewhat evergreen by providing additional summer water. Along the protected Southern California coast, supplemental water will keep the plants green year-round.

Propagate by seed, or by division in fall or winter.

PESTS AND PROBLEMS: Giant wild rye has no known pests or problems.

BOTANICAL NAME	*Elymus condensatus* 'Canyon Prince'
PRONUNCIATION	EL-lee-mus kon-DEN-sah-tus
COMMON NAME	'Canyon Prince' wild rye

DESCRIPTION: 'Canyon Prince' wild rye, discovered off the coast of California near San Miguel Island, was introduced by the Santa Barbara Botanic Garden. Some consider this outstanding blue-foliaged cultivar to be a natural hybrid of several wild rye species: It is superior in foliage, flower, and habit. Similar in most respects to the species, 'Canyon Prince' wild rye has a slowly spreading habit. The flowers rise 2 to 3 feet above the foliage and emerge powdery blue, maturing to a wheat color. Its hardiness is unknown. This cultivar should be propagated by division only.

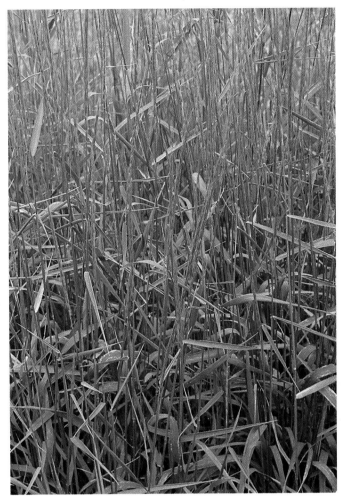

Elymus glaucus, blue wild rye.

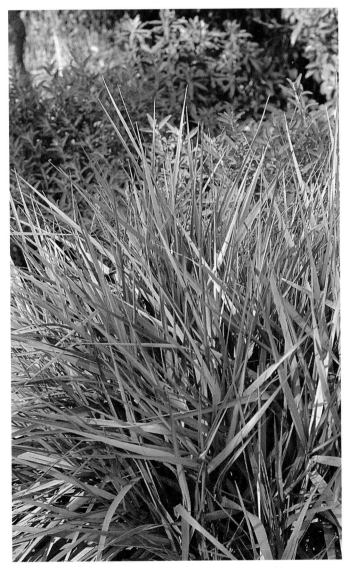

Elymus condensatus 'Canyon Prince', 'Canyon Prince' wild rye.

BOTANICAL NAME	*Elymus glaucus*
PRONUNCIATION	EL-lee-mus GLOU-kus
COMMON NAME	Blue wild rye
USDA HARDINESS ZONE	8 to 10 (hardiness untested; it may grow in Zone 7)
ORIGIN	North America
PREFERRED SITES	Open woods; dry hills mostly at 5,000 feet elevation or lower, primarily north-facing slopes

DESCRIPTION: This cool-season, semi-evergreen grass has a wide distribution over much of the western United States and is extremely variable in foliage and habit. Blue wild rye is often mislabelled as blue Lyme grass (*Elymus arenarius* 'Glaucus'), and plants most often offered as blue wild rye are indeed blue Lyme grass. Visual inspection immediately shows the two plants to be completely different because of the distinctive, metallic blue foliage of *E. arenarius* 'Glaucus'.

True blue wild rye is a far-ranging, mostly western, native American grass most often used as a large-scale ground-cover for erosion control. Its foliage is extremely varied, ranging from 2 to 4 feet in height, and from bright green to almost blue in color. Leaf widths vary from ⅜ to 1 inch wide and may be stiffly upright or weeping. The grass has a clumping habit. Plants begin growing actively with the first winter rains and flower from June to July. The flowers are borne in narrow, vertical spikes, 4 to 6 inches long and ¼ to ½ inch wide, emerging green and drying to a wheat color. Plants in arid western climates go summer dormant by July and remain dormant until the first rains.

LANDSCAPE USES: Blue wild rye is best used as a large-scale slope cover or groundcover for soil stabilization. Blue wild rye can grow under a canopy of high trees, but can withstand only light shade. Often, it is the primary ground-cover since it never becomes so dense as to prevent other plants, such as trees or shrubs, from maturing. It is often planted after fires for revegetation purposes.

CULTURE AND PROPAGATION: Blue wild rye adapts to a wide range of soils and climates. It seems to grow best in fertile soil on lightly shaded slopes. It will take full sun in areas near the coast, but in hot inland climates, it grows best in light shade or half-day sun. Regular watering will keep the foliage green until the onset of winter. In cold-winter areas the foliage becomes dormant by October or November. The plants are considered to be short-lived, with original clumps lasting two to three years; populations are renewed, however, through reseeding.

Propagate by seed, or by division in the spring or fall; it is easier to propagate by seed.

PESTS AND PROBLEMS: Blue wild rye has no known pests or problems.

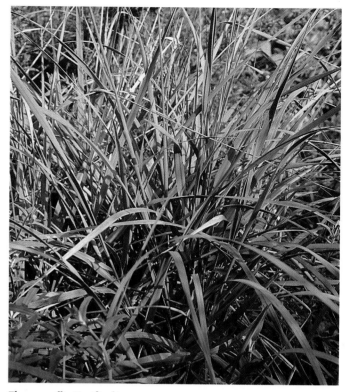

Elymus mollis, Pacific dune grass.

BOTANICAL NAME	***Elymus mollis* (also known as *Leymus mollis*)**
PRONUNCIATION	EL-lee-mus MOH-lis
COMMON NAME	Pacific dune grass, Pacific Lyme grass
USDA HARDINESS ZONE	7 to 10
ORIGIN	Coastal central California to Alaska
PREFERRED SITES	Sand dunes

DESCRIPTION: Pacific dune grass was the primary creeping dune grass of the western coast of the United States. Once found growing in broad expanses from Southern California to Alaska, it is now rarely found in the wild and has been largely replaced by the more aggressive European beach grass (*Ammophila arenaria*).

Primarily a pioneer plant, Pacific dune grass tends to be replaced by other coastal wildflowers and perennials as sandy dune areas become covered by vegetation. Its soft blue-gray foliage grows 2 to 3 feet tall but tends to stoop over, giving it an effective height of 1 to 2 feet. The leaves vary in width from ½ to 1 inch on spreading, rhizomatous stems. The plants go dormant in summer unless regular water is provided. Bluish green flower spikes emerge June through July, maturing to a wheat color. Though notice-able, the flower spikes are not particularly showy.

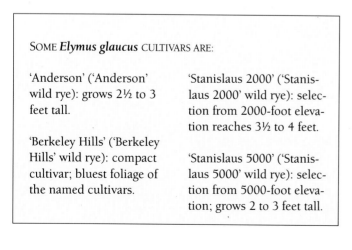

SOME ***Elymus glaucus*** CULTIVARS ARE:

'Anderson' ('Anderson' wild rye): grows 2½ to 3 feet tall.

'Berkeley Hills' ('Berkeley Hills' wild rye): compact cultivar; bluest foliage of the named cultivars.

'Stanislaus 2000' ('Stanis-laus 2000' wild rye): selec-tion from 2000-foot eleva-tion reaches 3½ to 4 feet.

'Stanislaus 5000' ('Stanis-laus 5000' wild rye): selec-tion from 5000-foot eleva-tion; grows 2 to 3 feet tall.

LANDSCAPE USES: Pacific dune grass is an excellent plant for coastal gardens as it will grow in dune sand or heavy clay. It helps stabilize sandy slopes. Its soft blue foliage is excellent in combination with other dune plants.

CULTURE AND PROPAGATION: Pacific dune grass grows best in sandy soil and full sun, although it tolerates heavier soils. A new crop of fresh blue foliage will appear if the grass is mowed or cut back to about 4 inches in midsummer, fertilized, and watered.

Propagate by seed or division. It is best to divide and plant this grass from November through April. Plantings are often specified as bareroot culms, meaning that the plant is grown in sandy beds, and when harvested the soil falls away. Because of this, culms are best planted in premoistened sand that must be kept moist until the culms have rooted.

PESTS AND PROBLEMS: Pacific dune grass has no known pests or problems.

BOTANICAL NAME	**Elymus racemosus 'Glaucus' (also known as Leymus giganteus 'Glaucus', L. racemosus 'Glaucus', and E. giganteus 'Glaucus'; mistakenly known as E. 'Vahl Glaucus')**
PRONUNCIATION	EL-lee-mus rays-MOH-sus GLOU-kus
COMMON NAME	Volga wild rye, Siberian wild rye, giant dune grass
USDA HARDINESS ZONE	4 to 10
ORIGIN	Siberia
PREFERRED SITES	Sandy and rocky soils

DESCRIPTION: This cultivar is virtually identical to blue Lyme grass (*Elymus arenarius* 'Glaucus'), differing only in that it appears more robust and grows about one-third larger in all respects. As indicated by the synonyms listed above, much confusion surrounds this species. Currently, two distinct clones of blue-foliaged wild rye appear to be in nurseries and garden centers. Nurseries are often unaware of their source, and the plants are often sold interchangeably. To further confuse the issue, plants in hot or arid climates often fail to grow as tall as they do in areas with cool to mild summers.

LANDSCAPE USES: Use volga wild rye wherever its blue foliage can be enjoyed. Its invasive, rhizomatous habit can be controlled in perennial borders by planting it in a drainage tile or concrete barrier. In dune plantings, its colonizing habit is useful as a dune stabilizer and for erosion control on coastal bluffs. It will tolerate both salt spray and ocean winds. It is a good drought-tolerant grass for dry coastal situations. Volga wild rye's foliage is striking against a dark background or combined with vibrant flower colors. Its blue foliage casts dramatic reflections along the water's edge.

CULTURE AND PROPAGATION: Volga wild rye grows in just about any soil type, in full sun or light shade, although it is less invasive in heavy clays and dry soils. In mild climates, it may never go completely dormant. Mowing or cutting it back will stimulate new growth and keep the foliage fresh and blue. In cold climates, a brief period of yellowish fall color precedes dormant winter foliage.

To retain its blue foliage, propagate the grass by division only, since it is variable from seed.

PESTS AND PROBLEMS: Volga wild rye has no known pests or problems.

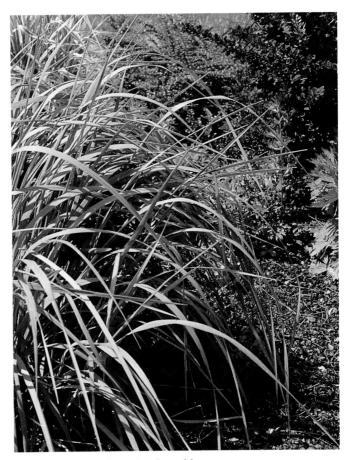

Elymus racemosus 'Glaucus', Volga wild rye.

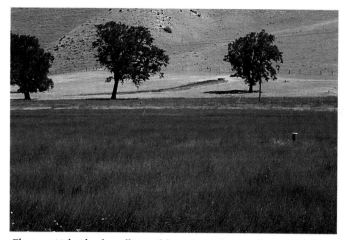

Elymus tritichoides, beardless wild rye, in native meadow in California.

BOTANICAL NAME	***Elymus tritichoides* (also known as *Leymus tritichoides*)**
PRONUNCIATION	EL-lee-mus trit-ih-KOY-deez
COMMON NAME	Beardless wild rye
USDA HARDINESS ZONE	7 to 10
ORIGIN	Western United States
PREFERRED SITES	Heavy soils, valleys, foothills, mountain flats

DESCRIPTION: Beardless wild rye is currently being selected and hybridized by plant enthusiasts and horticulturists throughout the West. The plant readily hybridizes in nature, and there is great interest in newly recognized clones and hybrids. Plants are being selected for drought tolerance, salt tolerance, color, foliage height, and a wide range of garden uses. Named cultivars are expected soon in nurseries and garden centers.

A dense, rhizomatous, creeping grass, beardless wild rye is an aggressive colonizer and a soil stabilizer. Though usually found in moist places, it tolerates considerable summer drought. Its green to blue-green foliage, 2 to 4 feet tall, grows in dense, spreading colonies. The leaves, ½ to 2 inches wide, vary in size depending on the cultivar. The flowers are narrow spikes, ¼ to ½ inch wide and 4 to 6 inches long. They emerge green in June and July and mature to a wheat color. The flowers are sporadic and rarely set seed. With irrigation, plants will stay green until the first frost. In winter dormancy they turn an attractive brown color that bleaches to gray as the season progresses.

LANDSCAPE USES: The dense, rhizomatous nature of beardless wild rye makes it an excellent choice for erosion control and mass plantings. Planted along the water's edge, it can help stabilize shorelines, levees, and water courses. It tolerates some shade and considerable drought when established in the fall or spring. Its invasive nature can be a detriment in small gardens and borders.

CULTURE AND PROPAGATION: Beardless wild rye tolerates a wide range of soils and climates, but it prefers moist, fertile soil in sun or light shade. Although naturally found in wet areas, beardless wild rye will sometimes survive hot, dry summers. If summer moisture is absent, plants go dormant. Watering and cutting back in midsummer will keep some measure of green in the plant into the fall.

Propagate by division and planting of rhizomes in spring or fall.

PESTS AND PROBLEMS: Beardless wild rye has no known pests or problems.

ONE CULTIVAR OF ***Elymus tritichoides*** IS:

'Gray Dawn' ('Gray Dawn' beardless rye): bluish gray leaves in midsummer.

ANOTHER SPECIES OF WILD RYE IS:

Elymus virginicus (Virginia wild rye): nearly identical to Canada wild rye (*E. canadensis*); found throughout the South.

EQUISETUM
HORSETAIL, SCOURING RUSH

This genus of annual and perennial herbs of the Equisetaceae family comprises primitive spore-bearing plants, their existence dating well back into the fossil record along with the dinosaurs. They grow mostly in wet areas in almost every part of the world. Horsetails have jointed, segmented stems that contain silica, making them unusually rough to the touch. Some varieties have branched foliage, while others are unbranched. The common name horsetail derives from certain varieties whose bushy, slender stems and weeping habit resemble a horse's tail. Its other common name reflects the strength of the silica in the stems of scouring rush (*Equisetum hyemale*), which were used to polish tin and wood.

Unless they are contained, most horsetails are too invasive and vigorous for small gardens. Given enough time, plants can easily escape most containers, so plant them in the strongest barriers available.

Listed are the better-known garden favorites. They range from 2-inch miniatures to 8-foot giants. Properly situated in the garden, they can be extremely dramatic, as their strong forms lend a unique and dynamic architectural quality.

BOTANICAL NAME	*Equisetum hyemale*
PRONUNCIATION	eh-kwih-SEE-tum heye-uh-MAWL-ee
COMMON NAME	Scouring rush
USDA HARDINESS ZONE	4 to 10
ORIGIN	Found throughout the Northern Hemisphere
PREFERRED SITES	Wet areas, marshes

DESCRIPTION: Scouring rush is found worldwide, and different varieties exist in nurseries and garden centers. Its jointed, rushlike foliage grows somewhat helter-skelter: The slender stems grow horizontally in youth, but the plant sends up thicker, vertical stems as it ages. At maturity, it grows 1 to 2 feet tall. The foliage is narrow, ⅛ to ¼ inch wide when young, and lies fairly prostrate. The stems of older plants grow ⅜ to ½ inch thick, and reach 3 to 6 feet in height. Even mature plantings will have some horizontally growing stems, giving them an animated effect. The evergreen foliage is grayish green, turning to greenish bronze in the winter. The spores are borne in conelike spikes at the tip of the stem.

LANDSCAPE USES: Scouring rush is a dramatic garden accent. Its stems have an architectural quality that create distinc-

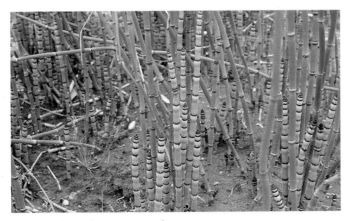

Equisetum hyemale, scouring rush.

tive silhouettes when backlit. The plants grow well in wet areas or shallow water. They make excellent pot or tub subjects. As a groundcover they need plenty of room and constant moisture. They can be grown in small gardens if contained in strong, undrilled pots, as they spread invasively from rhizomes and will colonize an area quite quickly. Scouring rush can also be planted alongside other shade-loving perennials such as brunnera, rodgersia, and bergenia. The foliage is stunning in both fresh and dried arrangements.

CULTURE AND PROPAGATION: Scouring rush prefers wet, fertile soil with full sun. Plants will generally grow where there is sufficient moisture, and they are extremely tolerant of soil type. They grow in water 4 to 6 inches deep and will spread into deeper water as they age. Scouring rush tolerates considerable shade, although it is somewhat less vigorous in deeper shade.

Propagate by division in spring or fall.

PESTS AND PROBLEMS: Scouring rush can take over small gardens, and plants can be difficult to eradicate. Eradication is best achieved by diligent, ongoing removal.

ONE VARIETY OF *Equisetum hyemale* IS:

Robustum (Giant scouring rush): similar to the species, with robust vertical growth 5 to 7 feet tall. Also sold as *E. hyemale*.

BOTANICAL NAME	*Equisetum scirpoides*
PRONUNCIATION	eh-kwee-SEE-tum skir-POY-deez
COMMON NAME	Dwarf horsetail, dwarf scouring rush
USDA HARDINESS ZONE	5 to 10
ORIGIN	Throughout North America
PREFERRED SITES	Moist places

DESCRIPTION: This miniaturized version of giant scouring rush resembles its giant cousin in almost every respect. It grows thin, wiry leaves, ¹/₁₆ inch wide, and reaches 6 to 8 inches tall in dense mats. The evergreen foliage is a dark olive green, blushing an attractive reddish brown in the fall and winter.

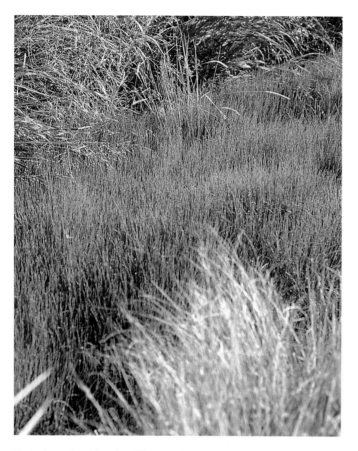

Equisetum scirpoides, dwarf horsetail.

BOTANICAL NAME	***Equisetum scirpoides* var. *contorta***
PRONUNCIATION	eh-kwee-SEE-tum sker-POY-dees kon-TOR-tah
COMMON NAME	Miniature contorted horsetail
USDA HARDINESS ZONE	7(?) to 10 (hardiness untested; may grow in Zone 7)
ORIGIN	Japan
PREFERRED SITES	Moist places

DESCRIPTION: This miniature is the smallest and finest-textured of all the horsetails. Its thin, wiry, contorted foliage grows 2 to 6 inches tall from slowly spreading rhizomes. The foliage is typical of the genus, with rough, grooved, silica-rich stems and joints ½ to 1 inch apart.

LANDSCAPE USES: Miniature contorted horsetail makes an excellent filler between stepping stones and in rock gardens. It is a good choice for small containers and makes an attractive bonsai subject. The plant is not as invasive or rapidly spreading as dwarf horsetail (*Equisetum scirpoides*). It grows in shallow water and so it is a good plant for moist cracks or other wet places.

CULTURE AND PROPAGATION: Miniature contorted horsetail prefers constant moisture and rich, fertile soil in full sun or partial shade. It will grow in shallow water 1 to 2 inches deep. Plants will not tolerate drying out and are quick to die if allowed to stay dry for too long.

Propagate by division.

PESTS AND PROBLEMS: Miniature contorted horsetail has no known pests or problems.

LANDSCAPE USES: Dwarf horsetail makes an attractive, low, grassy-looking groundcover in moist or boggy soil. Its vigorous habit allows it to quickly fill a low, wet spot in the garden. It is useful in small pots or tubs, and in small ponds, pools, or puddles. It tolerates light shade and thrives in both moist and shady situations.

CULTURE AND PROPAGATION: Dwarf horsetail grows best in moist, fertile soil in full sun or partial shade. It is extremely tolerant of a wide range of conditions, including sun, heat, cold, windy coastal conditions, and moderately shaded sites. It must be constantly moist to look its best. Plants are slower to invade drier soils and usually will not aggressively invade dry sites. Plants grow well in shallow water 2 to 4 inches deep. Dwarf horsetail resents drying out. A planting of dwarf horsetail that has dried out can usually be renewed by cutting it back to the ground, watering it thoroughly, and giving it a light feeding. A tray of water placed under potted plants will help keep the roots moist. In water or in the ground, its spreading nature can be controlled by planting in a pot or drainage tile.

Propagation is easy from division of rhizomes.

PESTS AND PROBLEMS: Dwarf horsetail has no known pests or problems.

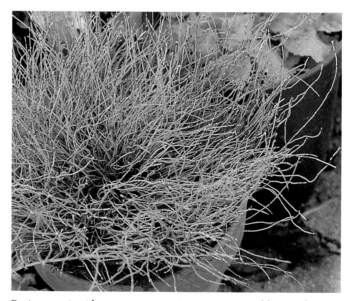

Equisetum scirpoides var. *contorta,* miniature contorted horsetail.

ANOTHER SPECIES OF HORSETAIL IS:

Equisetum diffusum (Himalayan horsetail): a subtropical species with branched foliage; grows 6 to 12 inches tall.

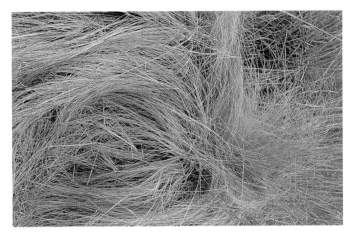

Eragrostis curvula, weeping love grass, in winter.

BOTANICAL NAME	***Eragrostis curvula***
PRONUNCIATION	air-ah-GROS-tis KURV-yew-lah
COMMON NAME	Weeping love grass, African love grass
USDA HARDINESS ZONE	7 to 10
ORIGIN	South Africa to Ethiopia
PREFERRED SITES	Sandy soils; now naturalized in large areas of the South and plains of the United States

DESCRIPTION: Introduced by the United States government in the 1930s for erosion control in the South, weeping love grass has now replaced native grasses in many areas of the South. The dark green, fine-textured, almost hairlike foliage of weeping love grass forms dense tufts. Its thin leaves, 1/16 to 1/8 inch wide, grow 2 to 3½ inches tall. The foliage blushes bronze-red after a hard freeze. Although evergreen in mild climates, it is deciduous in areas colder than Zone 9. The 2- to 3-foot-long flower clusters emerge on arching, weeping stems from August through September. They are blackish olive-purple, maturing to a grayish color. The flowers are quite airy and delicate and move easily in a breeze.

LANDSCAPE USES: Weeping love grass makes an interesting flowering accent planted alone or in groups. It provides erosion control and a tall groundcover on dry, steep banks. Extremely drought-tolerant, once established it will grow without summer water.

CULTURE AND PROPAGATION: Weeping love grass prefers sandy, well-drained soil with ample moisture and full sun. The plant's drought tolerance is legendary. In California, it withstands the worst of soils, including dry, heavy, and even serpentine soils. In marginal areas it is best planted in fast-draining, sandy soil in a warm, protected site.

Propagation is easiest by seed, or by division in spring or fall.

PESTS AND PROBLEMS: Weeping love grass reseeds readily in mild climates, a problem in small gardens. Plants may rot during a cold, wet winter or in heavy, wet clays.

BOTANICAL NAME	***Eragrostis spectabilis***
PRONUNCIATION	air-uh-GROS-tis spek-TAH-bil-is
COMMON NAME	Purple love grass
USDA HARDINESS ZONE	5 to 9
ORIGIN	North America, Maine to Florida, west to Arizona, north to Minnesota
PREFERRED SITES	Moist, sandy soil

DESCRIPTION: This showy, native American grass has colorful reddish purple flowers and a compact height that make it a worthy and versatile player in the garden. A clumping, warm-season grower, it forms tight, compact foliage 12 to

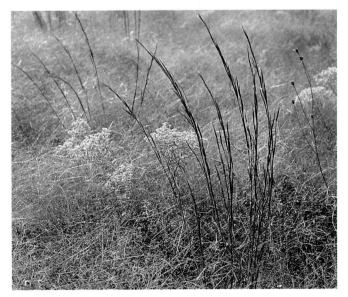

Eragrostis spectabilis, purple love grass.

18 inches tall and as wide. Its light green leaves, ¼ to ½ inch wide and 6 to 12 inches long, are soft and somewhat hairy. Its flowers appear red to purple from June through August in soft airy panicles that cover the foliage like a reddish cloud. The flowers reach 1 to 1½ feet above the foliage and mature to a soft cream color. Mature flowers often break off like a tumbleweed. The foliage turns reddish with the onset of fall.

LANDSCAPE USES: Purple love grass makes a fine accent, planted either as a specimen or in groups. Mass plantings are especially effective where a suitable backdrop, such as dark green leaves or broad-leaved perennials, sets off the grass's airy panicles. The relatively compact size of this grass makes it useful in the foreground of borders. Purple love grass is also good in coastal gardens and dry gardens. The flowers are excellent in fresh or dry arrangements.

CULTURE AND PROPAGATION: Purple love grass grows best in sandy, well-drained soil in full sun. Plants resent wet, heavy soil and damp, shady locations. Although tolerant of heat and drought, it does require summer water in arid southwestern climates.

Propagate by division or seed.

PESTS AND PROBLEMS: Plants grown in the South may not be cold-hardy in cold northern climates; seek locally grown plants for hardier strains.

BOTANICAL NAME	***Eragrostis trichoides* 'Bend'**
PRONUNCIATION	air-ah-GROS-tis trih-KOY-deez
COMMON NAME	'Bend' love grass, sand love grass
USDA HARDINESS ZONE	5 to 9
PREFERRED SITES	Sand barrens, open sandy woods

DESCRIPTION: Clumping, cool-season 'Bend' love grass has medium green foliage, 1 to 2 feet tall and wide. It is mostly deciduous in colder climates. Its leaves, ⅛ to ¼ inch wide, grow vigorously until the flowers emerge in late July. The flowers are showy, amethyst pink on large nodding panicles and almost obscure the foliage. They continue to bloom throughout August, then seem to cease growing until the fall. 'Bend' love grass's 3- to 4-foot-tall flower stems measure 6 to 8 inches across and will usually droop under their own weight.

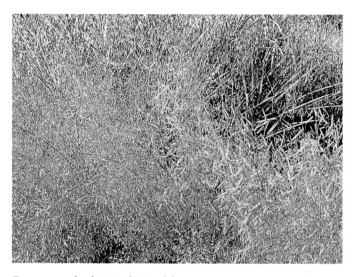

Eragrostis trichoides 'Bend', 'Bend' love grass.

LANDSCAPE USES: 'Bend' love grass provides a spectacular flowering accent when properly displayed. It is lovely planted alone or in groups. Its flowers are stunning in fresh or dried arrangements.

CULTURE AND PROPAGATION: 'Bend' love grass prefers moist, well-drained, sandy, fertile soil in full sun. It tolerates hot, dry sites but needs some summer water in hot, arid climates; a weekly watering will generally suffice. Strong, half-day sun is a minimum requirement for good flowering. Plants perform poorly in too much shade.

Propagation is easy from division or seed. Division is best in fall or spring. 'Bend' love grass will reseed readily in mild climates.

PESTS AND PROBLEMS: Heavy flowers may need the support of stakes, a low fence, or a trellis.

ERIANTHUS
PLUME GRASS

There are over 20 species of plume grass found in tropical and temperate climates in both hemispheres. Usually found in moist sites, they can be surprisingly adaptable. Most have distinctive spiky flowers which dry to showy, fluffy plumes. As a group, they tend to be effective naturalizers, spreading easily from seed. Mostly warm-season grasses, many have showy fall colors. Colors range from peach and orange through red and purple, and some have several colors. Cultivars of plume grass should be available in the near future. Their showy flowers, brilliant fall colors, and adaptability should increase their popularity among grass enthusiasts.

BOTANICAL NAME	*Erianthus contortus*
PRONUNCIATION	air-ee-AN-thus kon-TOR-tus
COMMON NAME	Bent awn plume grass
USDA HARDINESS ZONE	7 to 10
ORIGIN	Maryland to Florida, west to Texas, and north to southern Illinois
PREFERRED SITES	Moist, sandy pinelands, coastal plains

DESCRIPTION: This showy little southeastern native is as beautiful as it is tough. Its narrow, mostly upright foliage is an attractive bluish green, although seed-grown plants may vary from pale green to almost blue in color. Its leaves, ¼ to 1 inch wide, grow 1½ to 2 feet tall in mostly vertical clumps. A clumping, deciduous, warm-season grass, bent awn plume grass turns stunning shades of red and purple in the fall. Showy vertical flower spikes reach 3 to 4 feet above the foliage. They emerge silky purple and become fluffy and cottony with age. Cultivars selected for fall color may soon appear in nurseries and garden centers.

LANDSCAPE USES: Bent awn plume grass provides a striking foliage and flowering accent. Its narrow, upright habit makes it a useful plant for the back of borders. It is a good grass for coastal gardens because it tolerates sandy soils and ocean breezes. Its brilliant fall color is reason enough to plant this grass. It is stunning in fresh or dried flower arrangements.

CULTURE AND PROPAGATION: Bent awn plume grass grows best in well-drained soil in full sun, although it tolerates dry soil and light shade.

Propagate by seed, or by division in spring or fall. Plants may seed themselves in favorable conditions, although usually not invasively so.

PESTS AND PROBLEMS: Bent awn plume grass has no known pests or problems.

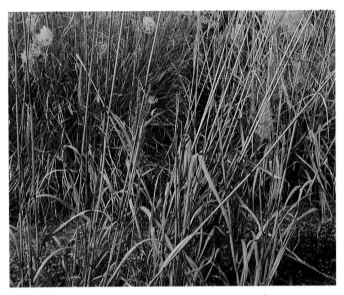

Erianthus giganteus, sugarcane plume grass, in winter dormancy.

BOTANICAL NAME	*Erianthus giganteus*
PRONUNCIATION	air-ee-AN-thus jeye-GAN-tee-us
COMMON NAME	Sugarcane plume grass
USDA HARDINESS ZONE	7 to 10
ORIGIN	Cuba; eastern United States from New York to Florida, inland from Kentucky to eastern Texas
PREFERRED SITES	Wet soils, bogs, ditches

DESCRIPTION: Tall, clumping, deciduous sugarcane plume grass has tall, showy plumes that rise up 9 feet above the foliage like a tall banner. The hairy leaves, ½ to ¾ inch wide, form dense clumps of foliage 3 to 5 feet tall and as wide. The large fluffy plumes, 8 to 16 inches tall and 5 to 8 inches wide, vary in color from purple to cream, silver, white, or red. They emerge from August through November and rise above the foliage in erect, persistent spikes. The onset of fall turns the plants orange, red, and finally straw-colored.

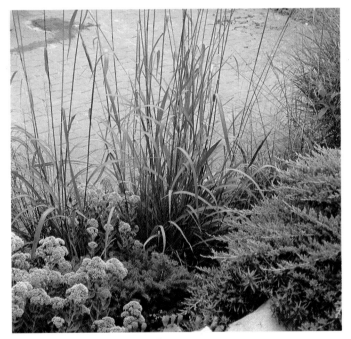

Erianthus contortus, bent awn plume grass.

LANDSCAPE USES: Sugarcane plume grass is a dramatic backdrop in a perennial border. The flowers make a beautiful display when backlit or placed against a dark background. This grass is a good choice for screening and windbreaks. It grows well near water, in bog gardens, or in tubs. The flowers are stunning in fresh or dried arrangements.

CULTURE AND PROPAGATION: Sugarcane plume grass prefers moist, fertile soil in full sun. It tolerates a variety of soil types from sand to clay, and thrives in coastal conditions and high heat. It tolerates boggy conditions. This grass may not bloom in cold-summer climates and should be overwintered in a greenhouse in areas of marginal hardiness. Plants may naturalize in moist soils and can be weedy in some situations. Thick rhizomes become quite tenacious with age, so plant with care in small gardens.
   Propagate by seed or division.

PESTS AND PROBLEMS: Sugarcane plume grass has no known pests or problems.

BOTANICAL NAME	***Erianthus ravennae***
PRONUNCIATION	air-ee-AN-thus ra-VEN-nay
COMMON NAME	Ravenna grass, hardy pampas grass, plume grass
USDA HARDINESS ZONE	6 to 10
ORIGIN	Southern Europe
PREFERRED SITES	Along stream courses; cultivated

DESCRIPTION: Clumping, deciduous ravenna grass is one of the giants of the ornamental grass world. Its robust, dense foliage grows 4 to 5 feet tall and as wide. Its tall flower spikes reach 8 to 12 feet above the foliage, creating dramatic towering forms in the garden. Its medium gray-green leaves, ½ to 1 inch wide and 3 to 4 feet long, are translucent if backlit by the sun. In the fall, the foliage turns shades of orange, beige, tan, brown, and purple, often with multicolors blended throughout. The brown winter skeleton looks dramatic against a dark green or snowy background. Silvery flowers with purple tones emerge in August, maturing to fluffy, cream-colored panicles that persist into winter.

LANDSCAPE USES: The amazing size and vigor of ravenna grass make it an ideal specimen or accent plant. It is stunning reflected in water and grows well along the water's edge and in coastal gardens. Its imposing size makes it ideal for use in parks, golf courses, highways, zoos, and other large-scale applications where a tall screen or windbreak is desired. Both flowers and foliage are used in fresh and dried arrangements.

CULTURE AND PROPAGATION: Ravenna grass prefers moist, well-drained, fertile soil in full sun. It is considerably drought-tolerant but looks better with constant moisture. As long as it has sun, it tolerates a wide range of conditions. The foliage can be cut back if the plants become too unattractive.
   Propagation is easy from seed, or by division in the spring. Plants may reseed themselves in favorable sites.

PESTS AND PROBLEMS: The flower spikes of ravenna grass may break in high-wind areas and usually look tattered by January. Its large size warrants careful consideration of its placement in the garden.

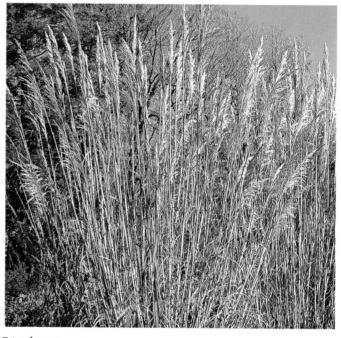

Erianthus ravennae, ravenna grass.

ANOTHER PLUME GRASS SPECIES IS:

Erianthus strictus (Narrow plume grass): similar to bent awn plume grass (*E. contortus*); a moisture-loving, deciduous U.S. native with brilliant fall color.

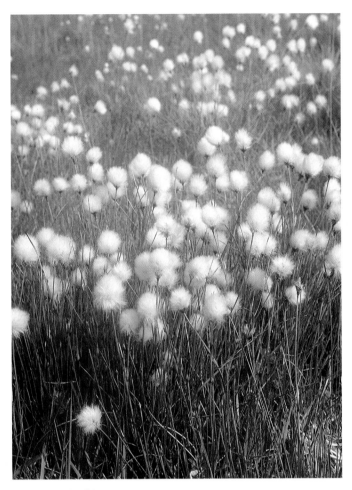

Eriophorum latifolium, cotton grass.

BOTANICAL NAME	***Eriophorum latifolium***
PRONUNCIATION	air-ee-OH-for-um
	lah-tih-FOL-ee-um
COMMON NAME	Cotton grass
USDA HARDINESS ZONE	4 to 7
ORIGIN	Europe, Asia, North America
PREFERRED SITES	Wet, marshy areas

DESCRIPTION: Cotton grass is similar to narrow-leaved cotton grass (*Eriophorum angustifolium*) except that it has a clumping habit and nodding seed heads. Its foliage grows 1 to 1½ feet tall, and flower spikes grow 1 to 1½ feet above the foliage. Its flowers emerge as showy, cottony heads from April through May and droop in pendulous, nodding tufts.

LANDSCAPE USES: Cotton grass is an excellent flowering accent for wet areas. It grows well in pots and tubs and is suitable for small gardens, where the spreading species of cotton grass might be unsuitable. Its handsome clumps and light green foliage make cotton grass a good choice for garden cultivation.

CULTURE AND PROPAGATION: Cotton grass grows best in wet or moist, peaty soil in full sun. It does not tolerate drought and will not bloom well in deep shade. Cotton grass struggles in hot climates.

Propagate by seed, or by division in the spring.

PESTS AND PROBLEMS: Cotton grass has no known pests or problems.

OTHER COTTON GRASS SPECIES ARE:

Eriophorum angustifolium (Narrow-leaved cotton grass): finer-textured species than *E. latifolium;* spreads from rhizomes.

Eriophorum vaginatum (Hare's tail cotton grass): grows 1 to 1½ feet tall with grayish foliage.

FESTUCA
FESCUE

To the considerable frustration of gardeners, reference works on ornamental grasses do not agree on the parentage, origin, nomenclature, or synonyms of the large and confusing genus *Festuca.* For example, many authorities consider some varieties and cultivars of *F. amethystina* (sheep's fescue) to belong to *F. cinerea* (blue fescue). Since botanists are still trying to decide, plant names in this book are based on a consensus of nursery growers, authors, and botanists. Whenever possible, synonyms will be given. Translations from German often vary; when more than one name exists, they will all be mentioned. Adding to the inconsistencies of nomenclature are the many nurseries throughout the United States selling fescues under incorrect names. This jumbled group of grasses is further confused by the improper propagation of plants from seed, the results of which can differ greatly from the species. This encyclopedia attempts to reduce the confusion.

Different cultivars and varieties of fescue differ in height, texture, and foliage color; flowers and flowering habits also vary. But the fescues have some cultural traits in common. Growth usually slows down in hot summer months. Many can look somewhat shabby in hot-summer climates, especially if grown in full sun.

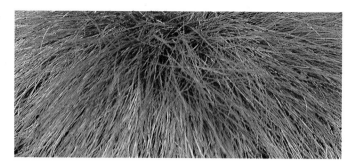

Festuca amethystina, sheep's fescue.

BOTANICAL NAME	***Festuca amethystina** (also known as **F. ovina** 'Glauca')*
PRONUNCIATION	fes-TOO-kah am-eh-this-TEE-nah
COMMON NAME	Sheep's fescue, fescue
USDA HARDINESS ZONE	4 to 9
ORIGIN	Alps, southeastern Europe
PREFERRED SITES	Open forested slopes, pine forests, dry sites

DESCRIPTION: Sheep's fescue is a clumping, cool-season, evergreen grass. Its soft foliage is fine-textured, somewhat weeping, and, for the most part, tends toward the blue side of green. Cultivars usually grow from 8 to 12 inches tall, with flower spikes that rise 12 to 18 inches above the foliage. The flowers usually emerge bluish to purplish from May through June, dry to a golden color as they mature, and then bleach grayish at maturity. Some cultivars are especially prized for their flowers. Sheep's fescue cultivars and the similar blue fescue and its cultivars offer gardeners over 25 different colors and textures from which to choose.

LANDSCAPE USES: Sheep's fescue is most often used as a groundcover or a single accent plant. Some cultivars have particularly showy flowers. The weeping ones are lovely when situated where the foliage can spill down a hill or slope. Sheep's fescue is a good choice for rock and trough gardens and does well in pots or tubs. Because the soft foliage and delicate flowers invite close inspection, the plants make effective edgings and fillers for foreground and spring borders.

CULTURE AND PROPAGATION: Sheep's fescue prefers cool, moist, well-drained soil in full sun; it rots easily in wet or poorly drained sites. Plants are primarily cool-season-growing and drought-tolerant in cool summer or coastal climates. They may perform poorly in hot, humid climates. Plants will tolerate coastal conditions, and in hot-summer climates will grow better along the coast. In arid western climates, plants require partial shade or half-day sun to avoid fading. In hot, humid climates, excellent drainage and partial shade are a must. The plants tend to look good for two to three years and then may begin to die out in the center. Cutting back yearly will stimulate new growth. Cut plants back to 3 to 4 inches tall in fall or early spring, taking care not to cut them too low to the crown. Sheep's fescue is best replanted every two to three years, either by division or with new plants.

Propagate by seed, or by division in fall or spring. Propagate named cultivars by division.

PESTS AND PROBLEMS: Sheep's fescue needs division or replacement every few years to remain attractive.

BOTANICAL NAME	***Festuca amethystina** 'Klose'*
PRONUNCIATION	fes-TOO-kah am-eh-this-TEE-nah KLOH-seh
COMMON NAME	'Klose' fescue

DESCRIPTION: 'Klose' fescue is named for the German nurseryman Heinz Klose. This compact grass grows to 8 inches tall with olive green foliage; new growth is an attractive blue-green. It has the finest foliage texture of all of the cultivars of sheep's fescue. One of the bluer of the greenish fescues, it does tend to turn brown in hot summer climates. Its flowers are not as showy as amethyst flowering fescue (*Festuca amethystina* 'Superba') and bronze luster fescue (*F. amethystina* 'Bronzeglanz').

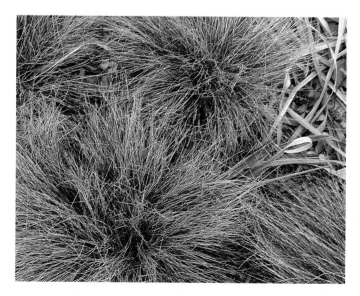

Festuca amethystina 'Klose', 'Klose' fescue, with winter bronze color.

OTHER *Festuca amethystina* CULTIVARS ARE:

'April Gruen' (April green fescue): grows 8 to 12 inches tall; bluish spring growth becomes olive green; showy blue-green flowers. Also sold as *F. cinerea* 'April Green'.

'Bronzeglanz' (Bronze luster fescue): less weeping; finer-textured; not as blue.

'Superba' (Blue sheep's fescue): fine-textured weeping blue-green foliage 8 to 12 inches tall; showy pink flowers in spring.

BOTANICAL NAME	***Festuca californica***
PRONUNCIATION	fes-TOO-kah cal-ih-FOR-nih-kah
COMMON NAME	California fescue
USDA HARDINESS ZONE	8 to 10
ORIGIN	California, native from Santa Barbara to north coast ranges; occasionally found in the Sierra Nevada mountains
PREFERRED SITES	Openings in woods, meadows

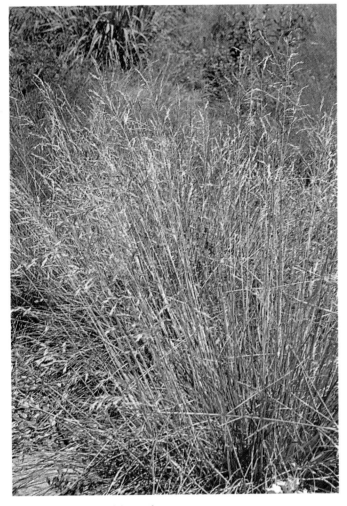

Festuca californica, California fescue.

DESCRIPTION: Clumping, cool-season, evergreen California fescue is admired for its rich foliage and showy flowers. Foliage color varies from greens to luminous blues. The handsome, graceful leaves, ⅛ to ⅜ inch wide and 1 to 2 feet long, form dense basal tufts 2 to 3 feet tall and as wide. Flowers emerge as green to bluish green showy panicles, 2 to 3 feet above the foliage, from April through June. They often turn purplish and mature to a golden color. The flower spikes are delicate and airy. Many blue-foliaged cultivars are currently being selected and named. These often turn purplish with the first frost and have generated great interest.

LANDSCAPE USES: California fescue provides a good groundcover for slopes in full sun or partial shade: A mass planting on a slope gives the illusion of falling water. In shady sites, it provides a good flowering accent. California fescue is stunning when combined with drought-tolerant ferns and other shade-loving perennials such as coralbells (*Heuchera*) and violets. It makes an excellent accent either alone or in groups, and its flowers are striking in fresh or dried arrangements.

CULTURE AND PROPAGATION: California fescue grows best in moist, well-drained, fertile soil in full sun or partial shade. Although it tolerates a wide range of conditions, including coastal slopes and windy sites, it performs poorly in too much shade. It is drought-tolerant in coastal climates.

Propagate by seed or division. Propagate blue cultivars by division only, as not all come true from seed.

PESTS AND PROBLEMS: California fescue has no known pests or problems.

ONE CULTIVAR OF *Festuca californica* IS:

'Salmon Creek' ('Salmon Creek' California fescue): stiff blue-gray foliage that has a distinctive burgundy blush.

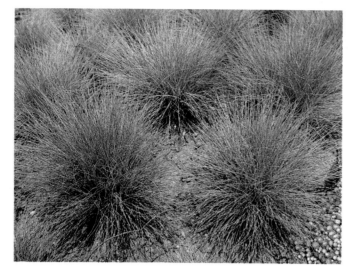

Festuca cinerea, blue fescue.

BOTANICAL NAME	***Festuca cinerea* (also known as *F. ovina, F. glauca, F. ovina* 'Glauca', and *F. arvernensis*)**
PRONUNCIATION	fes-TOO-kah sin-er-EE-ah
COMMON NAME	Blue fescue, blue sheep's fescue, sheep's fescue
USDA HARDINESS ZONE	4 to 9
ORIGIN	Europe, from Spain to the Caspian Sea and from Greece north to Norway and into the former U.S.S.R.
PREFERRED SITES	Mostly well-drained, open meadows

DESCRIPTION: Most American nursery growers and gardeners are familiar with the old garden plant *Festuca ovina* 'Glauca'. Usually grown from seed, this plant can take on various shades of blue or gray. Until recently, plants ordered under this name could arrive in almost any shade of blue or gray and were often mixed. During the last ten years, over 25 cultivars of different fescues have been introduced. These plants are propagated solely from division to protect their characteristic traits. Because blue fescue's range extends to so many climates and environments, considerable differences exist among the many cultivars, including differences in texture, color, flowering habit, and size. Many cultivars are new to U.S. nurseries, and their long-range performance in a given situation may be untested.

Blue fescue is a clumping, evergreen, cool-season grass. Some cultivars may become somewhat dormant in summer and require some summer dryness to thrive. Dense clumps of fine-textured foliage range from 4- to 6-inch miniatures to 18-inch tufts and are colored from bright blue to dark green. The flowers vary from merely noticeable to quite showy, and one cultivar is even selected specifically for its lack of flowers.

LANDSCAPE USES: Blue fescue and its cultivars are charming accents for their foliage color and texture. They make good groundcovers and are ideal in rock and trough gardens. Most make good pot or tub subjects. Their soft foliage is a good choice for edgings. The plants are solid performers in cool coastal climates.

CULTURE AND PROPAGATION: Blue fescue prefers moist, well-drained soil in full sun. It does not grow well in areas with hot, humid summers and must have good drainage in areas with high summer rainfall. In hot climates, provide plants with half-day sun or light shade. Blue fescue is drought-tolerant in areas with some summer moisture. Many cultivars slow their growth in the heat of summer. Some look shabby by August in hot climates and do not revive until the soil temperature cools down in late September. Trim the foliage yearly to help keep clumps tidy. Most clumps should be clipped 3 to 4 inches above the crown. Avoid cutting the plants back hard in the heat of summer, as they may not recover; it is best to cut them in fall or early spring.

Propagate by seed, or by division in spring or fall. Propagate named cultivars by division only.

PESTS AND PROBLEMS: Like the closely related sheep's fescue (*F. amethystina*), blue fescue may require replanting every two to three years. Old clumps often die out in the center, requiring replanting with either new plants or divisions of existing plants.

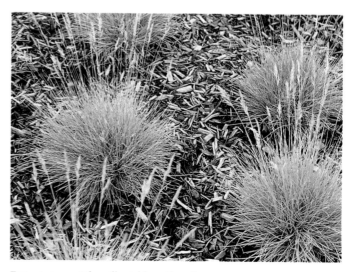

Festuca cinerea 'Blausilber', blue-silver fescue.

BOTANICAL NAME	*Festuca cinerea* 'Blausilber'
PRONUNCIATION	fes-TOO-kah sin-er-ee-AH BLOU-sil-ber
COMMON NAME	Blue-silver fescue

DESCRIPTION: The fine-textured foliage of blue-silver fescue grows to 6 inches tall. It is one of the finest blue fescue cultivars available. The foliage may burn somewhat in hot-summer climates.

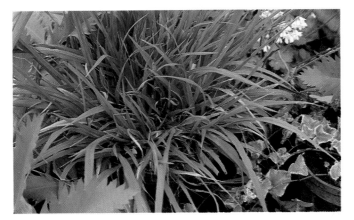

Festuca gigantea, giant fescue.

OTHER *Festuca cinerea* CULTIVARS ARE:

'Azurit' (Azure blue fescue): blue-gray foliage grows 12 to 16 inches tall; medium-textured foliage.

'Blaufink' (Bluefinch fescue): compact, fine-textured cultivar; grows 6 to 8 inches tall.

'Blaufuchs' (Blue fox fescue): blue, fine-textured; grows 6 to 12 inches tall.

'Daeumling' (Tom Thumb fescue): compact grower with silver-blue new spring growth, becoming green as the season progresses.

'Elijah Blue' ('Elijah Blue' fescue): soft powdery blue; medium-textured; grows to 8 inches tall.

'Fruehlingsblau' (Spring blue fescue): intense blue color; fine-textured; grows to 8 inches tall.

'Harz' ('Harz' fescue, Harz Mountain fescue): olive green; weeping; medium-textured; grows to 12 inches tall.

'Meerblau' (Ocean blue fescue): blue and green leaves on new growth; medium-textured; grows 6 to 12 inches tall.

'Platinat' (Platinum blue fescue): silvery platinum blue; 6 to 12 inches tall. Also sold as *F. amethystina* 'Platinat'.

'Sea Urchin' ('Sea Urchin' blue fescue): silvery blue-gray; medium-textured; grows 6 to 12 inches tall. Also sold as *F. cinerea* 'Seeigal'.

'Silberreiher' (Silver egret fescue): silvery blue; fine-textured; grows 6 to 12 inches tall.

'Soehrenwald' ('Soehrenwald' fescue): olive green, changes to blue-green as the season progresses; medium-textured; grows 8 to 12 inches tall.

'Solling' ('Solling' fescue): blue-gray; red-brown fall and winter color; fine-textured; grows to 8 inches tall with no flower spikes.

BOTANICAL NAME	*Festuca gigantea*
PRONUNCIATION	fes-TOO-kah jeye-GAN-tee-ah
COMMON NAME	Giant fescue
USDA HARDINESS ZONE	4 to 9
ORIGIN	Europe
PREFERRED SITES	Open woods, forest understory

DESCRIPTION: Clumping, cool-season, evergreen giant fescue is a strong performer in lightly shaded, damp locations. Its upright, arching leaves, ½ to ¾ inch wide and 2 to 3 feet long, are often twisted, revealing the undersides. The leaves are flat and somewhat V-shaped, dull green on top and glossy green below. The flowers bloom in July and August in loose, upright panicles rising 12 to 18 inches above the foliage. The flowers become a buff color and begin to spread and droop with age.

LANDSCAPE USES: Giant fescue is most valuable for massing and underplanting in wooded areas. Tolerant of moist sites, it will reseed and naturalize in damp locations. It is a good groundcover for lightly shaded slopes. Its foliage color is its most important asset, and it combines well with other shade-loving perennials such as ferns and hostas.

CULTURE AND PROPAGATION: Giant fescue prefers moist, well-drained, rich soil in partial sun. It does not respond well to hot, dry climates or highly alkaline soils. It tolerates full sun if it has sufficient moisture and also tolerates considerable shade if the soil is well drained. In sunny areas, you may prefer to use grasses that are more ornamental. Giant fescue is largely untested in the South and West.

Propagate by seed, or by division in fall or spring. It is easier to propagate giant fescue from seed.

PESTS AND PROBLEMS: Giant fescue has no known pests or problems.

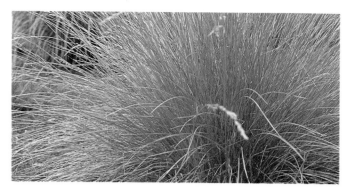

Festuca mairei, Maire's fescue, in winter dormancy in Maryland.

BOTANICAL NAME	***Festuca mairei***
PRONUNCIATION	fes-TOO-kah MAY-ree-eye
COMMON NAME	Maire's fescue, Atlas fescue, Moroccan fescue
USDA HARDINESS ZONE	5 to 10
ORIGIN	Northern Africa, including Morocco and the Atlas Mountains
PREFERRED SITES	Streamsides, rocky streams

DESCRIPTION: Dense, clumping, cool-season-growing Maire's fescue makes a handsome mound of unique evergreen foliage. Its narrow, flat leaves are ⅛ to ¼ inch wide and grow 2 to 3 feet tall. The glossy, pale gray-green foliage is useful in combination plantings in the garden. The noticeable but not particularly showy flowers bloom in June and are borne on stiff, slender stems that arch out from the foliage.

LANDSCAPE USES: Maire's fescue is effective planted alone or in groups and is an excellent blender and filler. Its pale foliage provides excellent contrast for darker plants. Grown for erosion control on slopes or open areas, it looks attractive in large-scale applications, such as in parks and zoos and along median strips.

CULTURE AND PROPAGATION: Maire's fescue prefers moist, well-drained, fertile soil in full sun. It is extremely tolerant of a wide range of conditions, including heat, drought, cold, moisture, seacoast exposure, and rocky or gravelly soils. A strong performer in the arid West, it needs summer watering to look its best.
    Propagate by seed, or by division in spring or fall.

PESTS AND PROBLEMS: Maire's fescue can develop rust. The foliage becomes almost orange if the infestation is severe. The rust never seems to hurt the plant, but simply discolors the foliage. It can be treated if desired (see page 23).

BOTANICAL NAME	***Festuca muelleri***
PRONUNCIATION	fes-TOO-kah MYOO-ler-eye
COMMON NAME	Mueller's fescue
USDA HARDINESS ZONE	5 to 9
ORIGIN	Europe
PREFERRED SITES	Rocky soils, mountain meadows

DESCRIPTION: Soft, fine-textured, hairlike foliage graces this compact, clumping evergreen. A cool-season grass, Mueller's fescue grows 6 to 8 inches tall and as wide. Its shiny foliage is green with a hint of bluish green. The flowers, not particularly showy or profuse, emerge bluish green in June and fade to a buff color at maturity.

LANDSCAPE USES: Mueller's fescue makes an excellent garden filler and groundcover. Planted in masses or groups, it creates soft hummocks of green, hairlike foliage. This grass is also well suited for rock and trough gardens. An ideal complement to dwarf conifers and other miniature evergreens, Mueller's fescue also provides a beautiful contrast to blue fescue selections.

CULTURE AND PROPAGATION: Mueller's fescue grows best in moist, well-drained, fertile soil in full sun. It does not like heavy, wet soils, especially in hot climates. Among the compact, clumping green fescues, this species has shown good heat tolerance in arid conditions. In hot, inland climates, part-day shade or light shade is best.
    Propagate by seed, or by division in spring or fall.

PESTS AND PROBLEMS: Mueller's fescue has no known pests or problems.

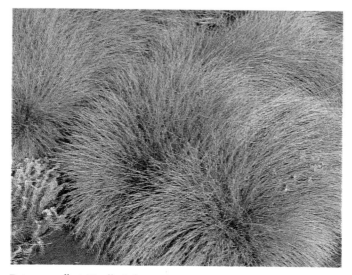

Festuca muelleri, Mueller's fescue.

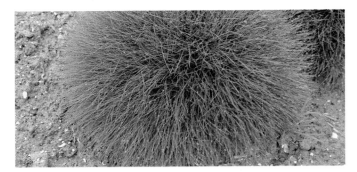

Festuca scoparia, bearskin fescue.

BOTANICAL NAME	***Festuca scoparia***
PRONUNCIATION	fes-TOO-kah skoh-PAH-ree-ah
COMMON NAME	Bearskin fescue
USDA HARDINESS ZONE	5 to 9
ORIGIN	Europe, Pyrenees Mountains
PREFERRED SITES	Rocky soil, alpine slopes

DESCRIPTION: Miniature, clumping bearskin fescue has sharp, prickly, bright evergreen foliage that forms dense, tight mats and grows 4 to 6 inches tall with needlelike leaves. The plants eventually form dense colonies, deceivingly sharp to the touch. The flowers emerge as fine, narrow, greenish spikes that mature to pale gold.

LANDSCAPE USES: Bearskin fescue is at its best in rock or trough gardens. Its dwarf mounding habit makes it a good choice for rocky slopes. It is a good pot and bonsai subject.

CULTURE AND PROPAGATION: An alpine grass, bearskin fescue is somewhat difficult to grow in cultivation. Plants prefer well-drained, rocky soil in full sun or partial shade. It is somewhat drought-tolerant in cooler climates; in hot, inland climates, plants need some moisture, excellent drainage, and partial shade. This grass does not tolerate heavy, wet soils and is not suitable for mass planting.
Propagate by division in the spring or fall.

PESTS AND PROBLEMS: Bearskin fescue has a tendency to die out in the center if it is crowded.

ONE CULTIVAR OF ***Festuca scoparia*** IS:

'Pic Carlit' (Dwarf bearskin fescue): sharp, prickly foliage grows 2 to 3 inches tall.

BOTANICAL NAME	***Festuca tenuifolia*** (also known as *F. capillata*)
PRONUNCIATION	fes-TOO-kah ten-yoo-ih-FOL-ee-ah
COMMON NAME	Fine-leaved fescue
USDA HARDINESS ZONE	4 to 9
ORIGIN	Continental Europe and England
PREFERRED SITES	Meadows

DESCRIPTION: Fine-textured and cool-season-growing, fine-leaved fescue is perhaps the greenest of the small clumping fescues. Its bright green, hairlike foliage grows 4 to 6 inches tall and becomes rather matlike with age. The flowers, 4 to 6 inches tall, are greenish upon emergence and turn beige as they mature. The flowers are noticeable but not particularly showy; the main attraction of this plant is its foliage.

LANDSCAPE USES: Fine-leaved fescue is a good rock and trough garden plant. An attractive groundcover, it is particularly striking in the early spring, when its new foliage is brightest. While it can be a lawn substitute, it tolerates only occasional foot traffic. Fine-leaved fescue is best used as filler between stones, along pathways, or in crevices.

CULTURE AND PROPAGATION: Fine-leaved fescue prefers moist, well-drained, fertile soil in full sun. Good drainage is essential for strong, healthy growth. Plants do not tolerate heavy, wet soil and languish in too much shade. This fescue is not well adapted to hot, inland climates; in such climates, plant it in half-day sun. If plants become too shabby, they may be dug and divided or replanted.
Propagate by seed, or by division in spring or fall.

PESTS AND PROBLEMS: Fine-leaved fescue is not well suited for large-scale mass plantings because the plants tend to die out in the center after a few years.

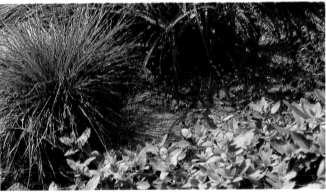

Festuca tenuifolia, fine-leaved fescue.

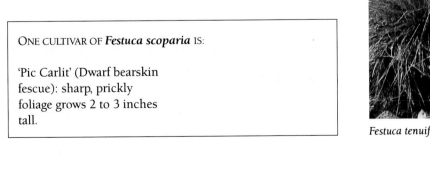

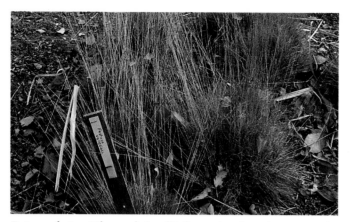

Festuca valesiaca 'Glaucantha', wallis fescue, in winter dormancy.

OTHER SPECIES OF FESCUE ARE:	
Festuca 'Czech' ('Czech' fescue): dark green foliage; showy flowers and good heat tolerance; the best green cultivar for mild climates.	*Festuca glacialis* (Glacier fescue): one of the most compact fescues with fine, blue-gray hairlike foliage; best in rock gardens.

BOTANICAL NAME	***Festuca valesiaca 'Glaucantha'***
PRONUNCIATION	fes-TOO-kah va-lee-see-AH-kah glou-KAN-thah
COMMON NAME	Wallis fescue
USDA HARDINESS ZONE	5 to 9
ORIGIN	Species origin: central Russia to the Pyrenees Mountains; central Germany to Greece
PREFERRED SITES	Rocky slopes, mountain meadows

BOTANICAL NAME	***Glyceria maxima 'Variegata' (also known as G. aquatica 'Variegata')***
PRONUNCIATION	GLIH-seer-ee-ah MAX-ih-mah var-ee-uh-GAH-tah
COMMON NAME	Variegated manna grass
USDA HARDINESS ZONE	5 to 10
ORIGIN	Species origin: Eurasia
PREFERRED SITES	Streamsides, wet sites

DESCRIPTION: Similar to clumping blue fescue cultivars, low, tight, evergreen wallis fescue has fine, weeping, powdery blue foliage. Its dense clumps of soft, hairlike leaves grow 4 to 6 inches tall and as wide. The powdery blue coating gives the leaves a rich look and feel. The flowers emerge bluish white and mature to a wheat color. They rise 4 to 6 inches above the foliage and are noticeable but not showy.

LANDSCAPE USES: Wallis fescue is best used as an accent in rock or trough gardens. It is also effective as a border or an edging or in combination with other blue fescue cultivars.

CULTURE AND PROPAGATION: Wallis fescue grows best in well-drained, rocky soils in full sun. Plants do not like heavy, wet, clayey soils. Drainage is essential, but plants resent drying out completely. This grass is not well adapted to hot, inland climates and is somewhat demanding in most garden situations.

Propagate by division only.

PESTS AND PROBLEMS: Mature plantings of wallis fescue tend to die out in the center.

DESCRIPTION: Deciduous, aquatic, variegated manna grass is a vigorous spreader with brilliantly variegated foliage. Its leaves, ¼ to ½ inch wide and 4 to 6 inches long, clothe culms that grow 2 to 3 feet tall and sometimes taller. New spring growth is decidedly pink, slowly changing to creamy yellow-white with thin green stripes by summer. The leaves become tinged with pink with the onset of fall. The foliage falls over in winter and is of no particular merit. The flowers are borne in noticeable, but not showy, loose panicles. In mild climates, flowering seldom occurs.

LANDSCAPE USES: Variegated manna grass is a wonderful foliage accent when combined with green-leaved wetland plants such as water lilies. It is suitable for ponds, pools, water gardens, pots, and tubs. Its spreading habit makes it naturalize along streamsides.

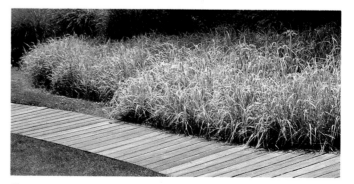

Glyceria maxima 'Variegata', variegated manna grass.

CULTURE AND PROPAGATION: Variegated manna grass grows best in moist, rich soils or shallow water in full sun. It grows well in hot climates as long as it is given constant moisture.

Propagate by division only.

PESTS AND PROBLEMS: To best contain its aggressive, spreading nature, plant variegated manna grass in a drainage tile.

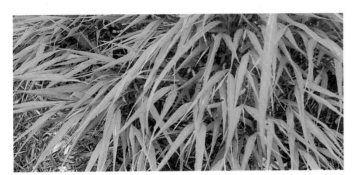

Hakonechloa macra, hakone grass.

BOTANICAL NAME	*Hakonechloa macra* (also known as *Phragmites macra*)
PRONUNCIATION	hah-koh-neh-KLOH-ah MAK-rah
COMMON NAME	Hakone grass
USDA HARDINESS ZONE	7 to 9
ORIGIN	Japan
PREFERRED SITES	Mountains, streamsides, cliffs

DESCRIPTION: Slow-spreading, deciduous hakone grass is prized for its delicate bamboolike foliage and rich fall color. Its bright green leaves clothe wiry stems that grow to 1 to 2 feet tall, much like a clumping dwarf bamboo. In hot climates, plants rarely reach 1 foot tall. The soft, glossy leaves, ¼ to ½ inch wide and 3 to 6 inches long, taper to a point. Although it spreads slowly from rhizomes, hakone grass is never invasive. The flowers bloom in late summer and early fall. The delicate, open panicles are not particularly showy but add a distinct airiness and lightness to the plant. In the fall, the leaves turn a wonderful pinkish red. In winter, dormant plants turn a beautiful bronze. Although 'Aureola', the variegated cultivar of hakone grass, is better known, the green-leaved species itself is a fine choice for most gardens. It tolerates mild-winter areas of California; other forms are not as accommodating. Hakone grass has been cultivated in Japan for some time but is a relatively new introduction to U.S. nurseries and may be hard to find.

LANDSCAPE USES: Hakone grass is perhaps one of the most elegant ornamental grasses for a shady site. It is attractive planted alone or in masses and is excellent in combination with other shade-loving perennials such as ferns and hostas. Hakone grass makes a good groundcover under a canopy of tall trees and is well suited for pots and tubs. Since the foliage and flowers tend to weep horizontally, it looks attractive on slopes. Its bamboolike foliage also makes it a good choice for oriental gardens.

CULTURE AND PROPAGATION: Hakone grass prefers moist, well-drained, fertile soil with light shade or half-day sun. Moisture and good drainage are the keys to good growth. The plants resent drying out and do not thrive in heavy, wet clay. The foliage tends to burn in full hot sun.

Propagate by seed, or by division in the spring.

PESTS AND PROBLEMS: Hakone grass has no known pests or problems.

BOTANICAL NAME	*Hakonechloa macra* 'Aureola'
PRONUNCIATION	hah-koh-neh-KLOH-ah MAK-rah aw-ree-OH-lah
COMMON NAME	Golden variegated hakone grass, golden variegated hakonechloa

DESCRIPTION: Similar in most respects to the species, golden variegated hakone grass is primarily distinguished by brilliant yellow foliage streaked with green lines. As with the species, the foliage turns an intense pink-red in the fall. This cultivar is not as vigorous as the species and prefers more shade to look its best. The foliage tends to burn in full hot sun but loses its yellow color in too much shade.

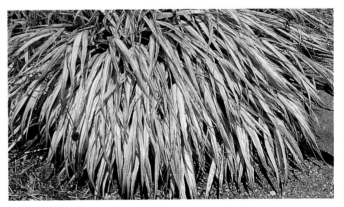

Hakonechloa macra 'Aureola', golden variegated hakone grass.

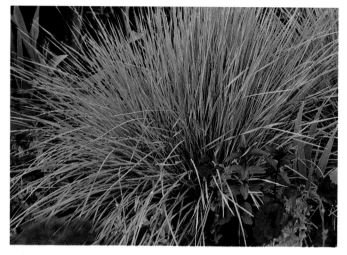

Helictotrichon sempervirens, blue oat grass.

BOTANICAL NAME	***Helictotrichon sempervirens***
PRONUNCIATION	hel-ik-toh-TREE-kon sem-per-VEYE-renz
COMMON NAME	Blue oat grass
USDA HARDINESS ZONE	4 to 9
ORIGIN	Eurasia
PREFERRED SITES	Meadows, dry hillsides

DESCRIPTION: Clumping, evergreen blue oat grass is noted for its bright blue foliage and showy flowers. The plants grow 12 to 18 inches tall and as wide. Its dense, tufted leaves, ⅛ to ⅜ inch wide, are an attractive metallic blue and are sharply pointed at the tip. The flowers are borne in an oatlike, one-sided panicle that appears in June and grows 1 to 2 feet above the leaves. Bluish white on emergence, the flowers dry to a golden wheat color. In cold climates, blue oat grass may be semievergreen.

LANDSCAPE USES: Blue oat grass is enjoyed primarily for its handsome blue foliage. It makes a fine accent planted alone or in masses. In mass plantings, plants need space to mature, fully display their foliage, and flower. The grass is useful as a flowering accent in borders and rock gardens and is a good choice for Mediterranean and coastal gardens.

CULTURE AND PROPAGATION: Blue oat grass prefers well-drained, fertile soil in full sun with good air circulation. In heavy, wet clays, it may be subject to root rot. An open, airy site is best for good foliage. The grass may not fare well during hot, humid summers. To grow in the less than ideal condition of high summer rainfall, plants need excellent drainage, and light or part-day shade.
Propagate by seed, or by division in spring or fall.

PESTS AND PROBLEMS: Since blue oat grass seems to require cold to bloom, it does not bloom dependably in mild climates. Blue oat grass may be prone to root rot in heavy or poorly drained soils, and in too much shade it may develop rust.

BOTANICAL NAME	***Holcus lanatus***
PRONUNCIATION	HOL-kus lah-NAH-tus
COMMON NAME	Velvet grass, Yorkshire fog
USDA HARDINESS ZONE	5 to 9
ORIGIN	Europe, Asia
PREFERRED SITES	Meadows, open fields; naturalized in North America

DESCRIPTION: Velvet grass is a spreading, cool-season grass valued for its soft, velvety foliage and silky white flowers. Its gray-green, semi-evergreen foliage grows 1 to 2 feet tall with soft leaves ¼ to ⅜ inch wide and 2 to 8 inches long. The plants tend to flop and spill. The flowers bloom on a spike 1 to 2 feet above the foliage in an open, loose panicle 3 to 4 inches long. The flowers, showy from June through August, are white and soft to the touch. The plants tend to become dormant in summer after they have flowered.

LANDSCAPE USES: Velvet grass is most often used for naturalizing in meadows and as a lawn substitute in areas of occasional traffic. Although it is attractive planted in borders, it tends to flop over and creep into adjacent spaces. Still, its soft foliage and attractive flowers make a fine groundcover in cool-summer areas. In coastal Mediterranean climates, velvet grass makes a suitable lawn substitute if given sufficient moisture and good drainage. The flowers are beautiful in fresh and dried arrangements.

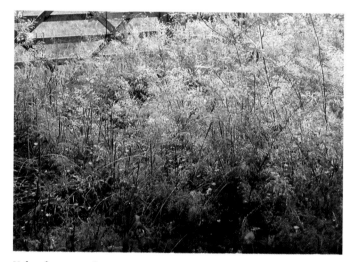

Holcus lanatus, velvet grass.

CULTURE AND PROPAGATION: Velvet grass grows best in moist, well-drained, fertile soil with full sun or partial shade. Plants do poorly in hot climates. Cut back and water after plants flower to keep foliage looking fresh in midsummer.

Propagate by seed or division.

PESTS AND PROBLEMS: Velvet grass may be prone to rust. Although rust is treatable (see page 23), it will rarely kill the plant.

BOTANICAL NAME	*Hordeum jubatum*
PRONUNCIATION	hor-DEE-um joo-BAH-tum
COMMON NAME	Foxtail barley, squirreltail
USDA HARDINESS ZONE	5 to 9
ORIGIN	North America, Alaska to Mexico, throughout the western United States into the Northeast
PREFERRED SITES	Open meadows, prairies

DESCRIPTION: Short-lived, perennial, cool-season foxtail barley has soft, feathery flower heads that sway rhythmically in the slightest breeze. Rather scruffy in foliage, it is treated as an annual in most garden situations. Its fine-textured, light green foliage forms loose clumps of leaves 1 to 2 feet tall and as wide. The flowers emerge greenish or purplish in June and become brown with maturity. The flowers, held on nodding stems 1 to 1½ feet above the foliage, are foxtail-like whisks, 2 to 4 inches long and as wide, with long awns that give them their characteristic wispiness. The plants decline rapidly after flowering, as they shatter and become windborne at maturity.

LANDSCAPE USES: Foxtail barley is best used as a flowering accent in perennial borders and for naturalizing in dry areas. Since it reseeds readily, it is a fairly invasive grass. It is beautiful in mass plantings. The flowers are useful in arrangements and often are grown solely for this purpose.

CULTURE AND PROPAGATION: Foxtail barley prefers moist, well-drained soil in full sun. It is tolerant of a wide range of conditions and exposures, including heat, wind, poor or rocky soil, and extreme temperatures.

Propagation is best by seed.

PESTS AND PROBLEMS: Foxtail barley is often considered a weed and is usually not the best choice for permanent plantings. Though tolerant of many climates, its flowers are damaged by heavy rain and wind.

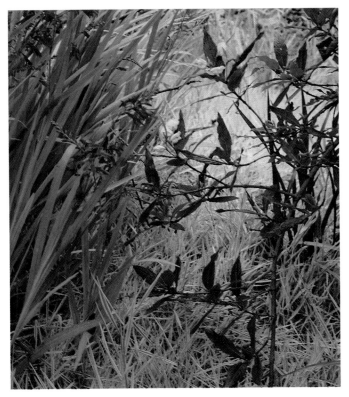

Holcus lanatus 'Variegatus', variegated velvet grass.

BOTANICAL NAME	*Holcus lanatus* **'Variegatus' (often confused with *H. mollis* 'Variegatus')**
PRONUNCIATION	HOL-kus lah-NAH-tus var-ee-uh-GAH-tus
COMMON NAME	Variegated velvet grass

DESCRIPTION: Soft, velvety foliage and bright white variegation distinguish variegated velvet grass from velvet grass. The variegated cultivar has a more compact habit, usually reaching 4 to 8 inches tall in a spreading, mat-forming clump. The pure white leaves have a wide central green stripe and several narrow green stripes. They grow ⅛ to ¼ inch wide and 3 to 5 inches long. Variegated velvet grass rarely flowers. This plant tends to overrun small gardens.

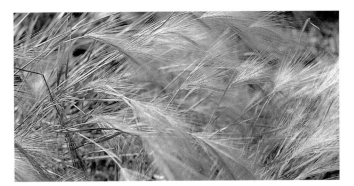

Hordeum jubatum, foxtail barley.

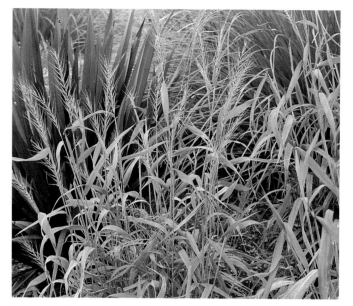

Hystrix patula, bottlebrush grass.

BOTANICAL NAME	***Hystrix patula***
PRONUNCIATION	HEYE-striks pah-TOO-lah
COMMON NAME	Bottlebrush grass
USDA HARDINESS ZONE	5 to 9
ORIGIN	East coast of the United States
PREFERRED SITES	Moist, rocky soils; a woodland native

DESCRIPTION: This clumping, cool-season grass is admired primarily for its showy, bristly flower heads that resemble bottlebrushes. Its dark olive-green leaves, ¼ to ½ inch wide and 4 to 8 inches long, form upright tufts of foliage 8 to 12 inches tall and as wide. Greenish flowers appear on the plant from June through August on a spike 1 to 2 feet above the foliage. The flowers usually mature to brownish and shatter by early fall.

LANDSCAPE USES: Bottlebrush grass is an attractive flowering accent for lightly shaded borders. It is effective planted alone or in groups and naturalizes in woodland gardens. Its attractive flowers are beautiful in fresh arrangements, provided the flowers are cut as soon as they are fully open to prevent shattering.

CULTURE AND PROPAGATION: Bottlebrush grass prefers moist, well-drained, fertile soil in light shade. It tolerates a wide range of conditions but resents hot, dry conditions in full sun. It tolerates more sun in moist, sandy soil.

Propagate by seed, or by division in fall or spring.

PESTS AND PROBLEMS: Bottlebrush grass has no known pests or problems.

BOTANICAL NAME	***Imperata brevifolia***
PRONUNCIATION	im-per-RAH-tah breh-vih-FOH-lee-ah
COMMON NAME	Satintail
USDA HARDINESS ZONE	7 to 9
ORIGIN	California, Arizona, New Mexico, Texas
PREFERRED SITES	Streamsides, sandy margins

DESCRIPTION: Satintail is a slowly creeping, warm-season grass that has attractive red fall color and cottony white plumes. Spreading from creeping rhizomes, satintail has vertical leaves, ½ to ¾ inch wide and 12 to 18 inches long, that taper to a point. The foliage is a translucent bright green that becomes red-stained as the season progresses. The flowers bloom on erect culms that are held 1 to 1½ feet above the foliage from May through June. They emerge satiny white and mature to fluffy, cottony heads. By fall, the foliage is entirely reddish purple. In mild climates, the foliage persists through the winter, until it is overgrown by new spring growth. In colder climates, foliage is deciduous.

LANDSCAPE USES: Satintail is a fine choice for naturalizing along streams or ponds. It is at its best planted in large masses at or near the water's edge. It is also a good pot or tub subject. The flowers are effective in fresh or dried arrangements.

CULTURE AND PROPAGATION: Satintail prefers fertile, moist, well-drained soil in full sun or partial shade. It tolerates considerable shade but will flower less and will not develop as good a fall color. It tolerates heat as long as moisture is present.

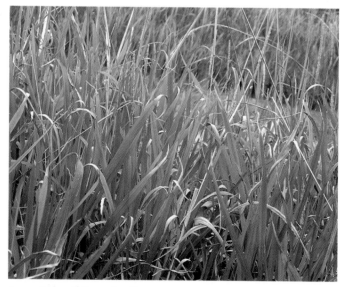

Imperata brevifolia, satintail.

Propagation by division is easy; propagation from seed is also possible.

PESTS AND PROBLEMS: Satintail may be somewhat invasive in ideal conditions, but will rarely spread into dry, unirrigated soils.

BOTANICAL NAME	***Imperata cylindrica* 'Red Baron' (also known as *Imperata cylindrica* var. *rubra*)**
PRONUNCIATION	im-per-AH-tah
COMMON NAME	'Red Baron' blood grass, Japanese blood grass, cranberry grass
USDA HARDINESS ZONE	6 to 9
ORIGIN	Japan
PREFERRED SITES	Moist, sandy streamsides

DESCRIPTION: 'Red Baron' blood grass is a warm-season grass with translucent, upright-growing foliage. The leaves, ⅛ to ¼ inch wide and 1 to 1½ feet tall, form slowly spreading colonies. Vertical leaves emerge bright green, with wine-red-stained tips, in the spring. The foliage becomes increasingly red as the season progresses. By fall, the foliage is blood red, creating stunning visual effects in early morning or late afternoon light. With the onset of winter, plants become dormant and the foliage takes on a pleasing copper color that makes a good winter show. 'Red Baron' blood grass does not produce flowers and appears to produce only vegetative growth.

LANDSCAPE USES: 'Red Baron' blood grass is effective planted as a specimen or in groups. The plants make fine specimens for pots or tubs. It it unsurpassed for fall color. It combines well with many perennials.

CULTURE AND PROPAGATION: 'Red Baron' blood grass prefers moist soil in full sun. It languishes in heavy, wet soils and resents hot, dry situations. It tolerates light shade, but the red coloring will be lessened. In hot southern and inland climates, 'Red Baron' blood grass looks best if given some shade during the hottest part of the day.

Propagate by division only.

'Red Baron' blood grass is also grown by tissue culture. This has proven to be a questionable practice, as the plants seem prone to mutation, becoming aggressively spreading, green-foliaged plants. Avoid tissue-culture-grown plants if possible.

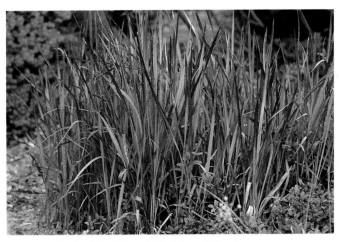

Imperata cylindrica 'Red Baron', 'Red Baron' blood grass.

PESTS AND PROBLEMS: A fine ornamental, 'Red Baron' blood grass has relatives that are feared worldwide as noxious weeds. *Imperata cylindrica*, its African relative, is an aggressively spreading grass that is outlawed in the United States. This cultivar is a diminutive, well-behaved, red-foliaged grass that seldom is a threat to the garden.

If 'Red Baron' blood grass should revert to a non-red form, remove it immediately. Reversions are usually aggressive spreaders.

JUNCUS
RUSHES

Close to 300 species of rushes are found throughout the world, most of them native to wet or moist sites in temperate regions. They usually have smooth, cylindrical leaves. Some are evergreen, while others become dormant with the first frost. Rushes can be found in sun or shade and in fresh or salt water. Although most are found along streams, in marshy areas, or in shallow water, some rushes tolerate seasonal drought.

Ranging in color from various shades of green through gray, rushes can be delicate miniatures 6 inches tall, or 6-foot giants. In the garden, rushes are at their best in or near water. They are excellent for naturalizing and stabilizing stream banks. Many are useful for providing habitat for birds and other wildlife.

In small gardens, rushes are excellent in tubs or small pools. Some have attractive flowers or foliage that are useful in fresh or dried arrangements.

Rushes have had a long association with man. Native Americans used rushes for basketry, crafts, housing, and transportation. Much of our original wetlands, home to most rushes, have been destroyed or are threatened with destruction. Only a concerted effort will reverse this sad trend.

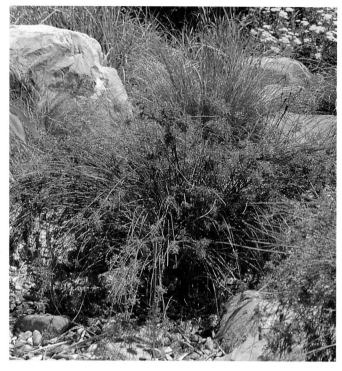

Juncus 'Carmen's Japanese', 'Carmen's Japanese' rush.

BOTANICAL NAME	***Juncus* 'Carmen's Japanese'**
PRONUNCIATION	JUN-kus
COMMON NAME	'Carmen's Japanese' rush
USDA HARDINESS ZONE	7 (?) to 9 (hardiness untested; may grow in zones colder than 7)
ORIGIN	Unidentified species from Japan—introduced by Ed Carmen, Carmen's Nursery, Los Gatos, California
PREFERRED SITES	Moist, boggy soil; shallow water

DESCRIPTION: Clumping, evergreen 'Carmen's Japanese' rush is distinguished by fine-textured, dark green foliage and showy seed heads. The cylindrical leaves, $1/16$ to $3/16$ inch wide, grow 18 to 24 inches tall. The flowers appear in early summer, maturing to clusters of fine seeds that cause the stems to bend in graceful arching curves. The showy seeds turn brownish at maturity.

LANDSCAPE USES: 'Carmen's Japanese' rush is useful in and around the water's edge. It grows in shallow water and makes a beautiful accent for pools and ponds. This grass is a choice selection for small water gardens, pots, and tubs. The flowers and seed heads are attractive in fresh or dried arrangements. 'Carmen's Japanese' rush is prized in Japan for making mats and baskets.

CULTURE AND PROPAGATION: 'Carmen's Japanese' rush grows best in moist, fertile soil in light shade or half-day sun. Plants will grow in shallow water 4 to 6 inches deep. Plants may sunburn in hot climates in full sun.

Propagate by seed, or by division in fall or spring.

PESTS OR PROBLEMS: 'Carmen's Japanese' rush has no known pests or problems.

BOTANICAL NAME	***Juncus effusus***
PRONUNCIATION	JUN-kus eh-FYOO-sus
COMMON NAME	Soft rush
USDA HARDINESS ZONE	4 to 9
ORIGIN	Worldwide
PREFERRED SITES	Wet areas, marshes, streamsides

DESCRIPTION: Clumping, deciduous soft rush is characterized by soft, round stems, $1/8$ to $1/4$ inch in diameter, that grow mostly vertically, $1\frac{1}{2}$ to $2\frac{1}{2}$ feet tall. Soft rush has medium green foliage. The plants turn yellowish brown with the first frost, becoming totally brown by late fall. Flowers are noticeable and are borne almost at the tip of the stem in early summer. They persist until dormancy in the fall.

LANDSCAPE USES: Soft rush is an effective foliage accent for pools, ponds, and streamsides. It grows in shallow water or moist, boggy soil, and is suitable for pots or tubs. Plants make a dramatic silhouette when backlit at night.

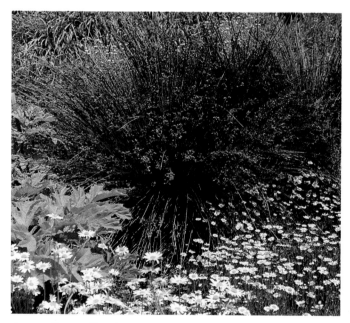

Juncus effusus, soft rush.

CULTURE AND PROPAGATION: Soft rush grows best in moist, peaty soils in light shade. It grows in shallow water and boggy soils with equal ease. The plants look better in light shade or part-day sun, especially in hot climates. Soft rush will naturalize readily in moist sites.

Propagate by seed or division.

PESTS AND PROBLEMS: Soft rush has no known pests or problems.

BOTANICAL NAME	***Juncus effusus* 'Spiralis'**
PRONUNCIATION	JUN-kus eh-FYOO-sus speer-AL-is
COMMON NAME	Corkscrew rush, spiral rush
USDA HARDINESS ZONE	7 to 9
ORIGIN	Horticultural selection from Japan
PREFERRED SITES	Wet areas, shallow water, moist or boggy soils

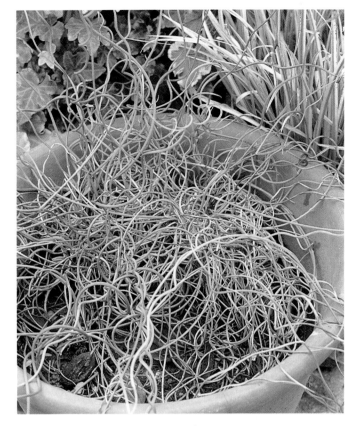

Juncus effusus 'Spiralis', corkscrew rush.

DESCRIPTION: This unusual semi-evergreen rush has cylindrical, twisted, coiling foliage; hence the common name corkscrew rush. In the spring, new leaves emerge tightly coiled and uncoil as they grow. The glossy, dark green, cylindrical leaves, ⅛ to ⅜ inch in diameter, grow into a whimsical sprawling clump 18 to 24 inches tall and as wide. The loose clump of spreading foliage has a slow to moderate growth rate. The flowers are borne in a cyme near the end of the stems and are noticeable but not particularly showy. Children and cats seem to love this plant. Give it a spot where its foliage can be appreciated.

LANDSCAPE USES: Corkscrew rush makes an attractive and comical addition to the garden. It grows well in pots and containers and thrives in moist locations and in water, particularly ponds and pools. Its foliage is beautiful in fresh or dried arrangements.

CULTURE AND PROPAGATION: Corkscrew rush grows best in moist, peaty soil in light shade. Its foliage has a tendency to burn in full sun, especially in hot climates. The plants do not tolerate drying out; to avoid brown tips, provide constant moisture. To keep plants in containers moist, place the container on a saucer filled with gravel and water.

Propagate by division. If you're prepared to cull seedlings, a large porton will come true when sown by seed.

PESTS AND PROBLEMS: Corkscrew rush has no known pests or problems.

BOTANICAL NAME	***Juncus mexicanus***
PRONUNCIATION	JUN-kus mek-see-KAHN-us
COMMON NAME	Mexican rush
USDA HARDINESS ZONE	8 to 10
ORIGIN	California, from Point Concepcion south into Mexico
PREFERRED SITES	Moist areas

DESCRIPTION: Creeping, evergreen Mexican rush spreads from underground rhizomes to create colonies of dark green foliage. Its narrow, somewhat flattened leaves, ¹⁄₁₆ to ⅛ inch wide, grow 12 to 18 inches tall, curving slightly at the tip. The flowers are very small and hardly noticeable.

LANDSCAPE USES: Mexican rush is effective planted at the water's edge and in moist, shady spots. It grows well in shade gardens, and in pots and tubs. It also makes a good groundcover in heavy, wet soils.

CULTURE AND PROPAGATION: Mexican rush likes moist, sandy soils in sun or shade. It tolerates a wide range of soil conditions as long as some moisture is present. Its foliage

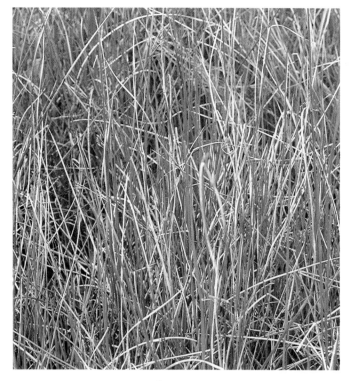

Juncus mexicanus, Mexican rush.

looks better in light shade. Mexican rush may go dormant in a hard freeze but will come up again in the spring. It tolerates considerable drought when established and is often found in nature in areas that are wet in the winter and dry in the summer.

Propagate by seed, or by division in fall or spring.

PESTS OR PROBLEMS: Mexican rush has no known pests or problems.

BOTANICAL NAME	***Juncus patens***
PRONUNCIATION	JUN-kus pah-TENZ
COMMON NAME	California gray rush
USDA HARDINESS ZONE	7 (?) to 9 (hardiness untested; may grow in Zone 7)
ORIGIN	Baja California north into Oregon
PREFERRED SITES	Moist, boggy areas, usually below 5,000 feet elevation

DESCRIPTION: California gray rush has handsome steel-gray foliage. A clumping, evergreen rush, it grows 1½ to 2½ feet tall. The slender, cylindrical leaves, ⅛ to ⅜ inch in diameter, are somewhat stiff and vertical. The flowers are inconspicuous.

LANDSCAPE USES: California gray rush makes an ideal accent for shady, moist spots. It grows in shallow water and makes an interesting groundcover massed along the water's edge or in dry streambeds. It also makes a fine pot subject.

CULTURE AND PROPAGATION: California gray rush prefers moist, fertile soil in light shade. It tolerates a wide range of conditions, from full sun to considerable shade, as long as moisture is present. Its foliage looks better if given some shade, but the plant will appear lanky and flop over in too much shade. California gray rush grows in shallow water 4 to 6 inches deep. It will also tolerate dry soil in summer, although foliage will show signs of drought stress.

Propagate by seed, or by division in spring.

PESTS AND PROBLEMS: California gray rush has no known pests or problems.

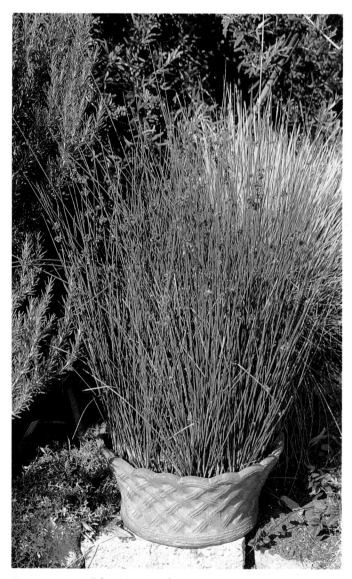

Juncus patens, California gray rush.

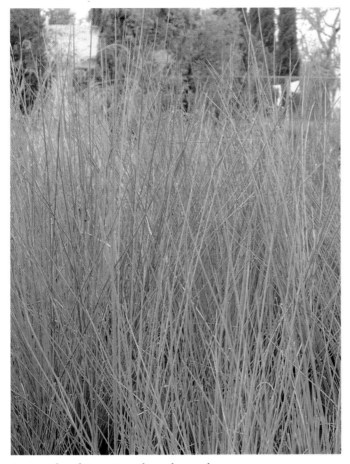

Juncus polyanthemos, Australian silver rush.

CULTURE AND PROPAGATION: Australian silver rush prefers moist, rich soil in full sun or light shade. It tolerates heavy soil and can be planted in shallow water 4 to 6 inches deep. The plant loses its blue color in too much shade. Although its cold-hardiness is unknown, its heat tolerance is excellent. It is worth trying this rush in colder climates.

Propagate by seed, or by division in spring or fall.

PESTS AND PROBLEMS: Australian silver rush has no known pests or problems.

KOELERIA
HAIRGRASS, JUNE GRASS

There are over 35 species of the tufted perennial grasses known as hairgrass or June grass. Found in the Northern and Southern hemispheres, usually in sunny locations on infertile or poor soils, these grasses usually resent rich, fertile soils and can be short-lived in many situations. Still, the species listed here are admired for their handsome foliage and flowers.

All cultivars of *Koeleria* should be propagated vegetatively.

BOTANICAL NAME	**Juncus polyanthemos**
PRONUNCIATION	JUN-kus pol-ee-AN-theh-mos
COMMON NAME	Australian silver rush
USDA HARDINESS ZONE	8 (?) to 10 (hardiness untested; may grow above Zone 8)
ORIGIN	South Australia
PREFERRED SITES	Moist areas, wet boggy sites

BOTANICAL NAME	**Koeleria argentea**
PRONUNCIATION	koh-LAIR-ee-ah ar-JEN-tee-ah
COMMON NAME	Silver hairgrass
USDA HARDINESS ZONE	7 to 9
ORIGIN	Europe
PREFERRED SITES	Dry meadows

DESCRIPTION: A new introduction to U.S. nurseries by Gary Hammer of Sunland, California, this grass is sure to find a place in warm-climate American gardens.

Stunning silver-blue Australian silver rush has graceful, clumping, evergreen foliage that grows 3 to 4 feet tall. Its long, slender leaves, ⅛ to ⅜ inch wide, create a delicate, arching sculpture in the garden; they move in the slightest breeze and seem to be constantly in motion. The flowers are insignificant.

LANDSCAPE USES: Australian silver rush makes a dramatic accent planted alone or in groups. It makes a good pot or tub subject. It will grow in shallow water and is effective planted along the water's edge or by ponds and pools.

DESCRIPTION: Clumping, cool-season-growing silver hairgrass has attractive two-toned leaves and slender, attractive flowers. The leaves, ⅛ to ¼ inch wide and 6 to 10 inches long, are grayish green on top and silvery underneath. Plants form dense tufts of foliage. The flowers bloom in late spring and early summer in narrow spikes held 10 to 12 inches above the foliage. The flower spikes emerge greenish and mature to a wheat color.

LANDSCAPE USES: Silver hairgrass is attractive planted in masses or groups. It makes an effective groundcover in sunny, well-drained sites and is a good choice for larger rock gardens and rocky slopes. Its interesting foliage is attractive and contrasts beautifully with other greens in the garden.

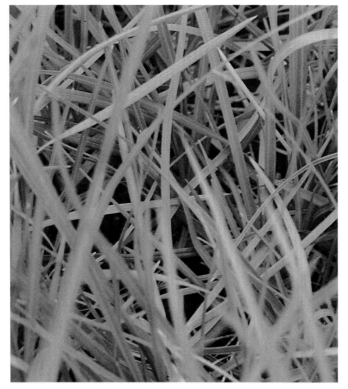

Koeleria argentea, silver hairgrass.

CULTURE AND PROPAGATION: Silver hairgrass prefers well-drained, infertile soil in a sunny location. It does not grow well in heavy, poorly drained soils or shady sites, and resents hot climates.

Propagate by seed, or by division in fall or spring.

PESTS AND PROBLEMS: Silver hairgrass can be short-lived and temperamental, but its handsome foliage is worth the trouble.

BOTANICAL NAME	*Koeleria brevis*
PRONUNCIATION	koh-LAIR-ee-ah BREH-vis
COMMON NAME	Blue hairgrass
USDA HARDINESS ZONE	6 to 8
ORIGIN	Europe
PREFERRED SITES	Dry, gravelly soils

DESCRIPTION: Blue hairgrass is somewhat similar to large blue hairgrass (*Koeleria glauca*), differing primarily in its diminutive size and softer foliage. Dense, compact tufts, 4 to 6 inches tall, form tight little clumps of blue-gray foliage. The attractive leaves, 1/8 inch wide and 3 to 4 inches long, are soft to the touch. The flowers emerge as slender blue-gray spikes and turn a wheat color at maturity.

LANDSCAPE USES: Blue hairgrass is best planted as a collector's specimen or an accent in rock and trough gardens. Its size makes it suitable for detail plantings, small gardens, and bonsai subjects.

CULTURE AND PROPAGATION: Blue hairgrass prefers sunny, well-drained sites in rocky or sandy soil.

Propagate by seed, or by division in spring or fall.

PESTS AND PROBLEMS: As with the other members of the genus *Koeleria*, blue hairgrass is short-lived and somewhat difficult to grow.

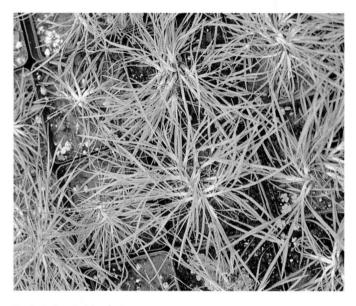

Koeleria brevis, blue hairgrass.

BOTANICAL NAME	*Koeleria glauca*
PRONUNCIATION	koh-LAIR-ee-ah GLOU-kah
COMMON NAME	Large blue hairgrass
USDA HARDINESS ZONE	6 to 9
ORIGIN	Central Europe to western Siberia
PREFERRED SITES	Sandy meadows, open coniferous forests

DESCRIPTION: Compact, clumping, cool-season-growing large blue hairgrass has attractive blue-gray foliage and showy flowers. Dense tufts of evergreen foliage emerge from the base of the plant and form clumps 6 to 12 inches tall and as wide. Its leaves are 1/8 to 3/8 inch wide and 6 to 8 inches long. The flower spikes emerge blue-green from May through June and mature to golden brown. The narrow flower spikes grow vertically, 8 to 12 inches above the foliage.

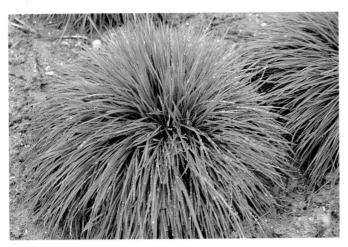

Koeleria glauca, large blue hairgrass.

LANDSCAPE USES: Large blue hairgrass makes an attractive accent plant for the foreground of a perennial border and is good for edging and massing. It is also well suited for rock gardens and small pots or tubs. Although short-spiked, the flowers are beautiful in fresh or dried arrangements.

CULTURE AND PROPAGATION: Large blue hairgrass prefers a sunny, well-drained site with infertile or slightly alkaline soils. It does not tolerate heavy, wet soil or shady sites. In moist, fertile soil, like that found in many perennial borders, large blue hairgrass performs well for only a short time, needing replacement after one to two years. It grows poorly in hot climates.

Propagate by seed, or by division in spring or fall.

PESTS AND PROBLEMS: Large blue hairgrass is perhaps best treated as an annual or a biennial. It has a tendency to be short-lived and to die out in the center. But this tendency is offset by its attractive foliage and charming flowers.

BOTANICAL NAME	**Koeleria macrantha**
PRONUNCIATION	koh-LAIR-ee-ah mah-KRAN-thah
COMMON NAME	June grass
USDA HARDINESS ZONE	4 to 9
ORIGIN	Circumpolar northern temperate zone
PREFERRED SITES	Dry meadows, poor soils

DESCRIPTION: Clumping, cool-season-growing June grass is widely variable and distributed all over the world. It is usually found in open prairies on poor or rocky soils, mostly in mixed stands with other perennial grasses. Un-

fortunately, the plant is rapidly disappearing from its native habitats. A tough grass accustomed to harsh environments, June grass is suitable for western and other dry gardens. Its blue-green foliage forms vertical tufts 1 to 1½ feet tall and 6 to 9 inches wide. The flowers, which grow 1 to 1½ feet above the foliage, emerge a glossy green and dry to a golden brown, narrow spike. The flowers appear in June and are showy until July, when they begin to shatter.

LANDSCAPE USES: June grass is ideal for drifts and masses in dry gardens and rocky soils and can provide effective groundcover and slope cover in hot, dry summer climates. It makes a good understory for tall pines and open meadows and is an excellent choice for naturalizing in large areas. Where its summer dormancy does not pose a fire concern, June grass is a good choice for western gardens.

CULTURE AND PROPAGATION: June grass prefers sunny, well-drained sites with sandy or rocky soils. It will take light shade and some moisture if drainage is good, but does not like heavy, wet soil, moist, fertile soil, or deep shade. The plants tend to become summer-dormant after July.

Propagation is easy from seed, and by division in the spring.

PESTS AND PROBLEMS: June grass has no known pests or problems.

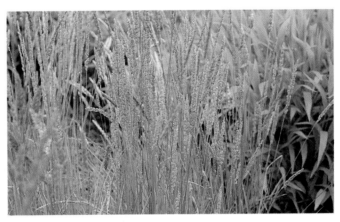

Koeleria macrantha, June grass.

ANOTHER SPECIES OF HAIRGRASS IS:
Koeleria albescens (Mediterranean June grass): similar to large blue hairgrass (*K. glauca*) with greener leaves and good heat tolerance.

LUZULA
WOODRUSH

Woodrushes are members of the rush family, Juncaceae, and constitute a group of plants found mainly in rich, moist woodlands in temperate climates. Many of the more than 80 species of woodrushes are welcome additions to any garden. As a group, they tend to be moisture and shade loving, their flowers blooming along with the earliest of the grasses and their allies.

Most woodrushes have grasslike leaves either edged or covered by soft, downy hairs. These hairs catch and hold morning dew, causing the plant to sparkle (hence the genus name *Luzula,* from the Latin *Luciola,* "glowworm"). Wood-rushes usually have showy flowers that bloom as early as February in some parts of the country. Their soft foliage makes a worthy companion for newly emerging bulbs, and they add charm to a woodland garden. Many areas of the United States contain native woodrush species, although most described here are European in origin. It can be hoped that more of our native woodrushes will find their way into American nurseries and garden centers.

BOTANICAL NAME	**Luzula nivea**
PRONUNCIATION	loo-ZOO-lah NIV-ee-ah
COMMON NAME	Snowy woodrush
USDA HARDINESS ZONE	4 to 9
ORIGIN	Northeastern Spain, central France, Italy, Yugoslavia
PREFERRED SITES	Open mountains; forests with moist, loamy humus

DESCRIPTION: Charming snowy woodrush has gray-green foliage covered by soft, downy hairs. Perhaps the most ornamental of all the woodrushes, its small size and ease of culture make it a fine addition to almost any garden. The leaves, ⅛ to ¼ inch wide and 6 to 8 inches long, form clumps of evergreen foliage 8 to 12 inches tall and as wide. Showy white flowers emerge on spikes 12 to 16 inches above the foliage. The flowers are fluffy white umbels, ½ to ¾ inch across, that dry to tannish brown and persist above the foliage.

LANDSCAPE USES: Snowy woodrush is a choice groundcover in moist, shady locations. While effective planted in masses and groups, snowy woodrush also makes a fine single specimen in a shady border. Some of the first blooms to appear in a spring border, the flowers are attractive in fresh or dried arrangements.

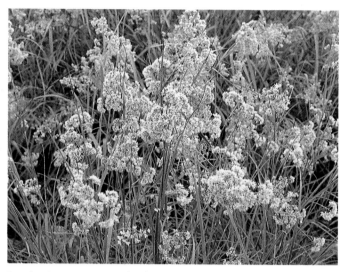

Luzula nivea, snowy woodrush.

CULTURE AND PROPAGATION: Snowy woodrush grows best in moist soil rich in humus in light shade. It is suprisingly tolerant of less than perfect conditions. Given adequate moisture and shade, it has performed well on the West Coast of the United States as far south as Los Angeles. While tolerant of full sun in colder climates, it will burn in hot inland climates if not given shade.

Propagate by seed, or by division in spring.

PESTS AND PROBLEMS: Snowy woodrush has no known pests or problems.

SOME **Luzula nivea** CULTIVARS ARE:

'Schneehaeschen' (Snow hare snowy woodrush): long-haired white flowers; grows to 18 inches tall.

'Snowbird' ('Snowbird' snowy woodrush): broader, hairy, gray leaves and pure white flowers.

ANOTHER SPECIES OF WOODRUSH IS:

Luzula pilosa (Hairy wood-rush): compact, evergreen foliage; grows 4 to 6 inches tall; clothed in downy hairs.

ONE CULTIVAR OF **Luzula pilosa** IS:

'Gruenfink' (Green finch woodrush): fresh green cultivar with improved color and foliage.

BOTANICAL NAME	***Luzula purpurea***
PRONUNCIATION	loo-ZOO-lah pur-PUR-ee-ah
COMMON NAME	Purple woodrush
USDA HARDINESS ZONE	6 to 8
ORIGIN	Europe
PREFERRED SITES	Woodlands, moist forest understory

DESCRIPTION: Similar to hairy woodrush (*Luzula pilosa*), purple woodrush is distinguished by reddish purple foliage in fall and winter. A compact, clumping plant that grows 4 to 6 inches tall and as wide, purple woodrush has glossy, medium green leaves ¼ to ½ inch wide and 4 to 8 inches long, edged with downy hairs. The foliage of purple woodrush darkens as the season progresses; by fall, it turns reddish purple or often somewhat mottled green and red. The flowers are noticeable but not showy, growing 3 to 4 inches above the foliage in April and May.

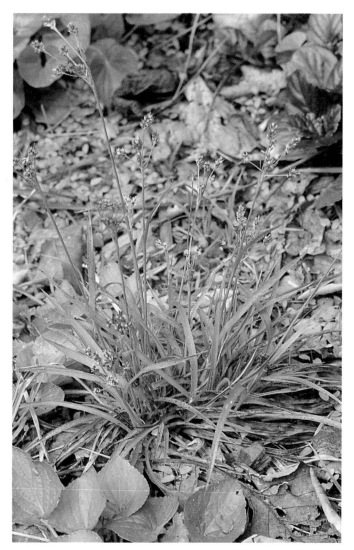

Luzula purpurea, purple woodrush.

LANDSCAPE USES: Purple woodrush makes a good groundcover under deciduous trees and shrubs. It is most effective planted in groups or masses and will naturalize in rock gardens and along pathways. Its reddish fall color makes a fine seasonal display.

CULTURE AND PROPAGATION: Purple woodrush prefers moist, acid, humus-rich soil in light to medium shade. Under these conditions, it will reseed itself copiously. It does not like hot climates in full sun; the hotter the climate, the more compact it will grow.

Propagate by seed, or by division in fall or spring; fall divisions need some protection from winter cold.

PESTS AND PROBLEMS: Purple woodrush has no known pests or problems.

BOTANICAL NAME	***Luzula sylvatica* (also known as *L. maxima*)**
PRONUNCIATION	loo-ZOO-lah sill-VAH-tee-kah
COMMON NAME	Greater woodrush, sylvan woodrush
USDA HARDINESS ZONE	4 to 9
ORIGIN	Southwestern and central Europe
PREFERRED SITES	Forest understory, humus-rich soils

DESCRIPTION: This clumping, evergreen woodrush forms lush mounds of matlike foliage 8 to 12 inches tall. Its leaves, ½ to ¾ inch wide and 8 to 10 inches long, are bright green on emergence in the spring. The flush of new spring growth is both showy and enchanting, as the leaves catch and hold droplets of water, causing them to sparkle in bright spring light. The glossy leaves are soft with fine, whitish hairs. As the season progresses, the leaves mature to medium green. The foliage is evergreen in all but the coldest climates, although hard freezes may turn it brown. Flowers emerge in March in warmer climates and in April through May in cooler climates. The yellow-green flowers are borne in erect spikes 12 to 18 inches above the foliage and mature to chestnut brown.

LANDSCAPE USES: Perhaps one of the best ornamental grasses for shady woodland sites, greater woodrush is both beautiful and utilitarian. Its soft green foliage is one of the first signs of spring. Its ability not just to survive, but to thrive, in shade, in moisture, and in competition with tree roots makes it an invaluable plant for the woodland setting.

Greater woodrush is a fine groundcover in light to medium shade. While interesting as a single specimen, it is most attractive when massed in groups. It is well-suited for naturalizing in moist, shady areas and as an understory for woody deciduous shrubs. Greater woodrush is an ideal companion plant for ferns and woodland displays, and it sets off the beautiful foliage of hostas.

CULTURE AND PROPAGATION: Greater woodrush prefers acid soil with plenty of moisture and light to medium shade. This grass is surprisingly tolerant of drier, less than ideal soil. Extremely cold-hardy, it can be successfully grown in Southern California if given light shade and moisture.

Propagate by seed, or by division in spring or fall; divisons not yet established by fall will need frost protection. Since cultivars are variable from seed, propagate them by division only.

PESTS AND PROBLEMS: Greater woodrush has no known pests or problems.

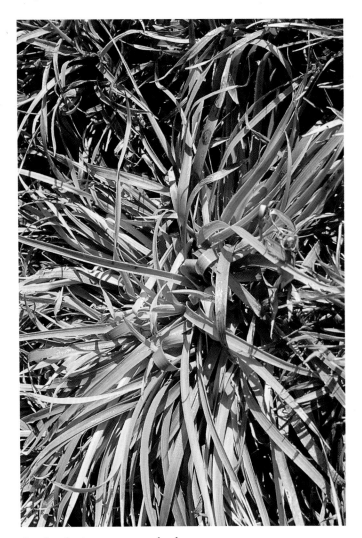

Luzula sylvatica, greater woodrush.

SOME *Luzula sylvatica* CULTIVARS ARE:

'Farnfreund' (Fern friend woodrush): compact cultivar of German origin.

'Hohe Tatra' (High tatra woodrush): a high-elevation selection; forms upright tufts, distinctly hairy leaves.

'Marginata' (Golden-edged woodrush): leaves have a thin, golden yellow edge.

'Tauern Pass' ('Tauern Pass' woodrush): matlike habit; resists winter browning.

BOTANICAL NAME	*Melica altissima*
PRONUNCIATION	MEL-ih-kah al-TIS-ih-mah
COMMON NAME	Siberian melic
USDA HARDINESS ZONE	4 to 8
ORIGIN	Central Europe into Russia
PREFERRED SITES	Open woods, meadows

DESCRIPTION: Siberian melic is a clumping, cool-season-growing, deciduous grass. Its glossy green foliage, ⅜ to ¾ inch wide and 8 inches long, forms loose tufts. The showy flowers are a narrow panicle that grows 1 to 2 feet above the foliage. The flowers vary from white to tawny to purple on emergence in June through July and flop over with age.

LANDSCAPE USES: Siberian melic is a showy flowering accent for lightly shaded woodland settings. Good for planting in groups and massing in clearings of deciduous woods, Siberian melic also makes an effective mid-border or back-of-the-border flowering grass for early summer appeal. It naturalizes well in woodland gardens.

CULTURE AND PROPAGATION: Siberian melic prefers moist, well-drained, humus-rich soil in light shade. It resents hot, dry situations or heavy, wet, poorly drained soil and does not grow well in hot-summer climates.

Propagation is easy by seed or division. Propagate cultivars from division, since they may not come true from seed.

PESTS AND PROBLEMS: Siberian melic has no known pests or problems.

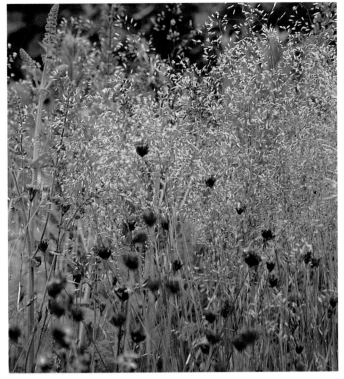

Melica altissima, Siberian melic.

SOME ***Melica altissima*** CULTIVARS ARE:

'Alba' (White Siberian
melic): pure white flowers.

'Atropurpurea' (Purple
Siberian melic): dark purple flowers in early sum-
mer.

BOTANICAL NAME	***Melica ciliata***
PRONUNCIATION	MEL-ih-kah sil-ee-AH-tah
COMMON NAME	Hairy melic, silky spike melic
USDA HARDINESS ZONE	5 to 8
ORIGIN	Europe, northern Africa
PREFERRED SITES	Rocky limestone slopes, sunny meadows

DESCRIPTION: Clumping, cool-season-growing, and deciduous, hairy melic has gray-green leaves, ¼ to ⅜ inch wide
and 8 to 12 inches long, forming loose tufts of foliage 10 to
12 inches tall and as wide. Showy flowers are spikelike,
fluffy white panicles arching 12 to 18 inches above the
foliage in early June, then covering the foliage and draping
out over the plant. Flowers fade by July.

LANDSCAPE USES: Hairy melic makes an excellent early
summer-flowering accent in the garden. It is especially
attractive when late afternoon light shines through the
flower heads, and is a lovely addition to cut flower arrangements.

CULTURE AND PROPAGATION: Hairy melic likes moist, well-
drained, fertile soil and sun. Good drainage is essential for
healthy growth, but plants resent completely dry soil and
full, hot sun. Hairy melic grows best in light shade or part-
day shade and stops growing in the summer heat.

   Propagation is easy by seed, or by division in spring or
fall.

PESTS AND PROBLEMS: Hairy melic's flowers tend to be somewhat weak and floppy. It may need staking if in a border.
Remove the flowers after they bloom, as they tend to look
shabby. Plant hairy melic where it will be hidden by
groundcovers or other plants by July.

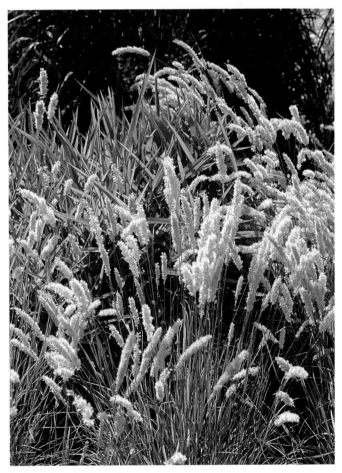

Melica ciliata, hairy melic.

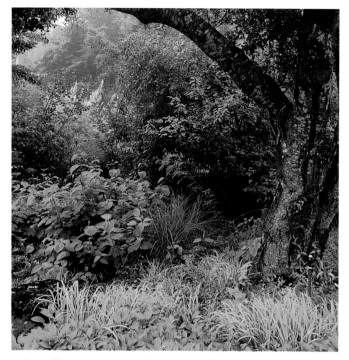

Milium effusum 'Aureum', golden wood millet.

BOTANICAL NAME	***Milium effusum* 'Aureum'**
PRONUNCIATION	MIL-ee-um eh-FYOO-sum AW-ree-um
COMMON NAME	Golden wood millet
USDA HARDINESS ZONE	6 to 9
ORIGIN	Species native to North America, Eurasia; 'Aureum' is a horticultural selection
PREFERRED SITES	Shady, moist meadows

DESCRIPTION: Golden wood millet is a loosely clumping, cool-season-growing, evergreen grass distinguished by golden yellow foliage and flowers. Its glossy leaves, ¼ to ½ inch wide and 12 inches long, form attractive clumps of foliage 6 to 18 inches tall. The flush of new spring growth is intensely yellow, fading to yellow-green as the season progresses. The flowers emerge 12 to 18 inches above the foliage from May through June. Golden yellow panicles look like delicate fountains that are transparent, yet shimmering. Plant growth tends to slow down after blooming.

LANDSCAPE USES: Golden wood millet is a stunning accent for both its foliage color and its graceful flowering habit. Effective planted alone or in groups, it can brighten up a dark area of the garden. It is a good choice for woodland gardens and perennial borders, and is a good plant to grow in rock gardens and in plantings that also contain ferns and hostas.

CULTURE AND PROPAGATION: Golden wood millet prefers cool, moist, fertile soil in light shade. It tolerates less than favorable conditions and considerable shade. Plants resent full sun in hot climates. One of the best ornamental grasses for shady sites, golden wood millet can be grown in hotter climates if properly situated and given at least partial shade, constant moisture, and good drainage.

Propagation is best by division, but plants will come mostly true from seed. Bright yellow plants are best propagated by division.

PESTS AND PROBLEMS: Golden wood millet has no known pests or problems.

MISCANTHUS
MAIDEN GRASS, SILVER GRASS, EULALIA

As a group, the genus *Miscanthus* includes some of the showiest and most beautiful of the flowering grasses. Selections from this genus, which is perhaps the royalty of the grass kingdom, range from 3-foot gems to 15-foot giants. Most are tough yet graceful performers—undemanding and satisfying garden subjects. The more than 20 species and 50 cultivars (with more arriving each year) assure maiden grass a place in almost any garden in America. A variety of hardiness characteristics, habits, sizes, and blooming periods gives gardeners a wide range of plants from which to choose.

Some species and cultivars spread from rhizomes; others make tight clumps. Some bloom in early spring; others bloom in the fall. Plants come in a wide array of variegations: white, yellow, or silver, with vertical banding. Some have brilliant fall colors: orange, red, yellow, purple, or mixtures of several colors.

This group is most appreciated, however, for its spectacular flowers. Emerging as silky tassels, pink, bronze, tan, silver, or multicolored, the flowers mature to fluffy plumes, showy and persistent well into winter. The plants are unsurpassed in providing a flowering accent, and their foliage and plumes add beauty and movement to the garden.

Many of the newer cultivars of maiden grass have been selected because they overcome the species' shortcomings: floppiness, flowers at foliage level, late flowering, and variable fall color. Yet despite these traits, maiden grass remains a choice ornamental grass where its billowy fine texture has the room to strut its stuff.

Many of the plants described here are currently or just now being offered in U.S. nurseries and garden centers. Many more may soon follow. Being new, many of these cultivars are untested in American gardens; when this is the case, it will be noted. Many may be hard to find and are available only through specialty nurseries (see Sources, page 180).

BOTANICAL NAME	**_Miscanthus giganteus_ (also known as _M. floridulus_)**
PRONUNCIATION	mis-KAN-thus jeye-GAN-tee-us
COMMON NAME	Giant Chinese silver grass
USDA HARDINESS ZONE	4 to 9
ORIGIN	China
PREFERRED SITES	Streamsides

DESCRIPTION: Giant Chinese silver grass is a clumping, warm-season-growing, deciduous grass prized for its huge column of robust foliage and tall silvery plumes. It is the largest *Miscanthus* species, sending up canes 2 inches thick and 10 to 14 feet tall. Mature clumps cut to the ground in March reach this height by July, becoming a vertical column of subtropical-looking foliage. Medium green leaves, ¾ to 1½ inches wide and 1 to 2½ feet long, arch out from the stout stems, giving an overall impression of falling water. In August or September, the 8- to 12-inch flowers appear on stalks 1 to 2 feet above the foliage. They emerge as reddish tan silky tassels and mature to fluffy silvery plumes. In cool-summer climates, flowers are often absent, but the foliage and winter effects alone are reasons for planting giant Chinese silver grass. The onset of fall brings a reddish purple stain to the green foliage. As winter progresses, leaves drop from the stout culms, leaving a

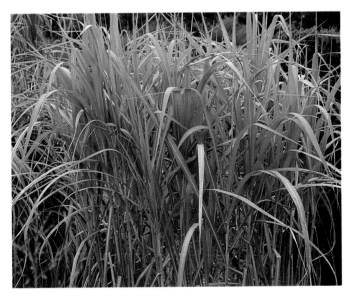

Miscanthus giganteus, giant Chinese silver grass.

striking vertical skeleton. Truly dramatic when thrusting through the snow or backlit against a winter sky, giant Chinese silver grass is a constantly changing player in the garden.

LANDSCAPE USES: Giant Chinese silver grass makes a fine hedge or tall screen in the garden. In hot-summer areas, it is one of the tallest flowering perennial accents available. It is stunning planted alone or in groups. In coastal gardens, it tolerates wind and salt spray. Giant Chinese silver grass grows well in containers as long as the pots or tubs are large. Plant this grass if you want a tropical effect, even in cold climates.

CULTURE AND PROPAGATION: Giant Chinese silver grass grows best in fertile, moist, well-drained soil in full sun. It is tolerant of less than perfect conditions, including partial shade. It will flop in too much shade and is good for windy and coastal sites.

Propagate by seed, or by division in the spring. Hard rhizomes may be difficult to divide, requiring a sharp axe and saw. You might have to use a tractor to remove old stands.

PESTS AND PROBLEMS: Giant Chinese silver grass usually loses its lower leaves by late summer. Plant a filler plant in front if the bare canes are undesirable.

BOTANICAL NAME	**_Miscanthus sacchariflorus_**
PRONUNCIATION	mis-KAN-thus sak-kar-ih-FLOR-us
COMMON NAME	Silver banner grass
USDA HARDINESS ZONE	5 to 9
ORIGIN	Northwestern China to central China, Korea, and Japan
PREFERRED SITES	Moist mountain meadows, streams

DESCRIPTION: Creeping, deciduous silver banner grass has aggressive, spreading rhizomes that form dense colonies. Its foliage grows 4 to 6 feet tall on stout, upright canes. The medium green leaves, ½ to ¾ inch wide and 8 to 10 inches long, are lush-looking. In the fall the color changes to an attractive orange-brown. The flowers bloom in August, rising 2 to 3 feet above the foliage. Whisklike and bright silver, the flowers remain showy into winter. Silver banner grass is one of the hardiest, most cold-tolerant species of *Miscanthus.*

LANDSCAPE USES: Silver banner grass is at its best massed along the water's edge. Its colonizing habit can be both a boon and a bane in the garden. Given plenty of room, silver banner grass is a fine choice; in smaller gardens it can easily become a pest. It is a good choice for water gardens since it will grow in shallow water.

CULTURE AND PROPAGATION: Silver banner grass grows best in wet, fertile soil in full sun. Plants do poorly in dry situations and may not flower. The grass grows slowly in heavy clays and will not spread as rapidly into dry areas. Plants seem to require cold and humidity to perform well. Large drainage tiles or pots will confine the rhizomes.

Propagate by seed, or by division in the spring.

PESTS AND PROBLEMS: Because of the warm, dry climate in Southern California, silver banner grass grows poorly there. Plants may only reach 2 to 3 feet tall and will languish without constant moisture.

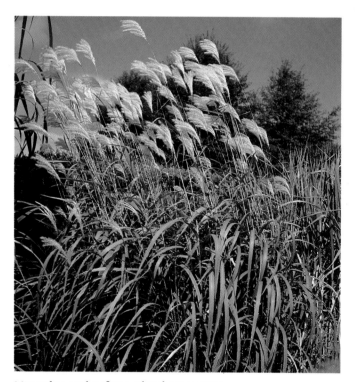

Miscanthus sacchariflorus, silver banner grass.

ONE CULTIVAR OF ***Miscanthus sacchariflorus*** IS:

'Robustus' (Giant silver banner grass): reaches 5 to 8 feet tall; a better bloomer for cool climates.

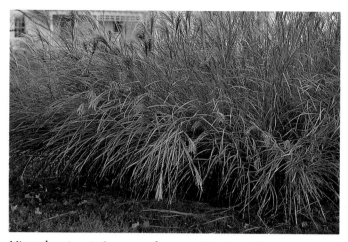

Miscanthus sinensis, Japanese silver grass, in winter dormancy.

BOTANICAL NAME	***Miscanthus sinensis***
PRONUNCIATION	mis-KAN-thus sin-EN-sis
COMMON NAME	Japanese silver grass, eulalia
USDA HARDINESS ZONE	5 to 9
ORIGIN	Cultivated in China and Japan. Some cultivars are reported to have been grown by the Japanese for hundreds of years.
PREFERRED SITES	Moist streamsides, meadows

DESCRIPTION: Japanese silver grass and its cultivars comprise some of the most desirable ornamental grasses grown today. Important cultivars will be described individually.

Japanese silver grass is a clumping, warm-season grass. Depending upon the latitude, plants begin to grow in March or April and begin to show their attractive foliage by May or June. Showy whisklike plumes begin to flower from July through September. Flowers range from silver to tan to reddish-purple on emergence, and dry to fluffy heads by fall. The fall foliage varies from tan and brown to brilliant red-orange and yellow. Except in mild climates, most cultivars are completely dry and dormant by December.

LANDSCAPE USES: Japanese silver grass makes an effective tall background, hedge, or screen. Its large-flowering accent provides exceptional fall color. Well-suited to water gardens at or near the water's edge, it also grows in shallow water and ponds. It is desirable for large-scale landscaping, such as along highways and on golf courses. Japanese silver grass makes a good coastal planting.

CULTURE AND PROPAGATION: Culture varies somewhat among cultivars, but most prefer moist, rich soil in full sun. Some are happy growing in water; others, once established, tolerate some measure of drought. Hardiness varies among cultivars, but most will tolerate Zone 6 with ease; some tolerate even colder temperatures. Plants struggle in hot, humid southerly climates; narrower-leaved varieties seem to handle heat and drought with greater ease.

Propagate by seed or division. It is best to propagate selected cultivars by division, since propagation by seed is variable.

PESTS AND PROBLEMS: Most Japanese silver grasses are pest- and trouble-free, with a few exceptions. Some have a tendency to flop with age and may require staking or tying to remain upright. Some tend to die out in the center and require lifting and dividing after four years or so. Some suffer from rust in periods conducive to rust disease; if left untreated, the rust will usually disappear with drier weather. Some may get mealybugs. Standard treatments (see page 23) will gain effective control, although only severe infestations seem to affect the vigor of the plants.

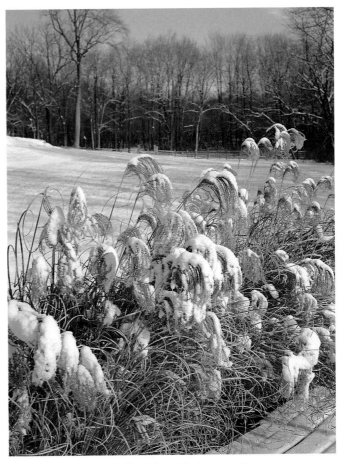

Miscanthus sinensis 'Gracillimus', maiden grass, with winter snow.

BOTANICAL NAME	***Miscanthus sinensis*** **'Cabaret'**
PRONUNCIATION	mis-KAN-thus sin-EN-sis
COMMON NAME	'Cabaret' Japanese silver grass

DESCRIPTION: 'Cabaret' Japanese silver grass has wide, ribbonlike foliage with milky white, linear-striped centers. The bright white centers and dark green leaf margins make a bold accent or focal point in the garden. The robust, upright, 6-foot-tall foliage is topped by copper-colored flowers in mid-September. The flower stems blush pink as they mature, and the flowers fluff to cream color with age. This introduction may be hard to find in nurseries, but is worth looking for.

BOTANICAL NAME	***Miscanthus sinensis*** **'Gracillimus'**
PRONUNCIATION	mis-KAN-thus sin-EN-sis gra-SILL-ih-mus
COMMON NAME	Maiden grass

DESCRIPTION: One of the oldest maiden grass cultivars in the nursery trade, the fine texture and showy flowers of *Miscanthus sinensis* 'Gracillimus' have made it one of the most popular of the ornamental grasses. The narrow, silver, midribbed leaves, ¼ to ½ inch wide, form stiffly erect clumps of foliage 5 to 6 feet tall. Depending on their location, the clumps tend to flop in the third or fourth year and require staking or division to stand upright. The fall foliage color varies from region to region: bright orange in the South and Southwest; green in fall, turning bright orange in December, in the West; and bleaching from green to almond, with relatively little orange in between, in the East. The copper-colored flowers appear in late September, rising 1 to 1½ feet above the foliage, although they often fail to bloom in areas with cool summers. The flowers mature to silver and remain showy into the winter months.

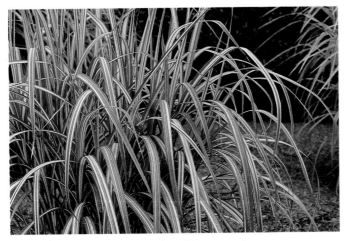

Miscanthus sinensis 'Cabaret', 'Cabaret' Japanese silver grass.

BOTANICAL NAME	***Miscanthus sinensis*** **'Morning Light' (also known as *M. sinensis* 'Gracillimus Variegatus')**
PRONUNCIATION	mis-KAN-thus sin-EN-sis
COMMON NAME	'Morning Light' Japanese silver grass

DESCRIPTION: The handsome foliage and showy flowers of 'Morning Light' Japanese silver grass are prized by gardeners across the country. Similar to *Miscanthus sinensis* 'Gracillimus' in leaf size and texture, 'Morning Light' Japanese silver grass has a narrow band of clear white on the leaf margins. The fine-textured leaves appear silver at a distance and give the plant an almost ghostly luminosity. The upright, arching foliage grows 4 to 5 feet tall, with flowers 5 to 6 feet tall. The flowers bloom late, usually in October, emerging reddish bronze and drying to fluffy cream. Many consider 'Morning Light' Japanese silver grass (introduced by the U.S. National Arboretum in Washington, D.C.) one of the finest cultivars of the recent ornamental grass introductions.

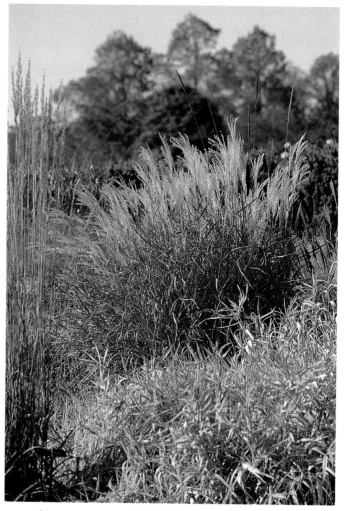

Miscanthus sinensis 'Purpurascens', flame grass, in blazing autumn color.

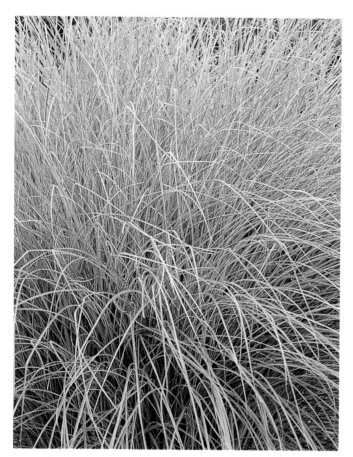

Miscanthus sinensis 'Morning Light', 'Morning Light' Japanese silver grass.

BOTANICAL NAME	***Miscanthus sinensis*** **'Purpurascens'**
PRONUNCIATION	mis-KAN-thus sin-EN-sis pur-pur-AH-senz
COMMON NAME	Flame grass, purple silver grass

DESCRIPTION: A handsome, compact selection, flame grass stands out in the garden with its brilliant orange-red fall color. Although weak-growing in hot climates, it is one of the best *Miscanthus* cultivars available when grown in preferred areas. Its compact, medium green foliage has a reddish tint. The leaves, ¼ to ½ inch wide, form tight, upright clumps 3 to 4 feet tall. Flowers emerge in July and August as showy silvery plumes 1 to 2 feet over the foliage. Flame grass begins to change color in September, eventually becoming a dazzling red-orange. Later in the fall, it darkens to a burnt reddish brown that remains attractive well into winter. It grows best in Zones 7 to 8.

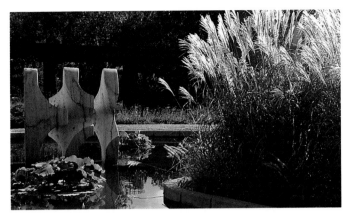

Miscanthus sinensis 'Silberfeder', silver feather maiden grass.

BOTANICAL NAME	***Miscanthus sinensis* 'Silberfeder'**
PRONUNCIATION	mis-KAN-thus sin-EN-sis SIL-ber-FEH-der
COMMON NAME	Silver feather maiden grass

DESCRIPTION: An older European selection, silver feather maiden grass remains one of the best maiden grass cultivars available today. Its rich green foliage has an attractive silver midrib. The foliage grows 5 to 6 feet tall and as wide in a graceful arching vase shape. The flowers are borne 2 to 3 feet above the foliage and are held well above the leaves, providing a distinct separation of foliage and flower. The flowers are silky and silvery upon emergence in August and make a fine show from summer well into winter. Stake older clumps to keep them upright.

BOTANICAL NAME	***Miscanthus sinensis* var. *strictus***
PRONUNCIATION	mis-KAN-thus sin-EN-sis STRIK-tus
COMMON NAME	Porcupine grass, banded miscanthus (incorrectly known as zebra grass)
USDA HARDINESS ZONE	4 to 9
ORIGIN	Horticultural selection
PREFERRED SITES	Moist, fertile areas

DESCRIPTION: Clumping porcupine grass is distinguished by bright yellow variegation in horizontal bands on the leaves. Its narrow, upright form is accented by stiff, upward-pointing leaves resembling porcupine quills. The foliage is similar to that of zebra grass (*Miscanthus sinensis* 'Ze-

brinus'). The two plants differ primarily in form and hardiness, zebra grass being lax and porcupine grass being tight, upright, and considerably hardier, surviving in Zone 4. The leaves of porcupine grass are ⅜ to ½ inch wide and 8 to 12 inches long, arching stiffly at a nearly 45-degree angle from the stems. The foliage grows 4 to 6 feet in neat, vertical clumps. The flowers bloom copper in September and rise 1 to 2 feet above the foliage. Porcupine grass's flowers dry to a fluffy tan, and the foliage turns straw-colored with the first frost.

LANDSCAPE USES: The foliage and flowers of porcupine grass provide a dramatic garden accent. The column of banded foliage is particularly effective when backlit by early morning or late afternoon light. Porcupine grass grows in or around ponds and pools and casts a beautiful reflection. It tolerates coastal conditions if the soil is sufficiently moist.

CULTURE AND PROPAGATION: Porcupine grass prefers moist, fertile soil in full sun. It grows in water up to 2 to 4 inches deep and tolerates wet, boggy soil. It also grows in light shade and in hot, inland climates and always looks better with light afternoon shade.

Propagate by division in the spring.

PESTS AND PROBLEMS: Porcupine grass has no known pests or problems.

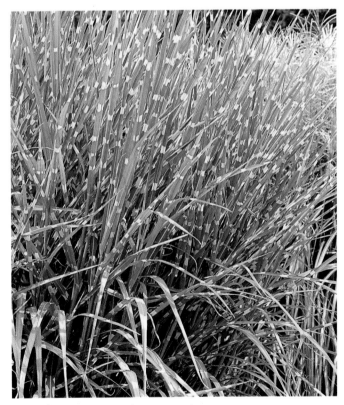

Miscanthus sinensis var. *strictus,* porcupine grass.

BOTANICAL NAME	***Miscanthus sinensis*** 'Variegatus'
PRONUNCIATION	mis-KAN-thus sin-EN-sis var-ee-uh-GAH-tus
COMMON NAME	Variegated Japanese silver grass

DESCRIPTION: One of the oldest cultivars of Japanese silver grass available, variegated Japanese silver grass has been used in gardens since 1900 and continues to be popular today. Its leaves, ¼ to ¾ inch wide, are white-striped. The loose, often flopping clumps reach 4 to 6 feet tall and as wide. The flowers rise 1 to 2 feet above the foliage in August and September. In fall, the foliage blanches almond. Variegated Japanese silver grass is widely adaptable, growing from San Francisco to Atlanta, and is surprisingly shade-tolerant. It will flop, however, if grown in too much shade. Older plants usually require staking. In hot southern and western climates, plant in light shade to prevent sunburned foliage.

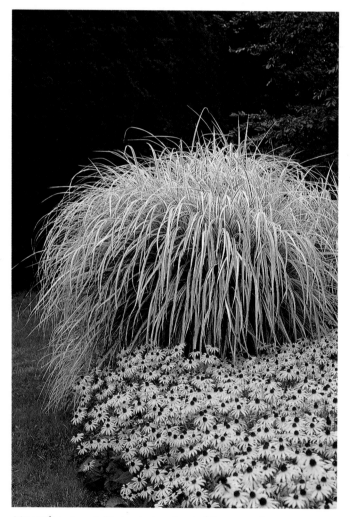

Miscanthus sinensis 'Variegatus', variegated Japanese silver grass.

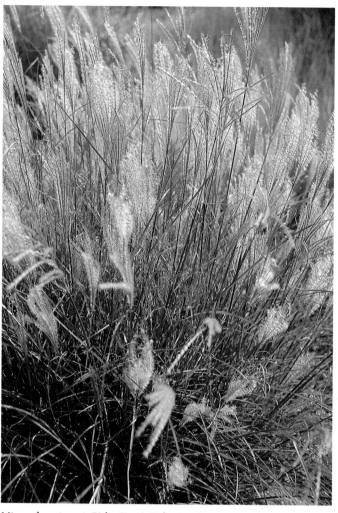

Miscanthus sinensis 'Yaku Jima', 'Yaku Jima' Japanese silver grass.

BOTANICAL NAME	***Miscanthus sinensis*** 'Yaku Jima'
PRONUNCIATION	mis-KAN-thus sin-EN-sis YAH-koo JEE-mah
COMMON NAME	'Yaku Jima' Japanese silver grass

DESCRIPTION: 'Yaku Jima' Japanese silver grass is a fine selection for small gardens. Its compact, fine-textured foliage, 3 to 4 feet tall, turns reddish brown in the fall, and the plant remains attractive well into winter. The reddish flowers are showy, though not quite as fluffy as most Japanese silver grass cultivars. They emerge in mid-September and often fail to rise much taller than the foliage, though they can grow 1 to 1½ feet above the leaves. One of the first compact *Miscanthus* cultivars, 'Yaku Jima' Japanese silver grass is now sometimes passed over for newer cultivars with showier flowers and better separation of foliage and flower, such as the dwarf 'Nippon' maiden grass (*M. sinensis* 'Nippon').

BOTANICAL NAME	**Miscanthus sinensis 'Zebrinus'**
PRONUNCIATION	mis-KAN-thus sin-EN-sis zeh-BREYE-nus
COMMON NAME	Zebra grass, banded miscanthus

DESCRIPTION: Zebra grass is a popular garden cultivar distinguished by its large, arching foliage and the yellowish white bands across the leaves. The leaves, ½ to ¾ inch wide and 1 ½ to 2 ½ feet long, arch lazily outward in broad, spreading clumps. The foliage clumps reach 5 to 6 feet tall and as wide, and turn brown with the first frost. The flowers bloom a pinkish copper in September, 1 to 2 feet above the foliage, and become fluffy as they mature. The large foliage and flowers of zebra grass make it a striking accent in the garden. Its size makes it effective as a single specimen, but it also looks attractive in groups, especially along the water's edge. The bright bands of variegation on the leaves sparkle like diamonds when backlit by early morning or late afternoon light. Plants usually flop with age and require staking to prevent sprawling. Yellow banding on this cultivar does not show on the foliage until early summer.

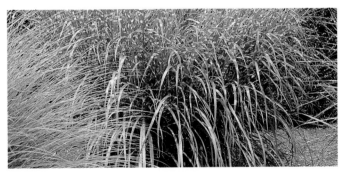

Miscanthus sinensis 'Zebrinus', zebra grass.

OTHER **Miscanthus sinensis** CULTIVARS AND VARIETIES ARE:

'Adagio' ('Adagio' Japanese silver grass): compact, silver-gray foliage grows to 2 feet tall; flowers emerge pink, becoming white.

'Arabesque' ('Arabesque' Japanese silver grass): compact grower.

'Autumn Light' ('Autumn Light' Japanese silver grass): robust grower; good yellowish fall color; extremely hardy.

Miscanthus sinensis var. *condensatus* (Purple-blooming Japanese silver grass): similar to *M. sinensis* with purplish-tinted flowers; early-blooming.

M. sinensis var. *condensatus* 'Silberpfeil' (Variegated silver arrow grass): similar to variegated Japanese silver grass (*M. sinensis* 'Variegatus') with brighter white variegation and less tendency to flop.

'Cosmopolitan' ('Cosmopolitan' Japanese silver grass): an improved form of *M. sinensis* 'Variegatus' with robust, wide leaves and a non-floppy habit; considered one of the best variegated maiden grasses.

'Emerald Shadow' ('Emerald Shadow' Japanese silver grass): velvety smooth 1-inch-wide leaves.

'Goldfeder' (Golden feather Japanese silver grass): green-centered, golden-edged leaves.

'Goliath' ('Goliath' Japanese silver grass): a vigorous selection; foliage grows 6 to 7 feet tall; flowers grow 2 to 3 feet above the foliage from August through September.

'Gracillimus Nana' (Dwarf Japanese silver grass): dwarf form.

'Graziella' ('Graziella' Japanese silver grass): foliage grows 4 to 5 feet tall; showy white flowers; good separation between foliage and flower.

'Grosse Fontaine' (Large fountain Japanese silver grass): cascading, fountainlike foliage; silvery plumes in August.

'Herbstfeuer' (Autumn fire Japanese silver grass): tall selection, grows to 4 feet; does poorly in hot climates of the South and West.

'Juli' (July Japanese silver grass): hybrid, producing a July-flowering plant; red flowers.

'Kaskade' (Cascade Japanese silver grass): cascading pink flowers; an outstanding new introduction.

'Kleine Fontaine' (Little fountain Japanese silver grass): compact grower.

'Malepartus' ('Malepartus' Japanese silver grass): robust-growing, with large flowers that emerge purplish pink and mature to silver; foliage bronzes in late summer.

'Nippon' ('Nippon' silver grass): exciting new compact selection; fine-textured foliage; good red-bronze fall color.

'November Sunset' ('November Sunset' Japanese silver grass): robust foliage; good yellow-orange fall color.

'Positano' ('Positano' Japanese silver grass): graceful, arching foliage with showy red flowers; good yellow-orange fall color.

(continued on next page)

'Puenktchen' (Little dot Japanese silver grass): an improved selection; fine-textured.

'Roland' ('Roland' Japanese silver grass): a large, robust cultivar blooming in August.

'Rotsilber' (Red-Silver Japanese silver grass): delightful 2- to 3-foot red flowers; attractive fall color to its silvery foliage.

'Sarabande' ('Sarabande' Japanese silver grass): fine-textured with silvery foliage.

'Silberspinne' (Silver spider Japanese silver grass): fine-textured, silvery foliage and unique spidery flowers.

'Silberturm' (Silver tower Japanese silver grass): upright, tall cultivar with silver flowers growing 8 to 10 feet tall.

'Sirene' (Siren Japanese silver grass): free-flowering, tall-growing; has a good separation of foliage and flower.

'Undine' ('Undine' Japanese silver grass): silvery white flowers on slender culms; noted for good fall color.

'Wetterfane' (Weather vane Japanese silver grass): distinct foliage with good reddish fall color.

'Zwergelefant' (Gnome elephant Japanese silver grass): free-blooming compact cultivar with silvery pink flowers.

plumes arch up and out 2 to 3 feet from the foliage, giving the plant a feathery, airy appearance. They become tan and fluffy with maturity. Though covered with flowers, the openness and delicacy of the spikes allow a view through the plant. In mild climates, the flowers are showy on the plant from May through November as flower production never seems to cease. In cold-winter areas, seeds are shed by November; the seed heads are not showy. Flower spikes often reach 7 feet under ideal conditions.

LANDSCAPE USES: Evergreen miscanthus makes an ideal large-scale groundcover and is gorgeous planted in groups. It makes an effective flowering accent for the middle or back of a perennial border and is also good in pots and tubs. It is one of the best maiden grasses for small gardens and for adding movement to the garden, since its airy flowers always seem to be in motion.

CULTURE AND PROPAGATION: Evergreen miscanthus prefers moist, fertile soil in full sun or light shade. It tolerates a wide range of conditions, from heavy to sandy soils and moist to dry situations. The plants resent long periods of drought but tolerate heat if soil is sufficiently moist. If the

BOTANICAL NAME	***Miscanthus transmorrisonensis***
PRONUNCIATION	mis-KAN-thus tranz-mor-ih-son-EN-sis
COMMON NAME	Evergreen miscanthus, Formosa maiden grass
USDA HARDINESS ZONE	7 to 10
ORIGIN	Taiwan
PREFERRED SITES	Moist areas, streamsides at higher elevations

DESCRIPTION: Evergreen miscanthus is an exciting new introduction that should have a great impact on western and southern gardens, where it will often remain wholly evergreen. Graced by showy flowers and hardy to Zone 7, this attractive, compact, clumping grass is bound to win over gardeners across the country. A warm-season grass, evergreen miscanthus has glossy green, narrow leaves, ¼ to ½ inch wide and 2 to 3 feet long, that form dense clumps 2½ to 3½ feet tall and as wide. In mild climates, flowers begin to appear in April; in cooler climates, in July and August. The silky, reddish brown, 6- to 8-inch-long flower

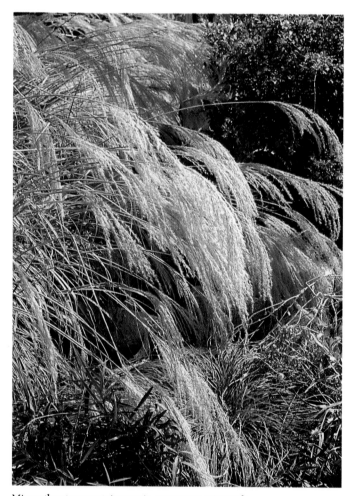

Miscanthus transmorrisonensis, evergreen miscanthus.

soil is too dry, the leaf tips will brown. Evergreen miscanthus takes light shade, but will not bloom as heavily in too much shade. It tolerates coastal conditions if moisture is sufficient.

Propagate by seed, or by division in spring or fall.

PESTS AND PROBLEMS: Evergreen miscanthus has no known pests or problems.

ANOTHER SPECIES OF MAIDEN GRASS IS:

Miscanthus oligostachys
(Small Japanese silver grass): a compact species with showy flowers reaching 3 to 4 feet; best in cool-summer climates.

MOLINIA
MOOR GRASS

This tiny group of Eurasian grasses has some of the showiest flowers of all ornamental grasses. Mostly warm-season grasses, moor grasses are easy to grow, and range in size from miniature to giant. In addition to showy flowers, most have handsome clumping foliage and brilliant fall colors. Most moor grasses have bright yellow to yellow-orange fall foliage that glows in the autumn light.

The flowers are borne in upright spikes that may be numerous and reach 6 to 7 feet tall. You can usually see through the mass of flowers, which creates a transparent curtainlike effect and adds drama to the garden.

Moor grasses differ from most other deciduous grasses. Most of these grasses go dormant but retain their strawy foliage over winter, whereas when moor grasses become completely dormant, the foliage detaches from hardened bulbous structures at the crown of the plant. This means the foliage shatters to the ground, especially in rainy or snowy weather. Though not showy in winter like many ornamental grasses, moor grasses are well worth using for their rich autumn colors and beautiful flowers.

Most moor grasses are slow to establish, and plants may not bloom well until their second or third year in the garden. Start with the largest possible plants for a quicker show. Most moor grasses prefer full sun, rich soil, and constant moisture to look their best. Moor grasses are never invasive. There are many cultivars for a variety of garden uses.

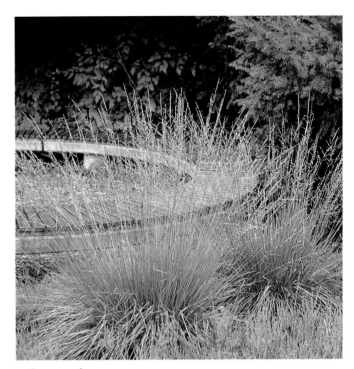

Molinia caerulea, moor grass.

BOTANICAL NAME	***Molinia caerulea***
PRONUNCIATION	moh-LIN-ee-ah ser-OO-lee-ah
COMMON NAME	Moor grass, purple moor grass
USDA HARDINESS ZONE	4 to 9
ORIGIN	Eurasia
PREFERRED SITES	Acid soils, boggy heaths, seasonally wet meadows, open woodlands

DESCRIPTION: Moor grass and its cultivars constitute some of the best ornamental grasses for American gardens. Their handsome foliage, showy flowers, easy culture, and brilliant fall color are welcome in many gardens.

This clumping, hardy, warm-season grass has upright, arching foliage. Its light green leaves are ¼ to ½ inch wide and 6 to 18 inches long, forming neat clumps 1 to 2 feet tall and as wide. Flowers emerge from late June to early July on long, stiff stems 1 to 2 feet above the foliage. The flowers are brownish, yellowish, or purplish on emergence, but fade to a tawny color. They are persistent and showy through fall. In late fall, old flowers and foliage break off at swollen bulbous structures at the base of the stems. Moor grass is one of the few grasses that will clean itself of last year's foliage.

LANDSCAPE USES: Moor grass is a useful accent plant for its flowers and fall color. Plant it either as a single specimen or in masses. It is a good choice for perennial borders. Its flowers enhance fresh or dried arrangements.

CULTURE AND PROPAGATION: Moor grass prefers moist, fertile, acid soil in full sun. It resents dry, alkaline conditions. The grass tolerates light shade and coastal conditions.

Propagate by seed, or by division in the spring. It is best, however, to propagate by division, as moor grass is extremely slow to grow from seed.

PESTS AND PROBLEMS: Moor grass is one of the slowest grasses to mature and flower; small divisions can take three to four seasons to reach maturity. To produce flowers the first season, use large, fist-sized divisions.

OTHER *Molinia caerulea* CULTIVARS ARE:

'Dauerstrahl' (Constant ray moor grass): a compact grower with arching flowers creating a rounded head.

'Heidebraut' (Heather bride moor grass): compact cultivar with erect flower stems.

'Moorflamme' (Moor flame moor grass): another good compact moor grass with good orange-red fall color.

'Moorhexe' (Moor witch moor grass): flowers purplish on emergence on fine-textured flower stems.

'Strahlenquelle' (Fountain spray moor grass): a good compact form with radiating flowers; more arching than the species.

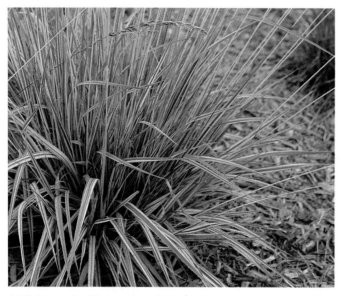

Molinia caerulea 'Variegata', variegated moor grass.

BOTANICAL NAME	*Molinia caerulea* 'Variegata'
PRONUNCIATION	moh-LIN-ee-ah ser-OO-lee-ah ver-ee-uh-GAH-tah
COMMON NAME	Variegated moor grass

DESCRIPTION: Variegated moor grass is, without a doubt, one of the most desirable small ornamental grasses for the perennial border. Similar to moor grass (*Molinia caerulea*) in most aspects, variegated moor grass is distinguished by leaves with creamy yellow-white, linear-striped variegation. The compact foliage grows 12 to 18 inches tall and as wide. Its purple flowers usually reach 6 to 12 inches above the foliage. Flowers fade to a brownish color and are persistent and showy on the plant. This grass is slow to establish and mature. Variegated moor grass is an excellent choice for lightly shaded borders and as an edging and accent.

Propagate by division only in the spring.

BOTANICAL NAME	*Molinia caerulea* subsp. *arundinacea*
PRONUNCIATION	moh-LIN-ee-ah ser-OO-lee-ah ah-run-din-AH-see-ah
COMMON NAME	Tall moor grass, tall purple moor grass
USDA HARDINESS ZONE	5 to 9
ORIGIN	Eurasia
PREFERRED SITES	Wet moorlands, boggy heaths, open woodlands

DESCRIPTION: Tall moor grass is similar in most aspects to moor grass (*Molinia caerulea*) but is distinguished by larger foliage and taller flowers. This warm-season grass has light gray-green foliage, ½ to ¾ inch wide and 12 to 18 inches long. It forms dense, upright, arching clumps 2 to 3 feet tall and as wide. The flowers emerge purplish or brownish in July on erect vertical spikes 3 to 4 feet above the foliage. In

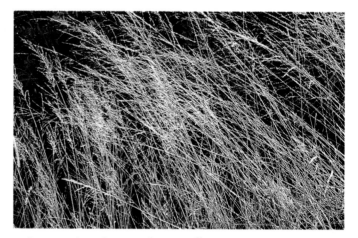

Molinia caerulea subsp. *arundinacea*, tall moor grass.

fall, the foliage and flowers turn bright yellow, providing a blazing autumn display, then they mature to tawny gold. By late fall the foliage and flower spikes shatter and break off at the ground at swollen basal nodes.

Tall moor grass is noted for its strong architectural form and tall, graceful flower stalks that sway in the slightest breeze. This grass is one of the better ornamental grasses for lightly shaded or full-sun borders. A dark background will show off its unique flower stalks. A major drawback is its slow growth rate. Small divisions take three to four seasons to produce good foliage and flowers. To overcome this slow growth rate, start with fist-sized or larger clumps.

BOTANICAL NAME	***Muhlenbergia dumosa***
PRONUNCIATION	myoo-len-BER-jee-ah doo-MOH-sah
COMMON NAME	Bamboo muhly
USDA HARDINESS ZONE	8 to 10
ORIGIN	Southern Arizona, northern Mexico
PREFERRED SITES	Dry, rocky slopes, below 4,000 feet elevation

DESCRIPTION: Clumping, cool-season-growing bamboo muhly has delicate fernlike foliage that resembles a fine-leaved bamboo. The evergreen foliage grows on woody canes that reach 3 to 6 feet tall in graceful, arching clumps. Its light green leaves, $1/16$ to $1/8$ inch wide and 2 to 3 inches long, clothe wiry, woody, branching stems. Small purplish flowers appear on inconspicuous spikelets in terminal branchlets, turning wheat-colored. When in seed, the plants have a wispy look, as though dusted with gold.

LANDSCAPE USES: The cloudlike, light, airy foliage of bamboo muhly provides a stunning accent, especially when planted where afternoon sun can backlight its leaves. This grass is an excellent substitute for bamboo in gardens

SOME *Molinia caerulea* SUBSP. *arundinacea* CULTIVARS ARE:

'Bergfreund' (Mountain friend tall moor grass): tall-growing flowers; bright yellow fall color.

'Karl Foerster' (Foerster's tall moor grass): tall cultivar with flowers 6 to 7 feet tall; an older but fine selection.

'Skyracer' ('Skyracer' tall moor grass): robust foliage.

'Staefa' ('Staefa' tall moor grass): flowers grow up to 4 to 5 feet tall.

'Transparent' ('Transparent' tall moor grass): tall-flowering; flowers appear almost transparent.

'Windspiel' (Windplay tall moor grass): tall-growing, golden flowers.

MUHLENBERGIA
MUHLY GRASS

This large and diverse group of grasses includes some of the most spectacular and durable ornamental grasses for western gardens. Encompassing over 125 species, this family is centered primarily in Mexico and the southwestern United States. The flowering forms range from the cylindrical gray spikes of deergrass (*Muhlenbergia rigens*) to the delicate, airy, violet-colored panicles of hairy awn muhly (*M. capillaris*). Bamboo muhly (*M. dumosa*) looks like a graceful clumping bamboo.

Relatively new to ornamental grass gardening, muhly grasses are especially important additions to western gardens, not only for their beauty, but also because most are heat- and drought-tolerant. On the whole, they remain untested in eastern and northern states; however, their showy flowers and foliage will certainly encourage further experimentation.

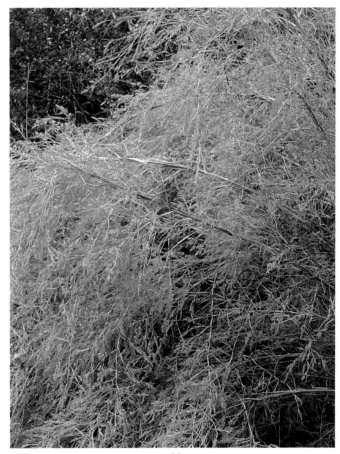

Muhlenbergia dumosa, bamboo muhly.

lacking sufficient water to support bamboo. Bamboo muhly is untested in much of the southern and eastern United States, although its grace and beauty may make it worth a try. A good pot and tub subject, bamboo muhly is also outstanding in fresh and dried flower arrangements.

CULTURE AND PROPAGATION: Bamboo muhly grows best in well-drained, fertile soil. It will take summer water but is extremely heat- and drought-tolerant. Once established, it tolerates coastal conditions and sandy or rocky soil. It doesn't seem to mind heavy, dry soils but may rot in heavy, wet soils. Bamboo muhly is a moderately fast grower.
Propagate by seed, or by division in spring or fall.

PESTS AND PROBLEMS: In extremely dry locations, the plants seldom reach over 3 feet tall.

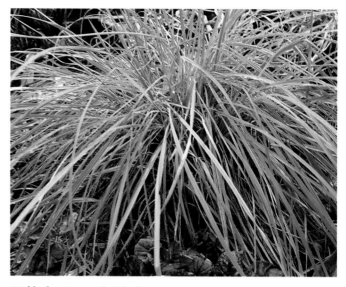

Muhlenbergia emersleyi, bull grass.

CULTURE AND PROPAGATION: Bull grass grows best in well-drained, fertile soil in full sun. It is tolerant of a wide variety of soils and climates, including extreme heat and cold, wind, and coastal conditions. It will tolerate moist soil as long as it has good drainage. This grass is untested in most eastern gardens.
Propagate by seed or division. Divisions are somewhat difficult, but since the grass is variable from seed, individuals with desirable characteristics should be propagated by division only.

PESTS AND PROBLEMS: Bull grass has no known pests or problems.

BOTANICAL NAME	***Muhlenbergia emersleyi***
PRONUNCIATION	myoo-len-BER-jee-ah ee-MER-slee-eye
COMMON NAME	Bull grass
USDA HARDINESS ZONE	5 to 9
ORIGIN	Texas to Arizona, Mexico
PREFERRED SITES	Medium and high elevations, rocky slopes, canyons, arroyos

DESCRIPTION: Handsome, clumping bull grass has glossy green foliage and attractive purplish tan flowers. A somewhat variable species, this semi- to wholly deciduous grass forms neat willowy tufts of medium green leaves ⅛ to ¼ inch wide and 1½ to 2 feet long. The flowers emerge from July through November and can be either short or long, drooping or vertical spikes 2 to 3 feet above the foliage. They range in height from 3 to 8 inches and are ½ to 1½ inches wide. Flower color varies from reddish to violet purple. The flowers can be either awned or awnless, depending on individual type. They then mature to a cream or tan color and are persistent and showy on the plant. In mild Mediterranean climates the foliage is evergreen. In cold inland climates and high elevations with prolonged hard freezing, the plants turn almond-colored. Cultivars should be available in the near future.

BOTANICAL NAME	***Muhlenbergia filipes***
PRONUNCIATION	myoo-len-BER-jee-ah FIL-lip-peez
COMMON NAME	Purple muhly
USDA HARDINESS ZONE	7 to 9
ORIGIN	North Carolina to Florida, along Gulf of Mexico to eastern Texas
PREFERRED SITES	Coastal plains, sand dunes, open coastal woodlands

LANDSCAPE USES: Bull grass is an odd name for such a delicate, handsome grass. It is a useful grass grown alone or in groups, and is good in rock gardens, dry gardens, and coastal gardens. Bull grass makes a good slope cover and erosion control, but it is slow to establish. Flowers are stunning in fresh or dried arrangements.

DESCRIPTION: The stunning violet purple panicles of purple muhly appear as clouds of purple over the foliage. This clumping, deciduous grass is thought by some to be a form of its close cousin, hairy awn muhly (*Muhlenbergia capillaris*). The two are quite similar and are chiefly distinguished by purple muhly's stouter flowering culms, longer awns, and later blooming time. Its delicate purple flowers emerge from October through November and mature to tan. They rise 2 to 3 feet above the foliage, are heavy on the plant, and often obscure the leaves.

LANDSCAPE USES: Among the most handsome of the native southeastern United States grasses, this showy bloomer makes a fine border specimen and is striking in large groups or masses. It is a good plant for coastal gardens and rocky or sandy soils. Its flowers are a stunning addition to fresh or dried arrangements.

CULTURE AND PROPAGATION: Purple muhly grows best in sandy or rocky soil in full sun. Good drainage is essential for good growth. It tolerates drought and wind but prefers some summer moisture. It tolerates light shade, but does not bloom as well in full sun.

Propagate by seed or division.

PESTS AND PROBLEMS: Purple muhly has no known pests or problems.

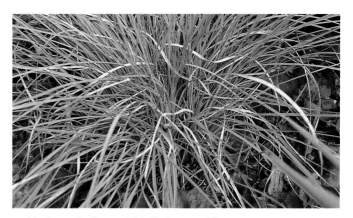

Muhlenbergia lindheimeri, Lindheimer muhly.

BOTANICAL NAME	*Muhlenbergia lindheimeri*
PRONUNCIATION	myoo-len-BER-jee-ah lind-HEYE-mer-eye
COMMON NAME	Lindheimer muhly
USDA HARDINESS ZONE	7 to 9
ORIGIN	Texas and northern Mexico
PREFERRED SITES	Rocky, usually calcareous soils in canyons, along streams, and in open areas

DESCRIPTION: Lindheimer muhly is a clumping, blue-foliaged grass noted for its handsome leaves and grayish flower spikes. Semideciduous in Mediterranean climates, it becomes wholly dormant in cold inland climates. Leaves of soft aqua blue, ⅛ to ¼ inch wide and 12 to 18 inches long, are V-shaped in cross section. The flowers are borne in a simple upright spike that rises 1½ to 2½ feet above the foliage. Showy and persistent on the plant, the flower spikes emerge purplish from September through December, becoming silver-gray at maturity.

LANDSCAPE USES: The beautiful flowers and foliage of Lindheimer muhly make it a fine specimen plant. Its neat growing habit makes it useful in perennial borders, and it is also effective in groups and as a ground cover or slope cover. The flowers are stunning in fresh arrangements.

CULTURE AND PROPAGATION: Lindheimer muhly prefers well-drained, moist, fertile soil in full sun. It tolerates a wide range of soil conditions, from rocky soil to heavy clay, and it tolerates drought and light shade.

Propagate by seed or division. Divisions are difficult; however, plants are variable from seed, so good blue selections should be propagated by division only.

PESTS AND PROBLEMS: Lindheimer muhly has no known pests or problems.

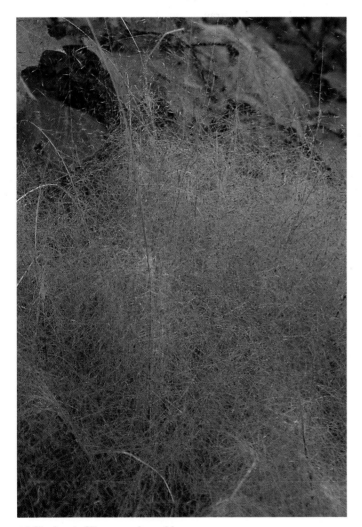

Muhlenbergia filipes, purple muhly.

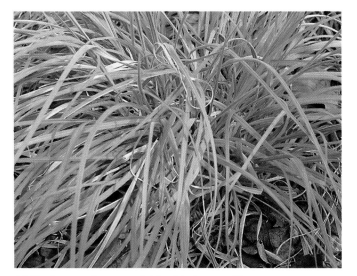

Muhlenbergia pubescens, soft blue Mexican muhly.

BOTANICAL NAME	*Muhlenbergia pubescens*
PRONUNCIATION	myoo-len-BER-jee-ah pyoo-BES-senz
COMMON NAME	Soft blue Mexican muhly
USDA HARDINESS ZONE	9 to 10
ORIGIN	Central Mexico
PREFERRED SITES	High-elevation rocky cliffs, canyons

DESCRIPTION: This clumping handsome grass has caught the attention of horticulturists and designers in the western United States. The blue-green foliage, ¼ to ⅜ inch wide and 8 to 12 inches long, is covered by soft downy hairs and forms tight clumps. With the first frosts, the foliage blushes reddish purple, further enhancing its year-round beauty. In hard freezes it may die back to the clump, emerging with new foliage in the spring. Flowers bloom in May and June on an upright spike 12 to 18 inches above the foliage. The flowers are an attractive amethyst-blue and soft to the touch; they dry to a wheat color.

LANDSCAPE USES: Soft blue Mexican muhly is an attractive accent alone or in groups. Situate it near pathways, where its soft foliage and flowers can be touched. It is a good choice for dry borders and rock gardens. Combine this grass with plants bearing white flowers or plants with silver or dark contrasting foliage, such as yarrow and artemisia.

CULTURE AND PROPAGATION: Soft blue Mexican muhly grows best in well-drained, fertile soil in full sun. It resents heavy, wet soils or deep shade. Plants tolerate light shade if drainage is excellent; they also tolerate coastal conditions and sandy or rocky soils.

Propagate by seed, or by division in spring or fall.

PESTS AND PROBLEMS: The hardiness of soft blue Mexican muhly is untested and untried in much of the South and East. It is hard to find in nurseries.

BOTANICAL NAME	*Muhlenbergia rigens*
PRONUNCIATION	myoo-len-BER-jee-ah rih-GENZ
COMMON NAME	Deer grass, muhly
USDA HARDINESS ZONE	7 to 9
ORIGIN	Texas, California from San Diego to Mount Shasta, northern Mexico
PREFERRED SITES	Streams, edges of meadows, dry hillsides, low elevations to 7,000 feet

DESCRIPTION: Deer grass is a clumping, cool-season grass of unusual beauty and adaptability. Heat- and drought-tolerant, it grows and flourishes in areas of little to no summer rainfall. Its gray-green leaves, ⅛ to ⅜ inch wide and 1½ to 2½ feet long, form dense clumps that grow 3 feet tall and as wide. The evergreen foliage holds its color in the summer even without additional summer water. Flowers are showy, slender, whiplike panicles, 2 to 3 feet tall, that emerge grayish in early summer and mature to buff later in the season. The flower spikes are vertical in youth, fan outward with age, and persist into winter.

LANDSCAPE USES: Deer grass is a fine choice as a specimen and an accent in dry western gardens. Its handsome foliage and showy flowers complement native western plants such as manzanita (*Arctostaphylos* spp.), wormwood (*Artemisia* spp.), and mountain lilac (*Ceanothus* spp.). A single plant

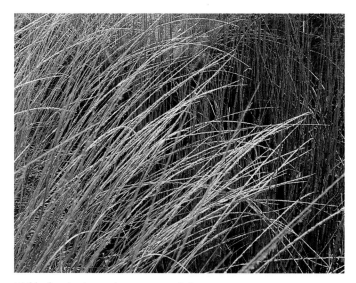

Muhlenbergia rigens, deer grass, at left.

provides a vertical accent, while a mass planting creates a horizontal effect. Deer grass is a useful slope cover for erosion control and does well in coastal gardens.

CULTURE AND PROPAGATION: Deer grass prefers moist, well-drained, fertile soil in full sun or partial shade. It tolerates extreme conditions, including hot, dry, rocky soil and alkaline and saline conditions. Found in nature in a wide range of climates and habitats, it thrives in most western gardens. Deer grass tolerates summer water, responding with faster, higher growth. If left unwatered in dry-summer areas, deer grass grows 2 to 3 feet tall; plants watered in summer can reach 3 to 4 feet tall.

Propagate by seed, or by division in spring or fall.

PESTS AND PROBLEMS: Deer grass has no known pests or problems.

ANOTHER SPECIES OF MUHLY GRASS IS:

'Muhlenbergia capillaris'
(Hairy awn muhly): nearly
identical to purple muhly
(*M. filipes*) with showy
violet-pink flowers.

BOTANICAL NAME	***Orysopsis hymenoides***
PRONUNCIATION	or-ee-SOP-sis heye-men-OY-deez
COMMON NAME	Indian rice grass
USDA HARDINESS ZONE	8 (?) to 10 (hardiness is untested; may grow above Zone 8)
ORIGIN	Northern Mexico, California, and throughout the arid southwestern United States, north into British Columbia
PREFERRED SITES	Open sandy hills, juniper woodlands

DESCRIPTION: This important western grass was a prime food source of Native Americans, who would grind the grain into flour to make bread. Both the leaves and grain have high nutritional value. Indian rice grass has been steadily destroyed in its native habitat since the 1800s; it is a grass worthy of restoration and preservation.

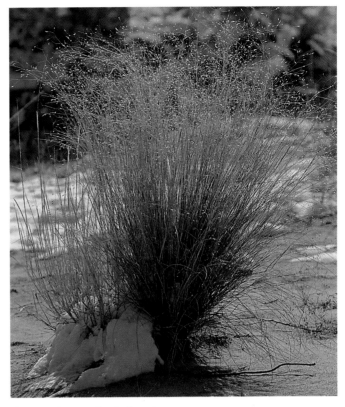

Orysopsis hymenoides, Indian rice grass.

Clumping and cool-season-growing, Indian rice grass grows in light, airy tufts 1 to 2 feet tall and as wide. Its long, slender, bright green leaves are $1/16$ to $1/8$ inch wide and 6 to 8 inches long. Its delicate, wiry flower stems are twisted and crinkled; flowers are borne in open panicles and form attractive seeds. The plant goes dormant by June, turning straw-colored, and remains this color until winter. Spring rains renew its growth.

LANDSCAPE USES: Indian rice grass makes a wonderful meadow plant in dry rock gardens and desert plantings, especially when planted in combination with desert annuals and perennials. Its airy form is an interesting accent in dry borders and sandy, dry creeks. The flowers and seed heads attract birds. An excellent specimen for flower arrangements, it is often found in flower markets; many people grow it specifically for cutting.

CULTURE AND PROPAGATION: Indian rice grass grows best in well-drained, sandy soil in full sun. It tolerates heavy soils and alkaline conditions, although it does not like heavy, wet soils, shade, or summer water. This grass is exceedingly drought-tolerant and can exist on 5 inches of annual rainfall. It can be difficult to grow in a container.

Propagate by seed only.

PESTS AND PROBLEMS: Indian rice grass has no known pests or problems.

BOTANICAL NAME	***Orysopsis milliacea***
PRONUNCIATION	or-ee-SOP-sis mil-ee-AY-see-ah
COMMON NAME	Smilo grass, rice grass
USDA HARDINESS ZONE	9 to 10
ORIGIN	Mediterranean region
PREFERRED SITES	Streamsides, canyons, low elevations; naturalized in California and Arizona

DESCRIPTION: This Mediterranean grass has naturalized throughout much of California, from San Diego to San Francisco. Introduced by the U.S. Forest Service, smilo grass was used extensively after fires for overseeding. It is now as entrenched as eucalyptus in the California flora.

Smilo grass is a cool-season, fast-growing, clumping, and drought-tolerant grass. Its shiny, bright green leaves, ½ to ¾ inch wide and 8 to 12 inches long, are borne on sturdy stems. New spring growth is often blushed purple-red on the leaf tips. The foliage forms lax, arching clumps 3 to 4 feet tall and as wide. The flowers emerge from May through October in silky green drooping panicles, 1 to 2 feet long, that arch up and out from the plant. The panicles mature to a silky golden yellow that shimmers in the sun. The flowers remain showy well into the winter. In the event of a hard freeze, smilo grass may go dormant.

LANDSCAPE USES: Smilo grass is useful as a slope cover and for erosion control. It will naturalize and is effective in large masses and groups. It tolerates considerable shade and makes a good groundcover under a high canopy of trees. Smilo grass's flowers are attractive in fresh or dried arrangements.

CULTURE AND PROPAGATION: Smilo grass prefers moist, fertile soil in full sun. It tolerates many extremes, from heavy, wet soil to dry, rocky soil. It is tolerant of coastal conditions and will grow in sand if moisture is sufficient. In hot, dry situations, smilo grass goes dormant in summer, resuming growth in late fall with the onset of cooler temperatures and fall and winter rains. Treat this grass as an annual in colder climates.

Propagate by seed, or by division in spring or fall.

PESTS AND PROBLEMS: Smilo grass will readily naturalize and can become aggressive in moist situations. In small gardens, this trait may be undesirable.

PANICUM
SWITCH GRASS

Over 600 species of switch grass can be found worldwide. In North America, switch grasses were a major constituent of the tallgrass prairie. *Panicum virgatum*, the most prominent of the prairie species, grows from Canada to Florida and from Maryland to Colorado. As these grasses are crowded out of their native habitats, switch grasses are increasingly colonizing wetter sites.

American nurseries are just now beginning to appreciate the varied forms and beauty of these native American grasses, long a staple of the German nursery trade. Many new and varied cultivars should soon appear, bred with an eye toward foliage color, habit, fall color, blooming time, and drought-tolerance.

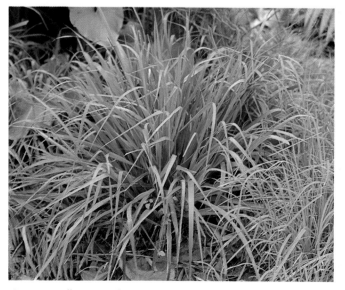

Orysopsis milliacea, smilo grass.

BOTANICAL NAME	***Panicum clandestinum***
PRONUNCIATION	PAN-ih-kum klan-DES-tih-num
COMMON NAME	Deer tongue grass
USDA HARDINESS ZONE	4 to 9
ORIGIN	North America: from Maine to Florida, Maryland to Kansas, Canada to Texas
PREFERRED SITES	Moist, open woods

DESCRIPTION: Clumping, warm-season-growing deer tongue grass has bright green bamboolike foliage that reaches 3 to 4 feet in arching mounds. Its leaves, ¾ to 1 inch wide and 6 to 8 inches long, clothe hairy stems that resemble bamboo. The foliage turns a mix of yellow and brown in fall and becomes almost prostrate under the

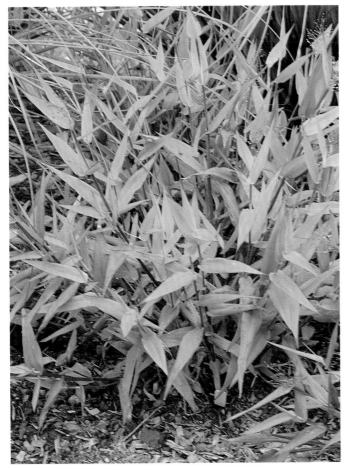

Panicum clandestinum, deer tongue grass.

BOTANICAL NAME	***Panicum virgatum***
PRONUNCIATION	PAN-ih-kum veer-GAH-tum
COMMON NAME	Switch grass
USDA HARDINESS ZONE	5 to 9
ORIGIN	Widespread over North America: Canada to Florida, Atlantic Ocean west to the Rocky Mountains
PREFERRED SITES	Prairies, open woods

DESCRIPTION: This wide-ranging native North American grass was one of the original components of the tallgrass prairie that once covered the vast interior of the United States. An extremely versatile grass, it tolerates a wide range of soil and climatic conditions. It is valued as an ornamental for its erect upright form, showy flowers, brilliant fall color, and interesting winter silhouette. Truly a grass for all seasons, switch grass is easy to grow and sure to please.

Switch grass is a clumping, warm-season grass. Leaf color ranges from deep green to gray-green. The leaves, ¼ to ½ inch wide and 18 to 24 inches long, clothe stiff, sturdy stems 4 to 7 feet tall. Its upright clumps begin to flower in July in airy panicles 1 to 2 feet above the foliage. The branched panicle is tightly ascending at first but becomes more airy as the branches spread open. The flowers emerge pinkish, reddish, or silvery, mature to grayish white or brown, and persist well into winter. In the fall, the plants turn various shades of yellow. The fall color is usually

weight of fall and winter rain and snow. The flowers are terminal panicles, 3 to 7 inches long, that emerge from July through August, blooming silvery and becoming brown and persistent at maturity. The weight of the flowers often causes the stems to bend toward the ground.

LANDSCAPE USES: Deer tongue grass is effective in mass plantings in moist woods, around pools or ponds, and along shady streams. Individual plants are good as specimens in water gardens. It is a fine choice for a large-scale groundcover and for naturalizing. Deer tongue grass is somewhat floppy and is usually at its best naturalizing on the fringe of the garden. The flowers add interest to fresh and dried arrangements.

CULTURE AND PROPAGATION: Deer tongue grass grows best in moist, fertile soil in medium to light shade. It suffers in hot, dry conditions. Although it will grow in full sun, it will usually be shorter and more yellow-green.

Propagate by seed, or by division in the spring.

PESTS AND PROBLEMS: Deer tongue grass has no known pests or problems.

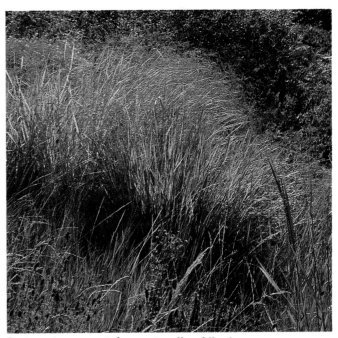

Panicum virgatum, switch grass, in yellow fall color.

strong and fades to beige with the onset of winter. Plants remain upright throughout the winter until cut back or overtaken by new foliage in the spring.

LANDSCAPE USES: Switch grass is effective planted alone or massed in groups. Tall cultivars make excellent background plants. Switch grass tolerates moist, wet soil and so makes a fine choice for water gardens, streamsides, and pond edges. It is also a good choice for naturalizing and attracting wildlife. Switch grass can be used along highways and roadsides, as a groundcover for erosion control, and for transition areas between garden and woods. The grass has one of the most beautiful fall color displays, usually yellow, but some cultivars turn red and orange. Because it holds its dormant form, switch grass is good for winter effects. The flowers and foliage of switch grass are stunning in fresh and dried arrangements.

CULTURE AND PROPAGATION: Switch grass prefers moist, fertile soil in full sun, although it tolerates extremes in soil conditions, from sand to heavy clay and from dry slopes to boggy areas. It thrives in seacoast conditions and tolerates wind and salt spray. It also tolerates light shade, but will flop if the shade is too heavy.

Propagate by seed, or by division in the spring. Propagate named cultivars by division only, since they do not come true from seed.

PESTS AND PROBLEMS: Switch grass can easily overtake a prairie seeding; it should make up no more than 10 to 15 percent of the seeding mix so that the other grasses can become established.

BOTANICAL NAME	*Panicum virgatum* 'Haense Herms'
PRONUNCIATION	PAN-ih-kum veer-GAH-tum HEN-suh HAIRMZ
COMMON NAME	Red switch grass

DESCRIPTION: Red switch grass is similar to switch grass (*Panicum virgatum*) in most aspects, differing mostly in its compact habit and bright red-orange fall color. Its foliage grows 3 to 3½ feet tall in a tight vertical column. Purplish red highlights on the leaf tips become redder as the season progresses. The foliage becomes reddish orange in October and matures to a gray-brown. With the foliage becoming redder and the seed heads maturing to a whitish gray, the plant resembles a fire with smoke rising above the flames.

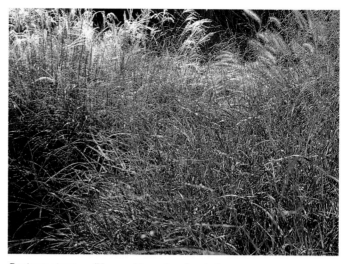

Panicum virgatum 'Haense Herms', red switch grass.

The flowers reach 12 to 16 inches above the foliage. As the delicate leaves and flowers are constantly in motion, a mass planting of this grass gives the impression of a small prairie fire. The onset of winter turns the dormant foliage a dark reddish brown.

BOTANICAL NAME	*Panicum virgatum* 'Heavy Metal'
PRONUNCIATION	PAN-ih-kum veer-GAH-tum
COMMON NAME	'Heavy Metal' switch grass

DESCRIPTION: A new introduction from Kurt Bluemel Inc. in Baldwin, Maryland, 'Heavy Metal' switch grass is already proving to be one of the most handsome switch grasses available. Its stiff, metallic blue leaves form a tight upright clump, 3 to 3½ feet tall, with flowers that grow 12 to 16 inches above the foliage. Its powder-blue foliage turns bright yellow in the fall.

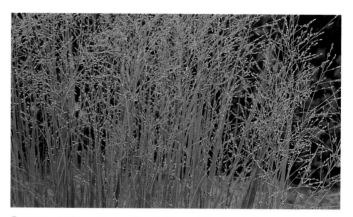

Panicum virgatum 'Heavy Metal', 'Heavy Metal' switch grass.

OTHER *Panicum virgatum* CULTIVARS ARE:

'Rehbraun' (Deer red-brown switch grass): a taller cultivar, not as colorful as others.

'Rotstrahlbusch' (Red rays switch grass): considered the reddest of the red switch grasses.

'Squaw' ('Squaw' red switch grass): grows 3 to 4 feet tall.

'Strictum' (Tall switch grass): a fine older cultivar with bluish green foliage; blooms early and has good vertical-growing foliage.

'Warrior' ('Warrior' switch grass): a strong-growing, tall cultivar with reddish brown foliage in late fall.

Some *Pennisetum* species naturalize readily from seed, becoming weedy or problematic. Some will become pests in certain climates, so look carefully for the cultural requirements of the plants on the following pages to gauge the possibility of weediness for your garden. Where fountain grass has the potential to reseed in your garden, remove the flower heads before maturity or before they shatter to prevent unwanted seedlings from appearing. However, you might be missing out on beautiful fall and winter effects by doing so.

Botanically speaking, the fountain grasses are somewhat of a mess. Botanists are currently examining this huge group of plants, and new botanical classifications are perhaps soon to follow. Considerable confusion exists, so check the synonyms at each entry for other names used in the past.

PENNISETUM
FOUNTAIN GRASS

Over 120 species of annual and perennial grasses are included in the genus *Pennisetum*, the fountain grasses. Widely distributed in both tropical and temperate regions, they grow in savannas, in woodlands, in the tropics, and along seashores. The genus includes pearl millet (*P. glaucum*), an important food source in many dry countries throughout the world.

The species and cultivars described here produce some of the showiest flowers of all the ornamental grasses. The flowers range from white to cream, pink to red, and black to brown.

The flowers of fountain grass are typically soft, bottle-brush-like foxtails. Their generally easy growth and long-lasting nature have made them favorites of ornamental grass enthusiasts.

Some fountain grasses are hardy into Zone 5, whereas others are perennial only in Zone 10. In colder climates, tender fountain grasses can be effectively grown as annuals. Some, such as tender fountain grass (*P. setaceum*) or feathertop (*P. villosum*), are extremely drought-tolerant, growing in arid western climates that get little or no summer water. Most fountain grasses are warm-season plants, going dormant with cool winter temperatures. In some temperate western climates or subtropical southern climates, plants stay essentially evergreen with little or no dormancy. Most fountain grasses are clump-forming, although two species, meadow pennisetum (*P. incomptum*) and feathertop (*P. villosum*), spread from underground rhizomes and are effective on banks and for erosion control.

BOTANICAL NAME	***Pennisetum alopecuroides (also known as P. japonicum)***
PRONUNCIATION	pen-ih-SEE-tum al-oh-pek-yur-OY-deez
COMMON NAME	Fountain grass
USDA HARDINESS ZONE	6 to 9
ORIGIN	Eastern Asia, Australia
PREFERRED SITES	Extensive and widely distributed in open meadows, openings in woods, streamsides

DESCRIPTION: This clumping, warm-season-growing fountain grass is one of the most versatile, dependable, and showy of all the ornamental grasses. It is graced by handsome, glossy, bright green foliage that grows 2 to 3 feet tall and as wide. The leaves, ¼ to ½ inch wide and 18 to 30 inches long, form a dense, upright mound. The foliage becomes streaked with yellow and brown with the onset of fall, becomes completely almond-colored in late fall, and continues to fade to a straw color as winter progresses.

The showy flowers begin to emerge in mid-July and continue into August. The stiff foxtail flowers, 1 to 3 inches wide and 4 to 10 inches long, are borne on somewhat arching stems, making a cascade of flowers. They emerge creamy white to light pink or tan. Mature flowers are generally reddish brown. Flower color may vary somewhat on seedling-grown plants. The flowers persist on the plant into mid-autumn, when the flower heads begin to mature and shatter. Shattered seeds drop to the ground; the flower stems persist into winter.

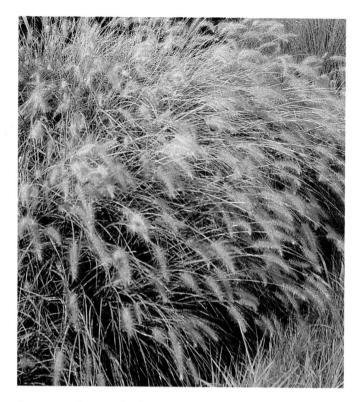

Pennisetum alopecuroides, fountain grass.

BOTANICAL NAME	***Pennisetum alopecuroides 'Hameln'***
PRONUNCIATION	pen-ih-SEE-tum al-oh-pek-yur-OY-deez HAH-muln
COMMON NAME	'Hameln' fountain grass

DESCRIPTION: 'Hameln' fountain grass differs from the species in its dark green, finer-textured foliage and compact whitish flowers. The leaves, ⅛ to ¼ inch wide and 12 to 20 inches long, grow in upright, mounding clumps. The greenish white flowers emerge a few weeks earlier than do the flowers of the species and mature to a creamy tan. The flowers, borne 12 to 18 inches above the foliage, are 1 to 2 inches wide, 3 to 4 inches long, and slightly curving. This is a good cultivar to plant where the species would get too large.

'Hameln' fountain grass does not reseed itself. It has been a poor performer in hot southern climates and mild, dry western climates, where it needs lots of moisture to grow at all. The plants require cold winters to perform well; the flowers are not as showy in mild or hot climates. 'Hameln' fountain grass is not recommended south of Zone 8.

LANDSCAPE USES: Fountain grass is attractive in mass plantings or groups and as a single specimen. Plants make excellent midborder or back-of-the-border candidates. The slightest breeze sets the foliage and flowers in motion. The plants are good for fall and winter effects, since they are at their prime when most other perennials in the garden have quit for the season. Fountain grass is ideally suited for planting around building foundations, particularly around modern, hard-edged architecture. It tolerates the wind and water edges of coastal gardens. Fountain grass is also good near lawns of schools, parks, golf courses, and marinas. Its flowers are handsome in fresh or dried arrangements.

CULTURE AND PROPAGATION: Fountain grass is extremely adaptable, growing in just about any soil that is moist, well-drained, and in full sun. It is happiest in moist, fertile loam but will tolerate a wide range of soil conditions. Drought-tolerant in colder climates, the plant requires weekly watering in dry, arid climates. It tolerates light shade but does poorly if there is insufficient light: Plants will not bloom if shade is too deep.

Propagate by seed, or by division in spring. Propagate named cultivars by division only. This grass will reseed moderately in most American gardens. In mild-climate areas, it will reseed only in irrigated gardens, as the plant must have additional summer water to thrive. In the West, plants rarely reseed invasively.

PESTS AND PROBLEMS: Fountain grass has no known pests or problems.

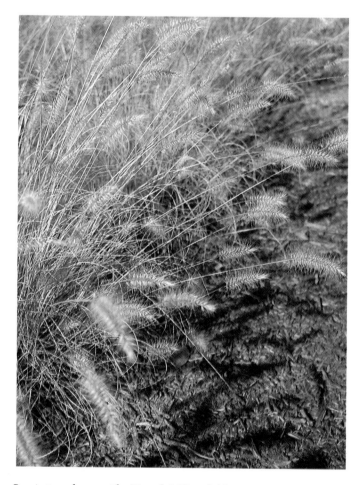

Pennisetum alopecuroides 'Hameln', 'Hameln' fountain grass.

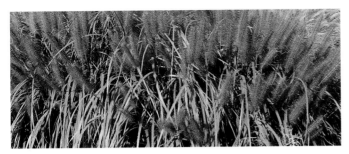

Pennisetum alopecuroides 'Moudry', black-flowering pennisetum.

BOTANICAL NAME	***Pennisetum alopecuroides 'Moudry' (also incorrectly known as Pennisetum alopecuroides 'Viridescens')***
PRONUNCIATION	pen-ih-SEE-tum al-oh-pek-yur-OY-deez MOU-dree
COMMON NAME	Black-flowering pennisetum, late-blooming fountain grass

DESCRIPTION: Black-flowering pennisetum is prized for its lush green foliage and large, almost black foxtails. Its dark green, glossy leaves, ½ to ¾ inch wide, form a dense, upright, mounded clump 18 to 26 inches tall and as wide. The foliage often contains a reddish purple tint. The flowers emerge a dark pearly brown in late August and early September; at their peak they appear almost black. They grow 6 to 8 inches long and 10 to 18 inches beyond the foliage. The fall foliage color varies from yellowish to pumpkin and matures to a straw color by winter. Black-flowering pennisetum is a prolific reseeder in almost any garden situation. However, it will not naturalize in arid western gardens that are not irrigated.

BOTANICAL NAME	***Pennisetum 'Burgundy Giant'***
PRONUNCIATION	pen-ih-SEE-tum
COMMON NAME	'Burgundy Giant' fountain grass
USDA HARDINESS ZONE	9 to 10
ORIGIN	Horticultural selection
PREFERRED SITES	Moist, well-drained areas

DESCRIPTION: This clumping, warm-season grass has wide burgundy leaves that form a pillar of colorful flowing foliage. The leaves, ¾ to 1 inch wide and 8 to 12 inches long, clothe sturdy stems that grow 4 to 5 feet tall in upright clumps. The rich burgundy red foliage appears almost tropical. The long, typically nodding foxtail flowers, 1 to 1½ inches wide and 8 to 12 inches long, arch out and above the foliage 1½ to 2½ feet. Blooms appear purple-red in mid-July, remain showy into the fall, and fade to cream color with age. Plants become dormant below 40°F and are killed at 32°F. 'Burgundy Giant' fountain grass may be hard to find in nurseries or garden centers.

LANDSCAPE USES: 'Burgundy Giant' fountain grass is a stunning accent in the back of a border, as a single specimen or planted in groups, and in fresh and dried flower arrangements.

CULTURE AND PROPAGATION: 'Burgundy Giant' fountain grass prefers moist, well-drained, fertile loam in full sun with protection from wind. It resents wet, boggy soil or too much shade. The leaves tatter and look ragged in windy sites, especially when winds are hot and dry. The plants love heat if moisture is sufficient but will not tolerate extended periods of drought. Plants can grow in coastal conditions if protected from heavy winds.

OTHER ***Pennisetum alopecuroides*** CULTIVARS ARE:

'Cassian' (Cassian fountain grass): a good new dwarf cultivar; bright fall color.

'Herbstzauber' (Autumn sorcery fountain grass): medium-sized fountain grass; good fall color.

'Little Bunny' ('Little Bunny' fountain grass): the smallest of dwarf fountain grasses; excellent rock garden choice.

'National Arboretum' ('National Arboretum' fountain grass): improved black flowers and foliage. A selection from the U.S. National Arboretum in Washington, D.C.

'Weserbergland' ('Weserbergland' fountain grass): almost identical to *P. alopecuroides* 'Hameln', only taller and having a more spreading habit.

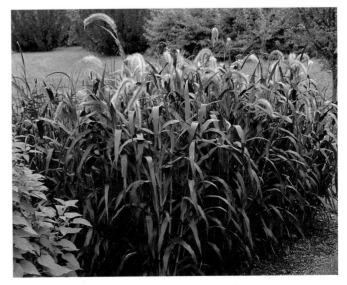

Pennisetum 'Burgundy Giant', 'Burgundy Giant' fountain grass.

'Burgundy Giant' fountain grass does not set viable seed. Propagate by division or from cane cuttings of thickened stems.

PESTS AND PROBLEMS: 'Burgundy Giant' fountain grass does not self-sow and will not naturalize in the garden. A tender subtropical grass, it must be either treated as an annual or dug and overwintered in a greenhouse at temperatures above 40°F.

BOTANICAL NAME	***Pennisetum caudatum***
PRONUNCIATION	pen-ih-SEE-tum cow-DAH-tum
COMMON NAME	White-flowering fountain grass
USDA HARDINESS ZONE	6 to 9
ORIGIN	Eastern Asia
PREFERRED SITES	Open meadows, streamsides

DESCRIPTION: This fountain grass differs from *Pennisetum alopecuroides* primarily in its silky white flowers that bloom early. The flowers are narrower than those of *P. alopecuroides* and are creamy white, fading to tan at maturity. The foliage can reach 3 to 3½ feet, with the flowers extending 1 to 1½ feet beyond. In all other aspects, white-flowering fountain grass is similar to, and in fact is thought by some botanists to be a variety of, *P. alopecuroides*.

LANDSCAPE USES: White-flowering fountain grass is charming planted alone or in groups. Its showy flowering habit is effective in borders and formal gardens. Mass plantings are particularly eye-catching, especially where flowers are placed against a dark background. It is good as a bank cover and for erosion control. Flowers are stunning in fresh and dried arrangements.

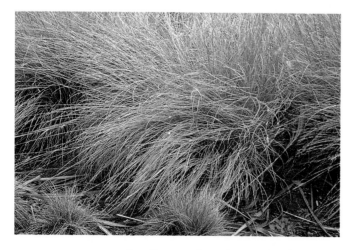

Pennisetum caudatum, white-flowering fountain grass, in winter.

CULTURE AND PROPAGATION: White-flowering fountain grass grows best in moist, fertile, well-drained soil in full sun. It tolerates light shade and other extremes, such as sandy soil, heavy clay, windy coastal conditions and heat, as long as adequate moisture is provided.

White-flowering fountain grass does not seed itself aggressively. It performs well in southern and western gardens but stays more compact in hot and arid climates. It blooms dependably in the South and West.

PESTS AND PROBLEMS: White-flowering fountain grass has no known pests or problems.

BOTANICAL NAME	***Pennisetum incomptum*** **(also known as *P. flaccidum*)**
PRONUNCIATION	pen-ih-SEE-tum in-COMP-tum
COMMON NAME	Meadow pennisetum
USDA HARDINESS ZONE	6 to 9
ORIGIN	Northeastern China to the Himalaya Mountains
PREFERRED SITES	Open woodlands, moist slopes

DESCRIPTION: Creeping, warm-season-growing meadow pennisetum is an aggressive spreader. Growing from runners and rhizomes, it quickly colonizes large areas. Its glossy, blue-green foliage reaches 2 to 3 feet in height. The leaves, ¼ to ⅜ inch wide and 12 to 18 inches long, clothe sturdy, upright stems. The flowers are purplish pink spikes that form vertical cylindrical foxtails and emerge as early as April in mild climates, June in cooler climates. The flowers mature to a creamy white and are showy from emergence into winter. Fall foliage ranges from brownish yellow to tan.

LANDSCAPE USES: Meadow pennisetum is best used in open areas such as parks, roadways, marinas, and golf courses to create large-scale meadow effects. It is also an excellent grass for soil stabilization and bank cover. It tolerates coastal conditions and is relatively drought-tolerant in Zones 6 to 8. The flowers are lovely in fresh and dried arrangements.

CULTURE AND PROPAGATION: Meadow pennisetum prefers moist, fertile soil in full sun to light shade. It will tolerate soil extremes from heavy clay to sandy and rocky soils. In summer, water it once or twice a week in arid southwestern gardens. It blooms poorly and flops in shady situations.

Propagation is easy by seed, and by division in spring or fall.

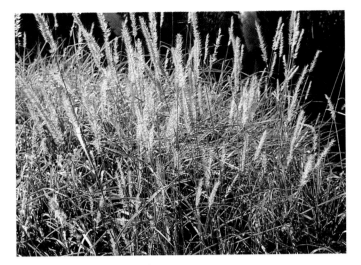

Pennisetum incomptum, meadow pennisetum.

PESTS AND PROBLEMS: Meadow pennisetum is an aggressive spreader able to take over a large area in a relatively short period of time. Carefully consider where you plan to use it in the garden. A drainage tile or root barrier of plastic, steel, or concrete to a depth of 2 feet will safely contain the rhizomes. Meadow pennisetum will also seed itself aggressively under ideal growing conditions. In western gardens, however, it will not reseed in unirrigated areas.

BOTANICAL NAME	***Pennisetum orientale***
PRONUNCIATION	pen-ih-SEE-tum or-ee-en-TAL-ee
COMMON NAME	Oriental fountain grass
USDA HARDINESS ZONE	7 to 9
ORIGIN	Central Asia to the Caucasus Mountains, northern and western India
PREFERRED SITES	Meadows, openings in woods

DESCRIPTION: Clumping, warm-season-growing oriental fountain grass is prized for its showy pink flowers and is considered by many to be the prettiest of the fountain grasses. It blooms early and continues to put on a show until mid-October. Its glossy, blue-green leaves, ⅛ to ¼ inch wide and 4 to 8 inches long, form handsome upright mounded clumps 12 to 18 inches tall and as wide. The flowers emerge in June in colder climates but bloom as early as late April in Southern California. Silky soft foxtails grow 3 to 4 inches long and ½ inch wide and arch out 12 to 16 inches from the foliage. The violet-pink flowers have an iridescent sheen that is especially lovely when lit by early morning or late afternoon light. They mature to a

creamy light brown and remain until shattering in mid-October. The foliage fades to yellow-brown in the fall, becoming straw-colored by early winter. The plants provide lovely winter effects, even in dormancy.

LANDSCAPE USES: Oriental fountain grass is one of the best small, clumping, blooming grasses for perennial borders and flower beds. It is certainly one of the longest-blooming grasses, and is attractive planted alone or in groups. Its compact habit makes it indispensable for small gardens and planters. Its flowers add color and texture to fresh and dried arrangements.

CULTURE AND PROPAGATION: Oriental fountain grass prefers warm, moist, well-drained loam in full sun or light shade. Plants languish in poorly drained soil or too much shade. It tolerates coastal conditions and sandy soils with adequate moisture. It is best to plant it in a protected location, and to give plants protection the first two seasons until they are fully established. Oriental fountain grass is not an aggressive self-seeder; occasional seedlings will appear, but never invasively. Oriental fountain grass needs some summer water; in areas of some summer rainfall it is somewhat drought-tolerant, but in areas with no summer rainfall, it needs some summer water.

Propagate by seed or division, although division is difficult and the percentage of loss is usually high. If dividing, spring is the best time.

PESTS AND PROBLEMS: Oriental fountain grass has no known pests or problems.

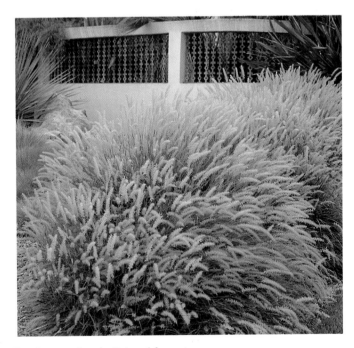

Pennisetum orientale, Oriental fountain grass.

BOTANICAL NAME	***Pennisetum setaceum*** (also known as *P. ruppelii*)
PRONUNCIATION	pen-ih-SEE-tum seh-TAY-see-um
COMMON NAME	Tender fountain grass, fountain grass
USDA HARDINESS ZONE	8 to 10
ORIGIN	Africa
PREFERRED SITES	Savannas, open prairies—widespread

DESCRIPTION: Clumping, warm-season-growing tender fountain grass has quickly become a favorite companion planting for flower and perennial beds. In colder climates, its fast growth and showy, pink, long-lasting flowers have made it a popular annual as well. Its glossy, light green leaves, ⅛ to ¼ inch wide and 1 to 2 feet long, form slender, upright, arching fountains of fine-textured foliage. The foliage forms dense tufts that reach 2 to 3 feet tall and as wide. The flowers emerge in May in warm climates, and in early summer in cooler climates. Long, soft, cylindrical, purplish pink plumes, the flowers are ¾ to 1 inch wide and 6 to 8 inches long and are borne 1 to 2 feet above the foliage. The flowers are showy and persist well into mid-October and even later in southwestern gardens. In mild climates, plants appear almost evergreen, although in the winter the foliage usually blanches to straw-colored before new winter or spring growth emerges. In cold climates and in the northern portion of Zone 8, tender fountain grass is killed by the first hard freeze. Leave the plants in the garden and enjoy their beautiful winter silhouettes.

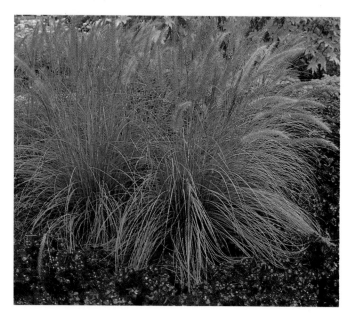

Pennisetum setaceum, tender fountain grass.

LANDSCAPE USES: Tender fountain grass grows best in moist, well-drained, fertile soil but tolerates wide extremes in soil and climate. It will grow in heavy clay or almost solid rock; in fact, it can grow in rock crevices or between paving stones. It tolerates light shade but flops in too much shade.

CULTURE AND PROPAGATION: Tender fountain grass is a moderately aggressive seeder which, in some instances, can be invasive. In Southern California, this grass has successfully colonized disturbed chaparral and is considered undesirable by local native plant societies. However, it is here to stay. Gardeners in areas adjacent to undisturbed pristine native areas should avoid this grass, since it overruns many of the native grasses and prevents their establishment. In cities or enclosed gardens, this naturalizing tendency is less likely to be a problem. In cold climates, winter temperatures will kill this grass, thereby rendering it noninvasive.

Propagate by seed only. Division is risky and usually unsuccessful. Seedling transplants are successful when plants are 2 to 3 inches tall and when care is taken to keep roots undisturbed.

PESTS AND PROBLEMS: In some areas, tender fountain grass can be an invasive seeder. Its aggressive nature can be problematic if seedlings are not removed. In mild climates, its tendency to reseed itself is inevitable, though it can be used to advantage in some situations, such as bank and erosion control.

BOTANICAL NAME	***Pennisetum setaceum* 'Rubrum'** (also known as *P. setaceum* 'Cupreum' and *P. setaceum* 'Atrosanguineum')
PRONUNCIATION	pen-ih-SEE-tum seh-TAY-see-um ROO-brum
COMMON NAME	Purple-leaved fountain grass, purple fountain grass, red fountain grass
USDA HARDINESS ZONE	9 to 10
ORIGIN	Horticultural selection
PREFERRED SITES	Moist, well-drained areas

DESCRIPTION: By whatever name, this fountain grass has quickly become one of the most popular ornamental grasses in the United States. Its clumping, warm-season-growing foliage is burgundy and topped by red-purple plumes. Used as an annual north of Zone 9, purple-leaved

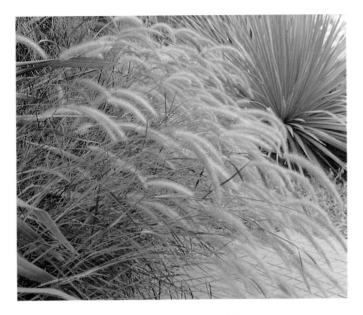

Pennisetum setaceum 'Rubrum', purple-leaved fountain grass.

fountain grass can be killed at 20°F. Its glossy foliage grows in upright, arching clumps 3 to 4 feet tall and as wide. Its leaves are ¼ to ½ inch wide and 8 to 12 inches long. The flowers emerge in June as soft red-purple nodding plumes, 8 to 12 inches long and ¾ to 1 inch wide, which arch up and out, 1½ to 2½ feet above the foliage. In Southern California, the flowers bloom as early as May. Their growth is rapid, and blooming continues throughout the summer. By late summer and early fall the plumes turn a soft brown and dance in the slightest breeze. The plants turn a straw color with the first hard freeze. The dried foliage provides winter interest.

LANDSCAPE USES: Both the foliage and flower of purple-leaved fountain grass make it a vivid accent. It is effective massed or in groups; on slopes, where its foliage can spill down a hill; or near water, where its form will be reflected on the water's surface. A one-season growth of 3 to 4 feet makes it a useful grass in parks, along roadsides, and at golf courses. If provided with sufficient moisture, it thrives in arid southwestern heat. It tolerates seacost conditions and will perform well in coastal gardens. Its flowers are attractive in fresh or dried arrangements.

CULTURE AND PROPAGATION: Purple-leaved fountain grass prefers well-drained, moist, fertile loam in full sun. It tolerates heavy, rocky, or sandy soil as long as water is regularly available. Plants will flop in too much shade and resent wet, boggy soils. Purple-leaved fountain grass tolerates windy coastal conditions. In cold climates, it is best used as an annual.

Propagate by division only, since plants do not set viable seed. Make divisions in late spring. Purple-leaved fountain

grass does not usually self-seed. While an occasional seedling may be found, often it will not be purple-leaved. Some seedlings with varying degrees of green and bronze tints have been selected and named.

PESTS AND PROBLEMS: Purple-leaved fountain grass has no known pests or problems.

BOTANICAL NAME	***Pennisetum setaceum* 'Rubrum Dwarf'**
PRONUNCIATION	pen-ih-SEE-tum seh-TAY-see-um ROO-brum
COMMON NAME	Dwarf purple fountain grass, dwarf red fountain grass

DESCRIPTION: This dwarf cultivar is from Santa Barbara, California. It is nearly identical to purple-leaved fountain grass (*Pennisetum setaceum* 'Rubrum'), distinguished only by its compact size. It grows only 2½ to 3 feet tall and as wide. It is difficult to find in nurseries.

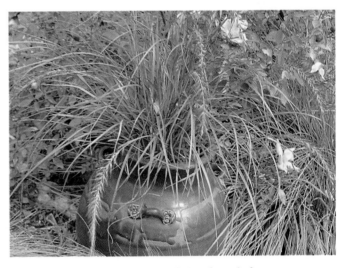

Pennisetum setaceum 'Rubrum Dwarf', dwarf purple fountain grass.

ANOTHER *Pennisetum setaceum* CULTIVAR IS:

'Olive Green' ('Olive Green' fountain grass): olive green-flushed bronze leaves; similar in form and flower to *P. setaceum* 'Rubrum'.

137

BOTANICAL NAME	***Pennisetum villosum***
PRONUNCIATION	pen-ih-SEE-tum vil-OH-sum
COMMON NAME	Feathertop, white-flowering fountain grass
USDA HARDINESS ZONE	9 to 10
ORIGIN	Africa
PREFERRED SITES	Dry savannas, open grassland—widespread

DESCRIPTION: Showy feathertop is an annual in most climates and an aggresive perennial weed in some southern and western climates. Feathertop is another example of a grass that is treasured in one area of the country and feared or disdained as a weed in others. Used properly, it is beautiful in any garden. Its bright, slightly blue-green leaves form spreading mats of creeping foliage 1 to 2 feet tall. The leaves are soft, and the stems are often clothed with downy white hairs. The bristly foxtail flowers look like white feather dusters. The flowers grow from 2 to 5 inches long and 2 to 4 inches wide. Flowers are silky greenish white as they emerge in July and August and become creamy white with age. The foliage goes dormant at temperatures below 32°F and can be killed below 20°F. In warm southern and western climates, feathertop can be mowed as a turf.

LANDSCAPE USES: Feathertop is a showy grass planted either alone or in groups. It masses well and thus makes a good groundcover on slopes or along streams. Feathertop is suitable for coastal gardens and will grow in sand dunes. Its flowers are lovely in fresh or dried arrangments.

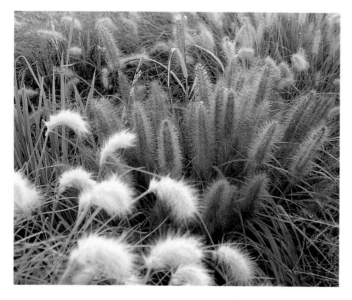

Pennisetum villosum, feathertop, with *P. alopecuroides* 'Moudry', black-flowering fountain grass.

CULTURE AND PROPAGATION: Feathertop grows best in moist, well-drained, fertile loam in full sun or light shade. It does not like deep shade, but seems to grow in just about any other exposure or soil. It tolerates heat, drought, wind, poor soil, and saline and alkaline conditions. Plants tolerate windy coastal conditions and salt spray. In cold climates, feathertop must be treated as an annual or dug and overwintered.

Propagation is easy by seed, or by division in spring or fall. Flower color may vary somewhat from seed, so propagate preferred clones vegetatively

PESTS AND PROBLEMS: Feathertop is an aggressive naturalizing grass. The plant self-sows prolifically in southern and western gardens and has invaded the Southern California coastal chaparral. For this reason, feathertop is considered a noxious weed by native plant enthusiasts. Plant feathertop with caution in mild climates, as it may become weedy with improper maintenance. Be sure to remove seeds before they shatter or remove unwanted seedlings to help prevent spreading. In mild climates plants also spread quickly by rhizomes. In areas of pristine native chaparral, other choices may be more appropriate for protection of the native grasses.

BOTANICAL NAME	***Phalaris arundinacea*** **'Dwarf Garters'**
PRONUNCIATION	fah-LAR-is ah-run-din-AH-see-ah
COMMON NAME	'Dwarf Garters', dwarf ribbon grass
USDA HARDINESS ZONE	4 to 9
ORIGIN	Horticultural selection
PREFERRED SITES	Streamsides, moist meadows, other moist areas

DESCRIPTION: Compact, white-foliaged, warm-season-growing 'Dwarf Garters' is a fine cultivar of the old variety ribbon grass (*Phalaris arundinacea* var. *picta*). The white-striped leaves of 'Dwarf Garters' are ¼ to ½ inch wide and 4 to 7 inches long, and have a refined upright habit. The foliage grows 12 to 15 inches tall and spreads slowly. The new spring growth is tinged pink, but this fades by early summer. The flowers are soft, white panicles that turn brown in late summer. They rise 6 to 12 inches above the foliage and are showy and persistent into the winter. This grass becomes tawny beige with the first frost and is dormant by late October or early November.

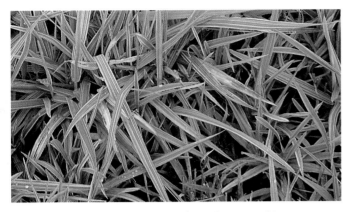

Phalaris arundinacea 'Dwarf Garters', 'Dwarf Garters' ribbon grass.

LANDSCAPE USES: 'Dwarf Garters' is an excellent choice for perennial borders since it does not spread aggressively or flop over. One of the best plants for white foliage in the garden, its white leaves are brighter white than the old variety (var. *picta*) and much more refined in habit. (The species itself, *P. arundinacea*, is extremely vigorous to the point of being invasive.) 'Dwarf Garters' makes an effective groundcover for moist or boggy soils. The plants grow well in tubs and pots and are suitable for small ponds or pools since they tolerate shallow water.

CULTURE AND PROPAGATION: 'Dwarf Garters' prefers moist, rich loam in light shade or half-day sun. It tolerates windy coastal conditions and will grow in sandy or rocky soil if moisture is sufficient. 'Dwarf Garters' grows in shallow water 1 to 2 inches deep. It does not bloom vigorously in mild climates.

Propagate by division only, in spring or fall.

PESTS AND PROBLEMS: 'Dwarf Garters' has no known pests or problems.

BOTANICAL NAME	***Phalaris arundinacea*** **'Feesey's Form'**
PRONUNCIATION	fah-LAR-is ah-run-din-AH-see-ah
COMMON NAME	'Feesey's Form' ribbon grass, strawberries and cream ribbon grass
USDA HARDINESS ZONE	4 to 9
ORIGIN	Horticultural selection
PREFERRED SITES	Rich, moist soil

DESCRIPTION: Spreading, warm-season-growing 'Feesey's Form' ribbon grass is prized for its white-striped foliage blushed with pink, and for its showy flowers. It is a major improvement on the older variety ribbon grass, *Phalaris arundinacea* var. *picta*. Its bright white leaves with green stripes, 6 to 8 inches long and ¾ to 1½ inches wide, clothe spreading stems that reach 1½ to 2½ feet tall. The new growth has a delicate pink blush that looks painted on. The pink tends to bleach out by summer. The flowers, soft white panicles that appear in June and mature to pale brown, grow 12 to 18 inches above the foliage and are showy into winter. The plants fade to beige with the first frost, and the bleached, upright foliage skeleton makes a striking winter accent.

LANDSCAPE USES: 'Feesey's Form' ribbon grass is an exceptional foliage accent. Its pink and white leaf color is particularly bright with new spring growth; even the flower spikes take on a pink blush. The showy flowers are an appealing accent, planted alone or in groups. This grass grows well near ponds and in moist or boggy borders. Both the flowers and foliage provide color in fresh arrangements and are often used in Easter baskets.

CULTURE AND PROPAGATION: 'Feesey's Form' ribbon grass grows best in moist, fertile soil in light shade or half-day sun. It also grows in boggy soil and shallow water 1 to 2 inches deep. Plants tolerate sandy or rocky soils if moisture is present; they resent drying out. The grass also tolerates windy coastal conditions. In hot inland climates, protect plants from full sun.

Propagate by division only, in spring or fall.

PESTS AND PROBLEMS: Occasionally, plants will revert to a nonvariegated form. Weed out such plants when they appear.

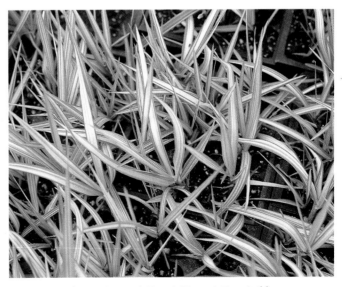

Phalaris arundinacea 'Feesey's Form', 'Feesey's Form' ribbon grass.

BOTANICAL NAME	***Phalaris arundinacea* 'Luteo-Picta'**
PRONUNCIATION	fah-LAR-us ah-run-din-AH-see-ah LOO-tee-oh PIK-tah
COMMON NAME	Golden ribbon grass, golden variegated ribbon grass
USDA HARDINESS ZONE	4 to 9
ORIGIN	Horticultural selection
PREFERRED SITES	Rich, moist soil

DESCRIPTION: Spreading, warm-season-growing golden ribbon grass is similar to the old variety ribbon grass (*Phalaris arundinacea* var. *picta*) but has pale gold-yellow variegation instead of white. Its leaves, ⅜ to ¾ inch wide and 4 to 7 inches long, create a spreading mass of foliage 1½ to 2½ feet tall. The soft white panicles bloom in June, 1 to 1½ feet above the foliage. They are showy and persist into winter. Variegation in the foliage tends to fade by late summer; new spring growth has the best coloring. In the fall the foliage turns beige and dries to a brownish white winter skeleton.

LANDSCAPE USES: A rapidly spreading groundcover, golden ribbon grass is a particularly suitable cover for moist, lightly shaded banks. It also grows well near pools and ponds and in shallow water. It is a fine choice for shady borders as a filler and spiller.

CULTURE AND PROPAGATION: Golden ribbon grass prefers moist, fertile soil in light shade or half-day sun. It grows in rocky or sandy soil as long as moisture is sufficient. Plants tolerate windy coastal conditions, and will grow in water 1 to 2 inches deep.
  Propagate by division only, in fall or spring.

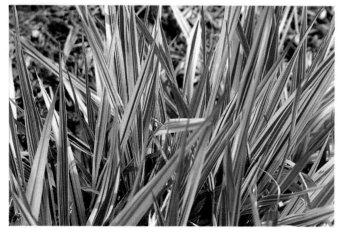

Phalaris arundinacea 'Luteo-Picta', golden ribbon grass.

PESTS AND PROBLEMS: Aggressively spreading golden ribbon grass may become invasive in favorable situations. Plant it in a drainage tile or root barrier to control spreading. This cultivar has the bad habit of reverting to a wholly green form without golden variegation. Reversions should be removed, because the green form is more aggressive and will eventually dominate the planting if allowed to remain unchecked.

BOTANICAL NAME	***Phalaris arundinacea* var. *picta***
PRONUNCIATION	fah-LAR-is ah-run-din-AH-see-ah PIK-tah
COMMON NAME	Ribbon grass, gardener's-garters
USDA HARDINESS ZONE	4 to 9
ORIGIN	Widespread throughout North America and Eurasia
PREFERRED SITES	Moist areas, streamsides

DESCRIPTION: Spreading, warm-season-growing ribbon grass has white variegated foliage and showy white flowers. The leaves, ¾ to 1 inch wide and 5 to 7 inches long, are striped green and white and taper to a point. New spring growth is often tinged pink. The foliage reaches 2 to 3 feet tall and often flops. The flowers appear in June as soft, white spikes 12 to 18 inches above the foliage and mature to pale brown. Plants bleach to beige with the first frost; the bleached foliage is attractive into winter.

LANDSCAPE USES: Ribbon grass is an old garden favorite and is often found in older gardens and abandoned farm sites. This spreading grass is effective as a groundcover and bank cover. It makes a desirable foliage and flowering accent in borders and formal plantings. Ribbon grass is good in or near ponds, as the grass will grow in shallow water. Plants also thrive in pots and tubs. Flowers and foliage are attractive in fresh and dried arrangements.

CULTURE AND PROPAGATION: Ribbon grass grows best in moist, fertile soil in light shade or half-day sun. Plants tolerate sand or rocky soil as long as moisture is present. The grass grows in shallow water 2 to 4 inches deep. In hot inland climates, the foliage will burn in full, hot sun. In such climates, half-day sun or filtered shade is best.
  Propagate by division only, in spring or fall.

PESTS AND PROBLEMS: Ribbon grass forms dense, very aggressive colonies that can overtake a garden. Confine it in a drainage tile to control its aggressive, spreading nature. However, in Mediterranean and dry southwestern climates, this plant is not aggressive or spreading.

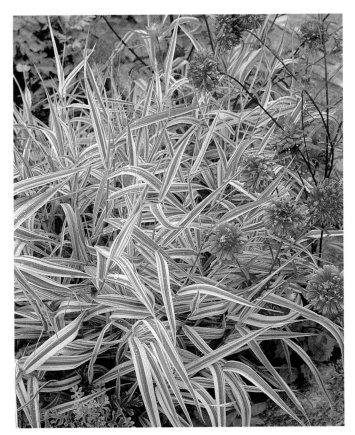

Phalaris arundinacea var. *picta,* ribbon grass.

BOTANICAL NAME	***Phragmites australis***
PRONUNCIATION	frag-MEYE-teez aw-STRAL-is
COMMON NAME	Common reed
USDA HARDINESS ZONE	4 to 10
ORIGIN	Large worldwide distribution, found in Northern and Southern hemispheres
PREFERRED SITES	In or near water, extensive wetland areas

DESCRIPTION: Common reed is an aggressive colonizer that can escape to become a noxious weed, crowding out native plants. A pioneer plant, it will eventually fill in small ponds and shallow water. The thick canes of this warm-season grass were originally used for thatching and roof construction. The plant is valuable for cleaning up polluted soil and water. Like cattails, common reed assimilates pollutants such as heavy metals. A massive grass reaching 10 to 18 feet tall, common reed is a commanding presence in the garden.

The ½- to 1-inch-wide, pointed leaves of common reed grow 8 to 12 inches long. The foliage is bluish green to medium green and the leaves clothe thick, stout stems, ½ to ¾ inch in diameter. The flowers are showy one-sided panicles borne 2 to 4 feet above the foliage. They emerge pinkish or purplish in late August and September, mature to a tawny color, and are showy well into winter. Silky at first, they fluff to a brown tassel and turn beige or russet in the fall. The foliage often turns golden yellow after the first frost.

LANDSCAPE USES: Common reed is perhaps best in large gardens or parks where it has plenty of room to grow. The plant is at its best naturalized along lakes or ponds, where its tall canes can arch out over the water's edge. An aggressive colonizer, it must be contained by root barriers. Carefully contained, it can make a beautiful tall accent for the back of a perennial border. Used in mass, it makes an effective screen or windbreak. Common reed does well in coastal plantings.

CULTURE AND PROPAGATION: Common reed prefers moist or boggy, rich soil in full sun, although it tolerates extreme soil conditions from pure sand to heavy clay. It tolerates salinity and alkalinity. It also tolerates light to medium shade but will flop if too shaded.

Propagate by seed, or by division in spring or fall.

PESTS AND PROBLEMS: Common reed usually is a vicious weed; its ability to spread invasively should not be underestimated. It can be contained in a drainage tile 3 to 4 feet long. Plants can be held in check along lawn areas by constant and close mowing.

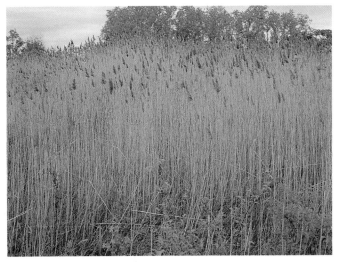

Phragmites australis, common reed.

BOTANICAL NAME	***Poa costineata***
PRONUNCIATION	POH-ah cos-tin-ee-AH-tah
COMMON NAME	Australian blue grass
USDA HARDINESS ZONE	8 to 10
ORIGIN	Southern Australia
PREFERRED SITES	Open meadows, grasslands

DESCRIPTION: A recent introduction to American nurseries, Australian blue grass has great beauty and an inherent toughness that lends itself to a variety of garden situations. A clumping, cool-season grass, it forms dense tufts of medium green foliage 1 to 2 feet tall and as wide. This fine-textured foliage, $1/16$ to $1/8$ inch wide, has rolled edges that almost conceal a powdery blue covering on the underside of the leaf. This coloring imparts a hint of blue to the foliage, giving the plant a charming sparkle. The flowers emerge greenish on vertical spikes 8 to 12 inches above the foliage in late spring. The open, airy panicles mature to a rich golden color and are persistent and showy until mid-fall.

LANDSCAPE USES: Australian blue grass makes a fine accent and is good planted singularly or in masses. The long, fine-textured foliage becomes pendulous, making it useful for containers and attractive spilling down a slope. Its drought tolerance and overall toughness make it a good choice for dry gardens. Though not spectacular, the flowers are useful in fresh arrangements.

CULTURE AND PROPAGATION: Australian blue grass prefers a fertile, moist, well-drained, sunny location. It tolerates a wide range of soil and climatic variance, including heat, drought, wind, and coastal conditions. It tolerates medium shade but flops in too much shade. In hot, arid, western climates, weekly summer water is best to maintain its green color. Australian blue grass's hardiness is untested below 10°F. It may grow in lower temperatures.
   Propagate by division or seed.

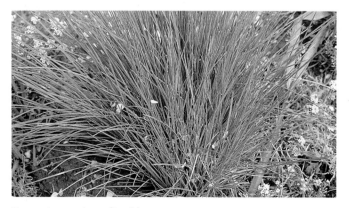

Poa costineata, Australian blue grass.

PESTS AND PROBLEMS: Australian blue grass has no known pests or problems.

OTHER SPECIES OF BLUEGRASS ARE:

Poa alpina var. *vivipara* (Alpine bluegrass): compact foliage; grows 6 to 8 inches tall; best in rock gardens.

Poa caesia (Greenland bluegrass): a diminutive, clumping evergreen rock garden grass with blue-green foliage; difficult in hot climates. Also sold as *P. glauca.*

Poa chaixii (Forest bluegrass): an evergreen grass growing 1 to 2 feet tall with bright green foliage; difficult in hot climates.

BOTANICAL NAME	***Rychelytrum neriglume***
PRONUNCIATION	ree-KEL-ee-trum ner-ih-GLOO-mee
COMMON NAME	Ruby grass
USDA HARDINESS ZONE	9 to 10
ORIGIN	South Africa
PREFERRED SITES	Open grasslands

DESCRIPTION: Clumping, somewhat cool-season-growing ruby grass is perhaps one of the showiest of the small flowering grasses. Its leaves, $1/16$ to $1/8$ inch wide, form tight clumps of soft foliage that grow 8 to 12 inches tall and as wide. The blue-green foliage blushes purple-red in the fall but remains evergreen in mild climates. The flowers emerge in May in mild climates and late June in colder climates. The narrow, silky, ruby-pink blooms, 3 to 4 inches long, are iridescent on emergence, maturing to creamy white. They are showy and persist into winter. The flowers grow on vertical spikes that rise 12 to 18 inches above the foliage. Ruby grass's cold hardiness is untested, but it is probably killed at 15°F. Ruby grass is hard to find in nurseries but is worth the search.

LANDSCAPE USES: Ruby grass is an excellent flowering accent for the front and middle of the perennial border. It is a good plant for coastal and rock gardens. Planted alone or in groups, it is especially effective when backlit by early morning or late afternoon light. Its flowers are stunning in fresh and dried arrangements.

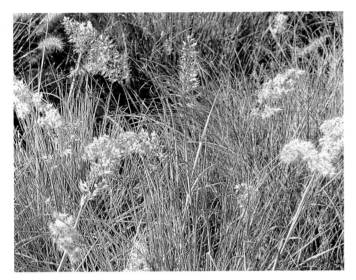

Rychelytrum neriglume, ruby grass.

CULTURE AND PROPAGATION: Ruby grass grows best in moist, well-drained soil in full sun. It tolerates heavy soil but resents wet, poorly drained sites. In addition, it will grow in coastal conditions and sandy soils. While it will tolerate light shade, plants languish in too much shade. Once established, ruby grass is somewhat drought-tolerant. Use it as an annual in cold climates.

Propagation by seed is best, as plants do not propagate easily by division.

PESTS AND PROBLEMS: Ruby grass has no known pests or problems.

BOTANICAL NAME	***Rychelytrum repens* (also known as *R. roseum*)**
PRONUNCIATION	ree-KEL-ee-trum REE-pens
COMMON NAME	Natal grass, ruby grass
USDA HARDINESS ZONE	9 to 10
ORIGIN	Southern Africa
PREFERRED SITES	Dry, rocky grasslands

DESCRIPTION: Natal grass is noted for its delicate pink flowers. The foliage of this creeping, warm-season grass reaches 1 to 2 feet tall. The glossy, bluish green leaves, ⅛ to ⅜ inch wide and 3 to 5 inches long, clothe floppy spreading stems. The flowers arch up and out from the foliage 1 to 1½ feet. They are borne in light, airy panicles that emerge silky rose-pink as early as May in mild climates and in July in cooler climates, and mature to pink, cream, and tan. Late in the season natal grass is usually a mix of colors. In mild climates, flowers bloom almost year-round and the grass is evergreen, but it becomes dormant in the summer

in dry climates. It is killed at temperatures below 20°F. Natal grass can be used as an annual in cold climates.

LANDSCAPE USES: The soft, fluffy, airy flowers of natal grass are spectacular in mass plantings, since even the slightest breeze sets them in motion. Almost without equal as a flowering accent when used in mass, the grass is a good choice for hot, dry slopes. Its floppy foliage looks stunning when spilling over walks and walls, and the fresh flowers are beautiful in arrangements.

CULTURE AND PROPAGATION: Natal grass prefers moist, fertile soil with good drainage and full sun. It tolerates a wide range of soil conditions, from heavy clay to dune sand, and also tolerates coastal conditions, wind, and salt spray. Plants tolerate light shade but flop badly in too much shade. Natal grass makes a fine annual, growing rapidly and flowering until frost.

Propagate by seed or by division, although it is easier to propagate by seed.

PESTS AND PROBLEMS: Natal grass can be an invasive naturalizer in mild climates. It is not a good choice for gardens situated near pristine native habitats, although in colder climates its seeding habit is of no consequence.

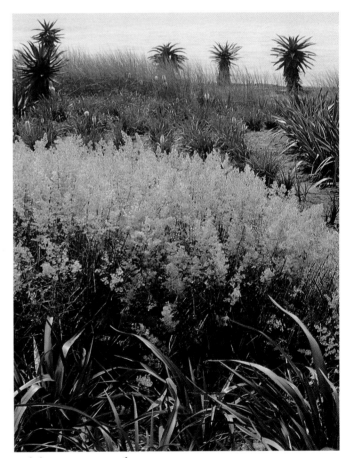

Rychelytrum repens, natal grass.

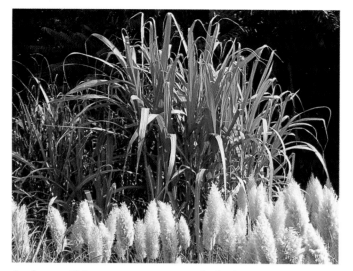

Saccharum officinarum, sugarcane, provides background for pampas plumes.

BOTANICAL NAME	***Saccharum officinarum***
PRONUNCIATION	sa-KAR-rum oh-fish-in-AR-rum
COMMON NAME	Sugarcane
USDA HARDINESS ZONE	9 to 10
ORIGIN	Tropical Southeast Asia; has been cultivated for centuries
PREFERRED SITES	Moist areas

DESCRIPTION: This robust clumping grass can grow as tall as 12 to 15 feet. Depending on the cultivar, sugarcane forms stout canes 1 to 3 inches in diameter with leaves 1 to 3 inches wide and 1½ to 5 feet long. Established plants form upright, arching clumps that can grow 8 to 10 feet in one season. Old leaves shed to show the varying colors of the smooth glossy canes. Sugarcane freezes back to mature cane at temperatures below 32°F. Some clones are killed below freezing, but some hardy clones have survived 10°F and show promise as selections for colder areas.

Sugarcane's flowers appear in fluffy panicles somewhat similar to a pampas grass plume. The 12- to 18-inch-long flowers bloom in September but rarely bloom in nontropical climates.

The recent surge in interest in the ornamental grasses is responsible for the appearance of several new clones of sugarcane. Many of these have unknown origins and have been passed down through generations of Hawaiian, Caribbean, Asian, and Latino families. It is hoped that more of these clones will be sorted out and given valid cultivar names. Much more research is needed to determine the hardiness and eventual heights in various climates. Several distinct clones of sugarcane deserve mention. More color forms, dwarf forms, and many other new and exciting varieties will soon find their way into American gardens.

Following is a list of unnamed clones now being grown in California:

Red cane, green leaves: cane thickness 1 to 2 inches; plants 6 to 12 feet tall.

Green cane, green leaves: cane thickness 1 to 2 inches; plants 6 to 12 feet tall.

Green and red variegated cane, green leaves: cane thickness 1 to 2 inches; plants 6 to 12 feet tall.

Green and yellow variegated cane, green leaves: cane thickness 1 to 2 inches; plants 6 to 12 feet tall.

Red cane, red leaves: cane thickness ¾ to 1 inch; plants 6 to 8 feet tall.

LANDSCAPE USES: Sugarcane provides a dramatic tropical accent for warm-climate gardens. An excellent screen and windbreak, it also grows well in pots and tubs. Colored cultivars make good foliage accents when used as annuals or potted plants. The canes are edible and are used for making refined sugar. Both the foliage and flowers are striking in fresh and dried arrangements.

CULTURE AND PROPAGATION: Sugarcane prefers moist, fertile soil in full sun. It tolerates a wide range of soil and climatic conditions, including coastal gardens, wet soil, and sandy soil if moisture is sufficient. It is drought-tolerant when established but does not like to be constantly dry. Plants love heat and will tolerate hot, dry winds if moisture is sufficient.

Propagate by seed, by division, or from cuttings of mature cane.

PESTS AND PROBLEMS: Sugarcane has no known pests or problems.

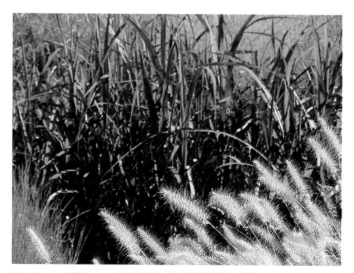

Saccharum officinarum 'Pele's Smoke', 'Pele's Smoke' sugarcane.

BOTANICAL NAME	*Saccharum officinarum* 'Pele's Smoke'
PRONUNCIATION	sa-KAR-rum oh-fish-in-AR-rum
COMMON NAME	'Pele's Smoke' sugarcane, red sugarcane

DESCRIPTION: Bold-textured, purple-foliaged 'Pele's Smoke' sugarcane makes a bold accent in the garden. Plants form a tall fountain of arching, purple foliage. The richly colored purple canes are as glossy and showy as the leaves. Plants rarely flower; blooming probably does not occur in non-tropical climates. Quart-sized clumps planted in spring can reach 6 feet tall by the end of summer. In cold climates, plant this sugarcane after the threat of frost has passed.

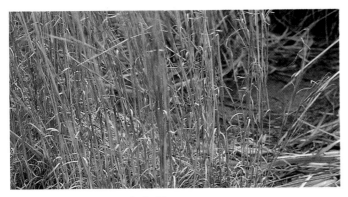

Schizachyrium scoparium, little bluestem.

BOTANICAL NAME	*Schizachyrium scoparium*
PRONUNCIATION	skits-ah-KEER-ee-um skoh-PAIR-ee-um
COMMON NAME	Little bluestem, prairie beard grass, broom sedge
USDA HARDINESS ZONE	3 to 10
ORIGIN	North America, from Canada to Florida, and Maryland to Utah. One of the most prevalent grasses in the eastern United States.
PREFERRED SITES	Prairies, open woods, dry hills

DESCRIPTION: A deciduous, clumping, warm-season grass, little bluestem is found throughout the eastern half of the United States. This grass can grow 2 to 5 feet fall, but usually grows to 3 feet. Its light green foliage, ¼ to ½ inch wide and 12 to 16 inches long, becomes darker with maturity. It has a medium texture and soft, somewhat hairy leaves. Most of its height is made up by flower spikes that emerge from July through September. Fluffy plumes of ripening seed heads catch the light beautifully. In the fall, little bluestem ranges from bronze to flaming orange. It will usually hold some measure of color well into winter.

LANDSCAPE USES: Little bluestem is effective as a large-scale groundcover for massing or naturalizing. Use it for transition areas between wood and pasture or for erosion and slope control. Single specimens are effective in borders and rock gardens. It also provides good cut flowers and fall color. Although named cultivars selected for outstanding fall colors are not yet available in nurseries or garden centers, they are sure to come.

CULTURE AND PROPAGATION: Little bluestem grows best in full sun and tolerates almost any soil except those that are boggy, wet, or mucky. Dependably drought-tolerant, it looks better with some summer water in arid southwestern climates. Little bluestem is a heavy seeder and can become a pest in certain situations.

Propagate by seed or division.

PESTS AND PROBLEMS: Little bluestem has no known pests or problems.

ONE CULTIVAR OF *Schizachyrium scoparium* IS:
'Blaze' ('Blaze' little bluestem): originally developed for forage, it has intense fall color ranging from pinkish orange to red-purple; blazing color lasts through winter.

SCIRPUS AND SCHOENPLECTUS
BULRUSHES/RUSHES

Bulrushes are native to almost every area of the United States where water is found. Gardeners would do well to investigate their own native bulrush species. Your local native plant society can help identify important species for your area. Although some bulrushes are aggressive spreaders, most are easily contained by root barriers or are held in check by the extent of their moist habitat. Many native bulrush habitats have been greatly reduced. This is unfortunate because these habitats are important to wildlife and they filter and clean polluted water.

BOTANICAL NAME	***Schoenplectus tabernaemontana 'Zebrinus' (also known as Scirpus lacustris* var. *tabernaemontana 'Zebrinus')***
PRONUNCIATION	show-en-PLEK-tus tab-er-nay-mon-TAN-ah zeh-BREYE-nus
COMMON NAME	Banded bulrush, zebra rush
USDA HARDINESS ZONE	7 to 9
ORIGIN	Horticultural selection from Japan
PREFERRED SITES	Shallow water, moist areas

DESCRIPTION: A spreading, warm-season-growing rush, banded bulrush produces cylindrical leaves variegated with horizontal bands. The effect is somewhat similar to zebra grass (*Miscanthus sinensis* 'Zebrinus'). The hollow leaves grow ¼ to ½ inch wide and 2 to 4 feet tall and are marked with greenish yellow or yellowish white bands, ¼ to ½ inch wide. The banding is most pronounced on new spring growth and tends to fade by late summer. The foliage forms slowly spreading colonies, usually in moist boggy soil or in shallow water. With the onset of cool temperatures, the foliage turns yellow, becoming brown and dormant by October or November. The flowers are typical conelike, brownish spikes. Although not showy, they are noticeable and make an interesting accent to the foliage. The terminal flowers appear from late June through August and persist into the winter.

LANDSCAPE USES: Banded bulrush looks lovely in pools and ponds, particularly where early morning and late afternoon

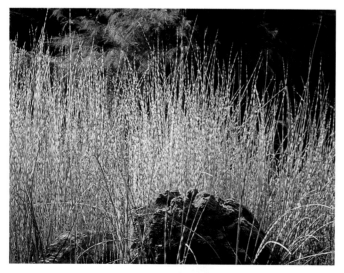

Schoenplectus tabernaemontana 'Zebrinus', banded bulrush.

sun can backlight the foliage and reflect in the water. It also does well in pots and tubs. The foliage is striking in fresh and dried arrangements.

CULTURE AND PROPAGATION: Banded bulrush grows best in rich, moist or wet soil or shallow water 2 to 6 inches deep, in full sun. The plants resent drying out and grow poorly in dry situations. Too much shade also results in weak growth. In hot, inland climates, half-day sun keeps the plants from yellowing.

Propagate by division only, in the spring.

PESTS AND PROBLEMS: Banded bulrush has no known pests or problems.

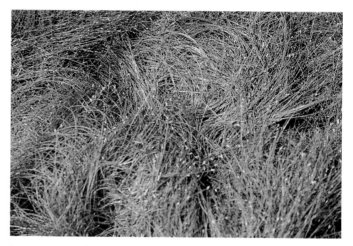

Scirpus cernuus, fiber optics grass.

BOTANICAL NAME	***Scirpus cernuus* (also known as *Eleocharis cernuus*)**
PRONUNCIATION	SKIR-pus SER-noo-us
COMMON NAME	Fiber optics grass, nodding scirpus
USDA HARDINESS ZONE	9 to 10
ORIGIN	Europe
PREFERRED SITES	Wet sites, saltwater marshes, brackish water

DESCRIPTION: A curious grasslike rush relative, fiber optics grass has fine, bright green, hairlike leaves capped by a terminal flower spike; the overall effect resembles the thin threads of fiber optics. This clumping warm-season rush bears cylindrical, bright, iridescent green leaves, ¹/₃₂ to ¹/₁₆ inch in diameter and 12 to 18 inches long. The plants form dense tufts of foliage 6 to 12 inches tall and, with age, form tussocks, with new green leaves emerging from old dead

146

foliage. The flowers are small white spikes, 1/16 to 1/8 inch long, that mature to a brown conelike structure and persist on the leaf tips throughout the winter. The leaves bend under the weight of the flowers. In colder areas of Zone 9 the plants freeze back to the crown. In mild or subtropical climates, the foliage stays evergreen.

LANDSCAPE USES: Fiber optics grass is ideal for ponds, pools, and water gardens, planted either on the water's edge or in shallow water. It is also attractive in shady wet spots of the garden. The plants are best displayed where the weeping foliage can spill over rocks, walls, or the edges of pots. This grass makes an interesting hanging basket and will grow indoors in strong direct light.

CULTURE AND PROPAGATION: Fiber optics grass prefers moist, fertile soil in full sun or light shade. It grows well in shallow water and resents drying out. In hot inland climates, plants grow best in half-day shade; in dry, arid climates, plants will yellow in full hot sun. Fiber optics grass may require cutting back. If cut back yearly, it responds with new foliage. If the grass has not been cut back for a year or more, cut it back no closer than 2 to 3 inches above the old crown line.

Although you can propagate fiber optics grass by seed or division, propagation is easier by division.

PESTS AND PROBLEMS: Fiber optics grass has no known pests or problems.

OTHER BULRUSH SPECIES AND CULTIVARS ARE:

Schoenplectus tabernae-montana 'Albescens' (White-striped bulrush): similar to banded bulrush (*S. tabernaemontana* 'Ze-brinus') with white-striped foliage; a choice selection.

Scirpus lacustris (Bulrush): deciduous, tubular, dark green foliage; 4 to 6 feet tall; a creeping bog-lover.

SESLERIA
MOOR GRASS

Another grass with the common name of moor grass, this genus contains several of the best ornamental grasses for mass plantings and groundcovers. Their ease of care, adaptability, and resistance to pests and problems make moor grass useful in a variety of situations. All species are evergreen and cool-season grasses. Most have handsome foliage though somewhat nondescript flowers; thus they are planted mainly for their foliage.

Moor grasses, with their noninvasive habits, make good fillers in the garden. They do quite nicely planted between perennials and as an understory for shrubs and trees.

BOTANICAL NAME	***Sesleria autumnalis***
PRONUNCIATION	sez-LAIR-ee-ah aw-TUM-nal-is
COMMON NAME	Autumn moor grass
USDA HARDINESS ZONE	5 to 9
ORIGIN	Eastern and northern Italy to Albania
PREFERRED SITES	Alkaline soils, margins of woods

DESCRIPTION: A tough but beautiful evergreen, autumn moor grass is admired for its bright yellow-green foliage and attractive flower spikes. Its yellow-green to almost chartreuse leaves form an upright tufted mound of foliage 16 to 18 inches tall and as wide. The narrow V-shaped leaves are 1/8 to 1/4 inch wide and 8 to 12 inches long. Flower spikes occur primarily in the fall, although they will bloom in May and June in mild climates. The flowers, 4 to 6 inches long and 1/8 to 1/4 inch wide, emerge as a narrow upright spike 6 to 8 inches above the foliage. They emerge purplish black and are covered with white silky stamens. They are noticeable but not particularly showy, maturing to brown and persisting throughout the winter.

LANDSCAPE USES: Autumn moor grass makes a fine large-scale groundcover. It is effective in large masses, on slopes, under the light shade of trees, and in coastal gardens and rocky sites. Autumn moor grass tolerates root competition from woody plants.

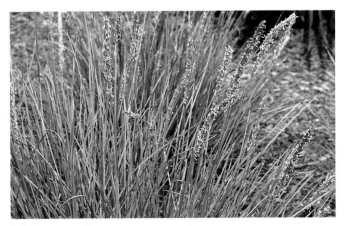

Sesleria autumnalis, autumn moor grass.

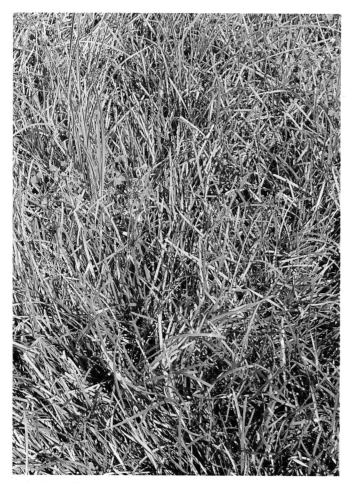

Sesleria caerulea, blue moor grass.

BOTANICAL NAME	***Sesleria caerulea***
PRONUNCIATION	sez-LAIR-ee-ah ser-ROO-lee-ah
COMMON NAME	Blue moor grass
USDA HARDINESS ZONE	5 to 9
ORIGIN	Northwestern Russia, Sweden, Bulgaria, Yugoslavia
PREFERRED SITES	Calcareous soils, openings in woods, meadows

DESCRIPTION: Clumping, cool-season-growing, evergreen blue moor grass has soft, attractive two-toned leaves that form clumps 6 to 12 inches tall and as wide. The leaves, dark green on the top and powdery bluish white underneath, twist and curl to expose both sides of the leaf, giving the plant a unique cool blue-green look. The leaves are ⅛ to ⅜ inch wide and 3 to 4 inches long with a soft, boat-shaped tip. The flowers bloom from March through June as tiny flower spikes, ¼ inch wide and ½ to ¾ inch long, borne on thin, wiry stems 6 to 8 inches above the foliage. The flowers emerge purplish and mature to a golden wheat color. They shatter late in the season and are self-cleaning. The flowers are noticeable but not particularly showy.

LANDSCAPE USES: Blue moor grass is effective in mass plantings and as a large-scale groundcover. It makes a good filler and edging plant in perennial borders and rock gardens. Blue moor grass does well in light shade under tall trees or woody shrubs, between stepping stones, and in cracks and crevices. Blue moor grass makes a cool blue-green lawn substitute but tolerates only occasional traffic. It makes a fine meadow for small urban gardens when naturalized with dwarf bulbs. Easy to grow and easy to please, blue moor grass is interesting when viewed up close along pathways and by patios.

CULTURE AND PROPAGATION: Blue moor grass prefers moist, well-drained rich loam in full sun or light shade. Plants resent drying out and grow poorly in dry sites and dense shade. In hot inland climates, plants prefer ample moisture and half-day sun. The grass tolerates coastal conditions as long as moisture is sufficient.

Propagate by seed, or by division in spring or fall.

PESTS AND PROBLEMS: Blue moor grass has no known pests or problems.

BOTANICAL NAME	***Sesleria heuffleriana***
PRONUNCIATION	sez-LAIR-ee-ah HYOO-fleer-ee-AH-nah
COMMON NAME	Green moor grass
USDA HARDINESS ZONE	5 to 9
ORIGIN	Southeastern Europe
PREFERRED SITES	Shaded sites, open woodlands, lime soils

DESCRIPTION: Attractive, clumping, cool-season-growing green moor grass has rich, glossy green foliage and attractive flowers atop wiry stems. The somewhat soft leaves, ⅛ to ⅜ inch wide, are bright green on top and light, powdery bluish green underneath. They form an upright, tufting mound of foliage 12 to 18 inches tall and as wide. The dark brown to black flowers first appear in mid-March on long, wiry stems 6 to 8 inches above the foliage. Noticeable but not necessarily showy, the flowers shatter by late season.

LANDSCAPE USES: Green moor grass is effective planted alone or in mass. It makes a fine large-scale groundcover planted in the light shade of tall trees and makes a good rock garden plant. Plants tolerate coastal conditions with sufficient moisture. Green moor grass can create low evergreen meadows and looks lovely when naturalized with bulbs and other spring-blooming perennials.

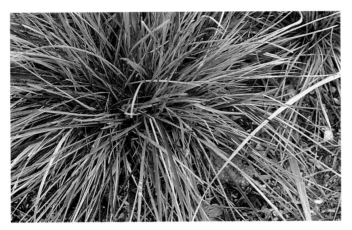

Sesleria heuffleriana, green moor grass.

CULTURE AND PROPAGATION: Green moor grass prefers moist, well-drained, rich loam in full sun or partial shade. It is drought-tolerant in all but the hottest arid inland climates, but looks better with regular water in southwestern gardens. It tolerates windy coastal conditions with adequate moisture. Plants always look nicer in light shade or half-day sun than they do in full sun.

Propagate by seed, or by division in spring or fall.

PESTS AND PROBLEMS: Green moor grass has no known pests or problems.

ANOTHER MOOR GRASS SPECIES IS:

Sesleria nitida (Gray moor grass): evergreen with blue-gray foliage, growing 12 to 18 inches tall; excellent for Mediterranean climates.

BOTANICAL NAME	***Setaria palmifolia***
PRONUNCIATION	seh-TAR-ee-ah palm-ih-FOL-ee-ah
COMMON NAME	Palm grass
USDA HARDINESS ZONE	9 to 10
ORIGIN	India, Africa
PREFERRED SITES	Grasslands, savannas

DESCRIPTION: Warm-season-growing, subtropical palm grass is admired for its bold foliage. Its deep green, pleated leaves, 2 to 3 inches wide and 1 to 3 feet long, resemble palm fronds and taper to a point. The foliage forms a

dense, upright, arching clump that can reach 3 to 6 feet tall and as wide. The flowers bloom from June through August. Their long, narrow spikes arch up and out from the foliage 2 to 3 feet and are tipped with fuzzy 3- to 5-inch-long foxtails. Both the sturdy flower stems and the wide, pleated leaves sway gently in the breeze. The foliage is evergreen in mild climates but is damaged below freezing. Some mature plants, however, have survived to 15°F.

LANDSCAPE USES: The bold foliage of palm grass provides a tropical garden accent. Even a single specimen can dominate the garden. Large specimens make a dense screen or background planting. Well-suited to pot and tub culture, palm grass is also appropriate at the water's edge, in shady situations, and in coastal gardens. Both the foliage and flowers are lovely in fresh and dried arrangements.

CULTURE AND PROPAGATION: While palm grass prefers moist, fertile soil in full sun or light shade, it is extremely adaptable. It thrives on moisture and tolerates wet soil but is considerably drought-tolerant once established. It also tolerates heavy clay and sandy soil. Well-suited to dry tropical sites, palm grass grows vigorously in dry shade. It tolerates the coastal conditions of wind, salt spray, and sandy soils as long as moisture is present. Palm grass thrives on the water's edge and can take occasional submersion. Its rapid growth makes it a good choice as an annual in cold climates. Plants can be dug in the fall and overwintered in a garage or other area where temperatures remain above 40°F.

Propagation is easy from seed; divisions should be done in late spring.

PESTS AND PROBLEMS: Since palm grass is a prolific seeder in mild climates, it can easily make a pest of itself if not carefully watched.

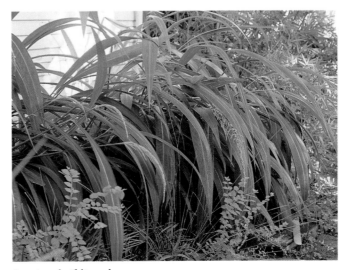

Setaria palmifolia, palm grass.

ONE CULTIVAR OF *Setaria palmifolia* IS:

'Variegata' (Variegated palm grass): similar to the species, with yellow-streaked leaves; rare.

BOTANICAL NAME	***Sorghastrum nutans* (also known as *Chrysopogon nutans*)**
PRONUNCIATION	sor-GAS-trum NOO-tanz
COMMON NAME	Indian grass, gold beard grass
USDA HARDINESS ZONE	4 to 9
ORIGIN	From Canada to Mexico and from Maine to Florida; New Jersey west to Colorado
PREFERRED SITES	Prairies, open woods

DESCRIPTION: Indian grass is one of North America's most beautiful native grasses. It was one of the major constituents of the tallgrass prairie that used to cover a sizeable portion of what is now the central United States; most of this prairie no longer exists.

Indian grass is an attractive, upright, clumping, warm-season grass. Although its foliage usually ranges from various shades of light to medium green, it may vary from gray-green to almost blue. Its leaves, ¼ to ½ inch wide and 8 to 12 inches long, branch off the stems at a 45-degree angle. In most situations, it grows between 2 and 3 feet tall, but in deep, fertile soil with plenty of moisture, it is capable of growing up to 5 feet tall. Late summer-blooming flowers are borne on stiff, erect spikes that grow 2 to 3 feet above the foliage. The flowers are borne in showy tan-yellow panicles 6 to 12 inches long and 1 to 3 inches wide on bright golden yellow stems. The paired spikelets have distinctive awns, giving them a soft, delicate, feathery quality. As the flowers mature, the bright yellow stamens turn bronze. As fall approaches, Indian grass becomes yellowish and then dries to an attractive burnt orange. Both the fall and winter colors are showy, reason enough for its use as an ornamental.

LANDSCAPE USES: Indian grass excels in mass plantings and prairie restorations. It is a good choice for naturalizing, for planting along highways, on slopes, and elsewhere for erosion control. A good flowering accent, it provides fall and winter color. It is also useful as a tall background grass. Even single specimens of Indian grass can be stunning. It is a must for fresh and dried flower arrangements.

CULTURE AND PROPAGATION: Indian grass tolerates a wide range of conditions. Although it grows best in deep, rich, moist loam in a sunny location, it tolerates far worse conditions and soil types, including light shade and sandy, gravelly, and wet soils. Drought-tolerant once established, Indian grass can benefit from additional water in the summer in arid western regions. In its native habitat, the grass grows in areas where it rains in summer.

Propagation is easy by seed, and Indian grass will readily reseed in the garden. From seed, plants need two seasons to become fully established. The grass may also be divided.

PESTS AND PROBLEMS: Indian grass will readily reseed itself in areas with adequate moisture, which may or may not be desirable.

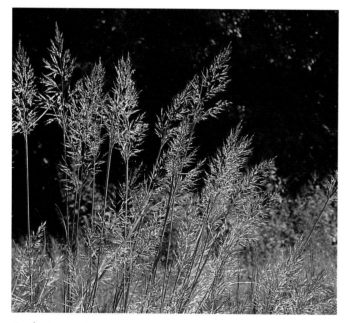

Sorghastrum nutans, Indian grass.

SOME CULTIVARS OF *Sorghastrum nutans* ARE:

'Holt' ('Holt' Indian grass): another prairie grass originally selected for forage purposes; superior ornamental qualities; distinguished by earlier blooms, prolific seed heads, and good fall color.

'Sioux Blue' ('Sioux Blue' Indian grass): similar in most respects to the species, with bright blue-gray foliage.

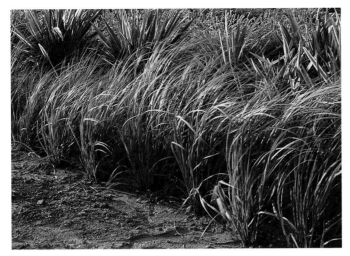

Spartina pectinata, prairie cord grass.

BOTANICAL NAME	**Spartina pectinata (also known as *S. michauxiana*)**
PRONUNCIATION	spar-TEE-nah pek-tin-AH-tah
COMMON NAME	Prairie cord grass
USDA HARDINESS ZONE	4 to 9
ORIGIN	Widespread, from Maine to eastern Oregon, south to North Carolina, and west to Texas
PREFERRED SITES	Low-lying moist areas, freshwater marshes

DESCRIPTION: Spreading, warm-season-growing prairie cord grass is one of the original grasses of the tallgrass prairie. Found primarily in low-lying, moist soils or on the margins of ponds and rivers, the plant produces graceful arching leaves that give the feeling of motion even when perfectly still; when moving in a breeze, the leaves sway in rolling waves.

An aggressive rhizomatous spreader, prairie cord grass has sharp-edged leaves ¼ to ¾ inch wide and 1½ to 2½ inches long. Its glossy green foliage grows 3 to 6 feet tall, usually to 3 feet in arid western climates. The flowers emerge in late July as one-sided brownish spikes that arch 2 to 3 feet above the foliage. Though noticeable, they are not particularly showy. In fall, the leaves turn a brilliant golden yellow, providing a good autumn display. The winter foliage holds its graceful arching quality, making it particularly attractive in snowy climates.

LANDSCAPE USES: Prairie cord grass is excellent planted on the water's edge in pools, ponds, and lakes, and it grows well in tubs and pots. Prairie cord grass controls erosion on river banks and streamsides, and provides an effective wildlife habitat. It is lovely in fresh or dried arrangements.

CULTURE AND PROPAGATION: Prairie cord grass prefers moist, fertile soil in full sun. Prairie cord grass is quite drought-tolerant when established and is heat-tolerant if moisture is sufficient. In dry gardens, plants spread slowly and rarely reach over 2 feet tall. Prairie cord grass tolerates heavy to sandy soils, fresh to brackish water, and windy coastal conditions. Plants flop in too much shade.

Propagate by seed or division. You can propagate it most easily by division or by cutting the rhizomes.

PESTS AND PROBLEMS: Prairie cord grass can spread aggressively in moist soils. Plant it in 3-foot drainage tiles or a concrete barrier to contain its spread.

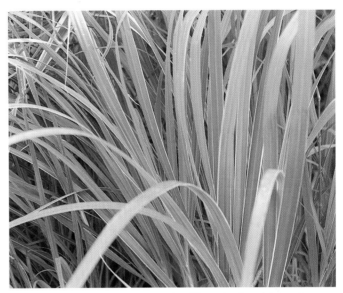

Spartina pectinata 'Aureomarginata', golden-edged prairie cord grass.

BOTANICAL NAME	**Spartina pectinata 'Aureomarginata'**
PRONUNCIATION	spar-TEE-nah pek-tin-AH-tah AW-ree-oh-mar-JIN-ah-tah
COMMON NAME	Golden-edged prairie cord grass

DESCRIPTION: Golden-edged priaire cord grass is similar to prairie cord grass in almost every aspect, except that the leaves have thin golden margins. The yellow edges are slight and usually only highlight the foliage; the plants do not appear golden or yellow. This highlight is an attractive trait and justifies planting this cultivar over the species. Plants will revert back to nonvariegated forms, but the variegation will usually reappear in time. Propagate by division only, in the spring or fall.

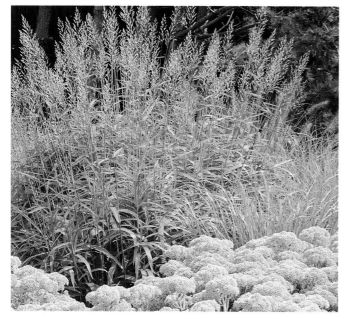

Spodiopogon sibericus, frost grass.

BOTANICAL NAME	***Spodiopogon sibericus (also incorrectly known as Muhlenbergia alpestris or Lasiogrostis splendens)***
PRONUNCIATION	spoh-dee-oh-POH-gon seye-BEER-ih-kus
COMMON NAME	Frost grass, graybeard grass
USDA HARDINESS ZONE	5 to 9
ORIGIN	Siberia, northern China, Korea, Japan
PREFERRED SITES	Grassy hillsides, openings in woods

DESCRIPTION: Frost grass is an attractive, small, flowering grass admired for its leaf, flower, and fall color. Its compact size and handsome habit make it a fine choice for smaller gardens and mixed borders. A warm-season grass, frost grass has a bamboolike quality: Its leaves angle up, becoming right-angled late in the season. The foliage creates bold architectural patterns and has great garden value. Bright green fuzzy leaves, ¾ to 1 inch wide and 6 to 8 inches long, form upright, clumping foliage 2 to 3 feet tall that spreads out with age. Foliage often displays purplish or wine tints, especially later in the season. The color is quite rich and blends nicely with other fall plantings. Flowers bloom from July through August in narrow, erect panicles, 3 to 4 inches wide and 8 to 12 inches long. The panicles rise 14 to 18 inches above the foliage; this separation of foliage and flower contributes to the flowers' airiness. Purplish at first, the flowers become fuzzy brown as they mature, remaining

showy and persistent on the plant into winter. With the first hard frost, the plant turns purplish brown. Its late-season form and color are most dramatic outlined with a coating of frost.

LANDSCAPE USES: Both the flower and foliage of frost grass provide effective accents, whether the plant appears alone or in groups. Its compact size makes it ideal for small gardens and perennial borders. It is also suitable for the margins of woods. Its striking fall color and winter character provide reason enough for planting it. It adds a tropical look to cold-climate areas and does well in lightly to moderately shady gardens.

CULTURE AND PROPAGATION: Frost grass grows best in moist, well-drained, fertile soil in full sun or light shade. It resents hot, dry sites and needs half-day sun in hot climates. It tolerates coastal conditions if moisture is sufficient. Although it also tolerates considerable shade, frost grass will flop if there is not enough light.

Propagate by seed, or by division in spring.

PESTS AND PROBLEMS: Frost grass grows slowly and poorly in hot climates, where it rarely reaches 2 feet. In these conditions its flowering is scant and not as showy. In borderline climates, you may need to move it around the garden until you find the right spot.

BOTANICAL NAME	***Sporobolus airoides***
PRONUNCIATION	spor-AH-boh-lus air-OY-deez
COMMON NAME	Alkali dropseed, alkali sacaton
USDA HARDINESS ZONE	7 to 9
ORIGIN	Mexico, California, Arizona, Texas north to Montana
PREFERRED SITES	Meadows and valleys, especially in moderately alkaline soil; sandy washes, heavy soils

DESCRIPTION: Clumping, warm-season-growing alkali dropseed was one of the major constituents of the great California central valley grasslands that have been destroyed by intensive agriculture. It is a tough, drought-tolerant grass with fine foliage and showy cloudlike flowers. Its narrow leaves, ¼ to ⅜ inch wide and 1 to 2 feet long, form dense clumps of somewhat sharp-edged grayish green foliage in upright, arching mounds 2 to 3 feet tall and as wide. The flowers emerge from June through July in delicate pink panicles, 5 to 10 inches long, that form a stiff pyramidal arrangement 2 to 3 feet above the foliage. The airy flowers first appear as pink clouds, then become golden late in the season, remaining showy until the first winter rains. The foliage turns yellowish with the first frost, becoming straw-colored in winter.

LANDSCAPE USES: Alkali dropseed is useful massed as a large-scale groundcover and for meadow applications, erosion control, and revegetation. Since the grass is extremely heat- and drought-tolerant, it also makes a fine specimen or accent in dry gardens. The flowers are stunning in fresh or dried arrangements.

CULTURE AND PROPAGATION: Alkali dropseed prefers moist, well-drained soil in full sun. It tolerates a wide range of soil and climatic conditions, including drought; heavy, sandy, and clay soils; alkaline and saline conditions; and even occasionally flooded lowlands. It can go without summer water in the arid West but would appreciate additional watering. This grass has a wide geographical range, and different cultivars may have different tolerances to minimum temperatures. In cold inland or northern climates, cultivars with proven local hardiness are best.

   Propagate by seed, or by division in spring or fall.

PESTS AND PROBLEMS: Alkali dropseed has no known pests or problems.

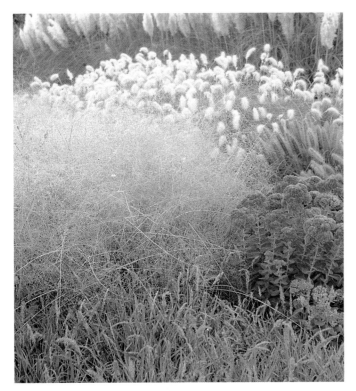

Sporobolus airoides, alkali dropseed.

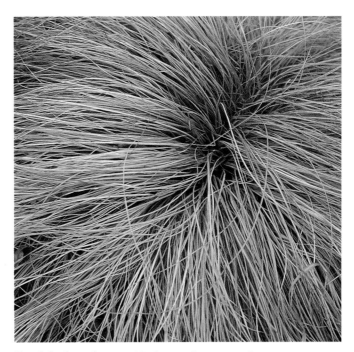

Sporobolus heterolepis, prairie dropseed, in winter dormancy.

BOTANICAL NAME	***Sporobolus heterolepis***
PRONUNCIATION	spor-AH-bol-us het-er-oh-LEP-is
COMMON NAME	Prairie dropseed, northern dropseed
USDA HARDINESS ZONE	3 to 9
ORIGIN	Prairie grasslands from Canada to Texas
PREFERRED SITES	Well-drained uplands

DESCRIPTION: Prairie dropseed was one of the major components of the American prairie, and its seeds were utilized as food by Native Americans. Once, its range was extensive, but prairie dropseed has been destroyed by overgrazing and farming; today, its presence in the wild is a good indication of undisturbed prairie.

   This handsome grass grows in upright, arching clumps. A slow grower, it is ranked somewhere between cool- and warm-season growing; emerging before many warm-season grasses, it slows down earlier than many other warm-season grasses. Its fine-textured, emerald green leaves, $\frac{1}{16}$ to $\frac{1}{8}$ inch wide and 2 to 3 feet long, form delicate hummocks of foliage 1½ to 2 feet tall. In the fall the foliage turns golden, often with orangish hues. The onset of winter turns the entire plant light creamy brown. Its August-blooming flowers smell distinctly sweet through September. The 6- to 8-inch-long airy panicles stand 2½ to 3½ feet above the foliage but tend to droop somewhat under the weight of the ripening seed.

LANDSCAPE USES: Prairie dropseed is useful for large-scale groundcovers, as a single specimen in dry borders, and as a flowering accent for hot, dry locations. It also attracts birds and other wildlife, and its delicate odor is a plus in any garden.

CULTURE AND PROPAGATION: Prairie dropseed prefers dry, rocky soil in full sun. It tolerates a wide range of conditions but grows best in well-drained soil. Prairie dropseed is extremely heat- and drought-tolerant. However, it does grow naturally in areas that receive some summer rainfall, and as such requires some watering in summer in arid western climates. It tends to flop in the shade.

Propagate by seed, or by division in spring or fall. Prairie dropseed does not seed invasively and infrequently self-sows.

PESTS AND PROBLEMS: Prairie dropseed tends to be slow-growing, usually taking three years to develop into mature flowering plants. If possible, plant two-year-old clumps.

BOTANICAL NAME	***Stenotaphrum secondatum 'Variegatum'***
PRONUNCIATION	sten-oh-TAF-rum sek-on-DAH-tum var-ee-uh-GAH-tum
COMMON NAME	Variegated St. Augustinegrass
USDA HARDINESS ZONE	9 to 10
ORIGIN	Horticultural selection native to Caribbean
PREFERRED SITES	Moist, sandy soil; tropical meadows

DESCRIPTION: This running, warm-season grass makes a bright yellow turf. A subtropical grass, it is identical to the common St. Augustinegrass of lawns (*Stenotaphrum secondatum*) except for its yellow-variegated leaves. This vigorous, creeping grass spreads rapidly and roots along the stem as it grows. The leaves, ¼ to ½ inch wide and 2 to 4 inches long, are glossy with creamy yellow-white stripes. The foliage lies flat on the ground but can reach 6 to 8 inches tall if confined and unmowed. The grass is evergreen in warm climates but is damaged at temperatures below 32°F; however, established turfs in protected areas have survived 18°F when mulched for winter protection. Insignificant flowers bloom in August and September.

LANDSCAPE USES: Variegated St. Augustinegrass is well-suited as a groundcover and foreground planting in annual

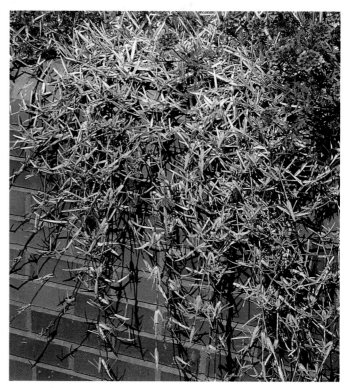

Stenotaphrum secondatum 'Variegatum', variegated St. Augustinegrass.

beds. It is attractive in coastal gardens as a lawn or groundcover. Basically a subtropical grower, variegated St. Augustinegrass is used as an annual in colder climates. In tropical and mild-winter climates, it makes an exciting lawn substitute: A golden yellow lawn is certain to turn a few heads in the neighborhood. It is used in parks, golf courses, and large-scale plantings to create patterns or pathways. The grass also grows well in hanging baskets and pots, and can be grown indoors in strong, indirect light.

CULTURE AND PROPAGATION: Variegated St. Augustinegrass prefers moist, well-drained soil in full sun or light shade. It tolerates a wide range of soil conditions, from heavy clay to dune sand, as long as moisture is sufficient. In areas with moderate to light summer rainfall, variegated St. Augustinegrass is drought-tolerant. In hot inland climates, it prefers light shade and weekly watering. It languishes in too much shade, but tolerates windy coastal conditions and saline and alkaline conditions.

Propagate by division or stem cuttings in spring or summer.

PESTS AND PROBLEMS: Variegated St. Augustinegrass is subject to typical lawn diseases and pests common to St. Augustine turfs: cinch bug, brown patch, dollar spot, and rust. Treat these diseases and pests with appropriate cultural controls. Plants may occasionally revert to nonvariegated leaves. If this occurs, remove the nonvariegated plants, or they may overtake the variegated parent plant.

STIPA
FEATHER GRASS, NEEDLE GRASS

This group of over 150 species of grasses includes some of the showiest flowering of all the ornamental grasses. Feather grass flowers are usually distinguished by long or prominent needlelike awns. These threadlike structures give feather grass its ethereal ability to catch light. In full glorious bloom, these feathery awns also impart movement rarely matched by other grasses. Feather grass plumes sway in the slightest breeze, and their silky awns glisten in early morning and late afternoon sunlight. These endearing qualities, along with their rugged adaptability, are what make feather grasses so popular.

Most feather grasses are native to open dry sites. Many are from the arid southwestern United States and the dry steppes of Europe and central Asia. They usually flourish in well-drained, sunny locations. Many have fine-textured, almost hairlike leaves. The foliage is often sparse, with the flowering culms comprising the bulk of the plant's mass. Most feather grasses are very showy in bloom, but decline quickly after flowering, becoming somewhat unattractive later in the season.

Feather grasses have other faults, too. Their long, needle-like awns can be hazardous to dogs, getting trapped in their ears and eyes. They can be difficult to propagate from division, and it can be hard to maintain attractive plants in nursery containers. Summer-dormant feather grasses can be flammable in areas where brush fires are a serious threat to homes and property: Take care when using summer-dormant grasses in high fire-risk areas. However, feather grasses are some of the most beautiful grasses to grow in hot dry climates.

feet above the foliage. The flowers bloom profusely in July and August. Plants become fully dormant in cold climates, but may remain evergreen in mild western climates.

LANDSCAPE USES: Feather grass makes a stunning flowering accent planted alone or in groups. It is an excellent grass for fresh or dried flower arrangements.

CULTURE AND PROPAGATION: Feather grass grows best in fertile, well-drained soil in full sun. Adapted to dry rocky slopes, it languishes in heavy, wet soil or shady sites.

Propagate by seed or division, although it is best to propagate by seed since divisions are unreliable.

PESTS AND PROBLEMS: Feather grass has no known pests or problems.

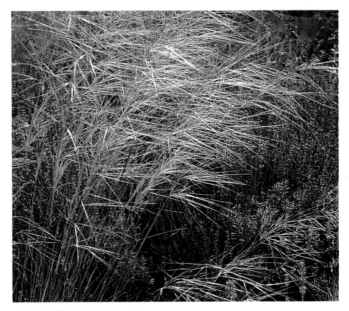

Stipa capillata, feather grass.

BOTANICAL NAME	***Stipa capillata***
PRONUNCIATION	STYE-pah kah-pil-AH-tah
COMMON NAME	Feather grass
USDA HARDINESS ZONE	6 to 9
ORIGIN	Widely distributed in Europe, from the Mediterranean to Siberia
PREFERRED SITES	Dry grasslands

DESCRIPTION: This semideciduous, clumping grass is noted for its upright silky panicles that form glistening masses of flowers. Its narrow leaves, ⅛ to ¼ inch wide and 1 to 2 feet long, are often rolled upwards. Feather grass has stiff, erect, gray-green powdery leaves 1 to 2 feet tall and as wide. The fine foliage is topped by upright panicles arching 1½ to 2

BOTANICAL NAME	***Stipa cernua***
PRONUNCIATION	STYE-pah SER-noo-ah
COMMON NAME	Nodding feather grass
USDA HARDINESS ZONE	8 to 9
ORIGIN	Originally found throughout California, from the Central Valley to the foothills
PREFERRED SITES	Dry grasslands

DESCRIPTION: Nodding feather grass once covered the state of California from top to bottom. Though mostly eliminated in its native habitats, it can still be found in small pockets throughout the state. Nodding feather grass is

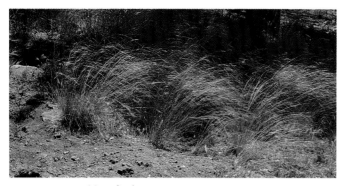

Stipa cernua, nodding feather grass.

almost identical to purple needle grass (*Stipa pulchra*). It differs from purple needle grass in that is has nodding awns, finer-textured leaves, more compact growth, and more flower spikes per plant. Its foliage grows 1 to 2 feet tall and as wide, with flowers that grow 1 to 1½ feet above the foliage. Flower spikes emerge from May through June and plants are usually dormant by July. The plant flowers more than other California native feather grasses.

LANDSCAPE USES: Nodding feather grass is best used in large masses or drifts. It is good for meadows and erosion control, and for hot inland valleys.

CULTURE AND PROPAGATION: Nodding feather grass prefers fertile, well-drained soil in full sun, but will grow in heavy, rocky, and sandy soils. Plants also tolerate light shade, wind, and heat. Water nodding feather grass until it is established; thereafter, it needs little or no summer water. It is best planted in fall or winter.

Propagate by seed, since division is rarely successful. When direct-seeding, make sure the seeds are pressed firmly into the soil. Plants are best from plugs.

PESTS AND PROBLEMS: Nodding feather grass has no known pests or problems.

BOTANICAL NAME	***Stipa gigantea***
PRONUNCIATION	STYE-pah jeye-GAN-tee-ah
COMMON NAME	Giant feather grass, golden oats
USDA HARDINESS ZONE	7 to 9
ORIGIN	Spain, mountainous regions of Portugal
PREFERRED SITES	Dry, grassy slopes

DESCRIPTION: Clumping, evergreen, cool-season giant feather grass is one of the showiest and most spectacular of all the flowering grasses. Its narrow rolled leaves, 1½ to 2

feet long and ¹/₁₆ to ⅛ inch wide, form dense tufts 1½ to 2 feet tall and as wide. The arching gray-green foliage is topped by flower spikes that can reach 3 to 4 feet above the leaves. The flower spikes emerge in May and are in full bloom by June. The loose, open panicle is held on stiffly erect culms that arch up and out from the foliage. The long golden awns, 4 to 5 inches long, dangle from the stems and move in the slightest breeze. Golden anthers increase this light-catching effect; plants are stunning even in moonlight. The flowers mature by late June, though spent flower stalks are persistent and showy well into fall.

LANDSCAPE USES: Giant feather grass excels as a specimen and as a tall flowering accent. It is useful in perennial borders, where its height can be used to full advantage. Giant feather grass is best displayed where early morning and late afternoon sun can backlight the spikes. Although tall, the flower spikes have a transparent quality that is useful even in small gardens. It is also a good plant for coastal gardens and windy sites. Its flowers are striking in fresh or dried arrangements.

CULTURE AND PROPAGATION: Giant feather grass grows best in well-drained, fertile soil in full sun. Plants resent heavy, wet soil and poor drainage. In colder climates, plants thrive in a warm, sunny, protected site. In areas of high rainfall, plants must have excellent drainage to survive. Plants grow and flower poorly in too much shade.

Propagate by seed, or by division in the early spring or fall. Division may be difficult. Germination can take 100 days or more.

PESTS AND PROBLEMS: Gophers seem to have a preference for this grass and can cause considerable damage in a short period of time. In areas where gophers are present, protect plants in wire cages or eliminate gophers. A mature plant can be eaten to the ground in less than a day.

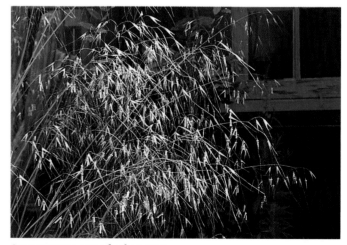

Stipa gigantea, giant feather grass.

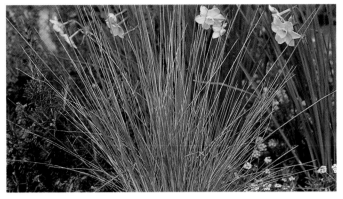

Stipa ichu, Peruvian feather grass.

BOTANICAL NAME	***Stipa ichu***
PRONUNCIATION	STYE-pah EE-choo
COMMON NAME	Peruvian feather grass
USDA HARDINESS ZONE	8 to 10
ORIGIN	Peru, Chile, Andean mountains and plains
PREFERRED SITES	Rocky soils, grasslands

DESCRIPTION: This clumping, evergreen grass makes a stiff, fine-textured tuft of bright green foliage 2 to 3 feet wide and as tall. The thin, $^1/_{16}$- to $^1/_8$-inch-wide leaves have rolled, somewhat sharp edges and a needlelike point. The upright divergent foliage is almost lime green, enhancing its overall beauty. Showy flowers appear in spring, with the glossy, silken awns typical of the feather grasses. The flowers emerge just above the foliage and mature to a golden color. Flowers shatter by midsummer.

LANDSCAPE USES: Peruvian feather grass is an extremely durable grass for hot southwestern areas. It is a useful groundcover and is good for massing, but is equally effective as a single specimen. It is a handsome companion plant for succulents and other drought-tolerant or Mediterranean plants. It is also good for coastal gardens. Peruvian feather grass will naturalize under favorable conditions, but is not considered an invasive grass.

CULTURE AND PROPAGATION: Peruvian feather grass prefers fertile, well-drained soil in full sun or partial shade. Plants will tolerate a wide range of soils and climates. Plants tolerate heavy clay, rocky or sandy soils, and coastal conditions. Plants tolerate light shade, but don't grow well in partial to full shade.
   Propagate by seed. Division is difficult but possible in the spring.

PESTS AND PROBLEMS: Peruvian feather grass has no known pests or problems.

BOTANICAL NAME	***Stipa lepida***
PRONUNCIATION	STYE-pah LEH-pih-dah
COMMON NAME	Foothill feather grass
USDA HARDINESS ZONE	8 to 9
ORIGIN	Coastal from San Diego to Northern California; also Sierra Nevada foothills
PREFERRED SITES	Brushlands, chaparral

DESCRIPTION: This native California grass is almost identical to purple needle grass (*Stipa pulchra*) and nodding feather grass (*S. cernua*). Together, these three grasses once comprised a large portion of the native California grasslands, most of which no longer exist today. Foothill feather grass is especially difficult to distinguish from purple needle grass, and the two are often confused. Foothill feather grass is generally more compact and has finer-textured foliage. These two plants are nearly identical in all other aspects.

LANDSCAPE USES: Plant foothill feather grass in groups in native, coastal, or dry gardens. It also makes a good groundcover and slope cover for dry sites.

CULTURE AND PROPAGATION: Foothill feather grass grows best in well-drained, fertile soil in full sun. Plants tolerate extremes in soil conditions from sand to clay, as well as light shade and coastal conditions.
   Propagate by seed.

PESTS AND PROBLEMS: Foothill feather grass has no known pests or problems.

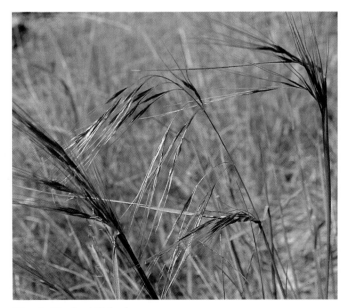

Stipa lepida, foothill feather grass.

BOTANICAL NAME	***Stipa pulchra***
PRONUNCIATION	STYE-pah PUL-krah
COMMON NAME	Purple needle grass
USDA HARDINESS ZONE	8 to 9
ORIGIN	Central valleys, foothills, coastal plains of California
PREFERRED SITES	Dry grasslands, open sunny areas

DESCRIPTION: Clumping, cool-season purple needle grass has gray-green leaves. Foliage is ⅛ to ¼ inch wide and 12 to 18 inches long, forming dense tufts. By April, green-flowering culms emerge 2 to 3 feet above the foliage. The 3- to 4-foot awns emerge purple, giving the plant its common name of purple needle grass. The plant is showiest from May through June as the flowers mature to a golden color. With the hot temperatures of July, the plant becomes dormant and ceases to grow. The return of the rainy season in November starts the cycle anew.

LANDSCAPE USES: Purple needle grass is excellent in mass plantings as a groundcover and for erosion control. It is effective in large areas for naturalizing and for meadows, for dry gardens and rocky slopes, for windy sites, and for coastal gardens. Extremely drought-tolerant, it is a must for any native California garden.

CULTURE AND PROPAGATION: Purple needle grass prefers a well-drained sandy loam in full sun. It will tolerate considerable extremes in soil and exposure, including heavy, serpentine, and sandy soils. It resents wet or shady condi-

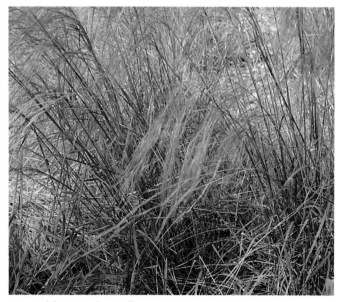

Stipa pulchra, purple needle grass.

tions, but will tolerate light shade if drainage is good. Purple needle grass will naturalize if conditions are favorable, but it is not invasive.

Propagate purple needle grass by seed, since divisions are rarely successful. Plants need to be drilled or pressed firmly into the soil to germinate readily. The seed for this grass is expensive and difficult to obtain. The best way to achieve large-scale plantings is by planting plugs or small starts.

PESTS AND PROBLEMS Purple needle grass can be difficult to maintain in containers, since plants seem to resent container culture. Unfortunately, this will limit its availability.

BOTANICAL NAME	***Stipa ramosissima***
PRONUNCIATION	STYE-pah ram-oh-SIS-sih-mah
COMMON NAME	Pillar of smoke, Australian plume grass
USDA HARDINESS ZONE	9 to 10
ORIGIN	Australia
PREFERRED SITES	Open grasslands

DESCRIPTION: Pillar of smoke is a stunning addition to the American nursery trade that has caused a sensation on the California horticultural scene sure to ripple across the country.

This cool-season-growing, evergreen grass has a columnar growth habit and showy flowers that bloom along its stems in such a way that the illusion of a pillar of smoke is created. Its heat- and drought-tolerance make it a versatile and hardy plant for southern and western gardens. Pillar of smoke's bright green foliage, ⅛ to ¼ inch wide and 8 to 10 inches long, clothes woody, vertical culms that can reach pencil thickness and can grow over 6 feet tall. Mature clumps can grow 3 feet wide and 6 to 7 feet tall in a vertical bamboolike clump. The stems may branch with the leaves emerging from internodes along the height of the culms. The flowers, branched panicles 6 to 8 inches long in radiating whorls like a Christmas tree, emerge from late winter through the summer in almost unending procession. Silky bronze on emergence, the flowers mature to a cream color, then fade to gray. Since flowers bloom on newly arising culms and terminal culms, the illusion of a plume of smoke is uncanny. Though the typical *Stipa* awn is only ½ inch long, the flowers are so numerous on the spike that it is quite showy. Plants remain evergreen in mild climates and have withstood 18°F without damage. Its hardiness in colder climates is largely untested.

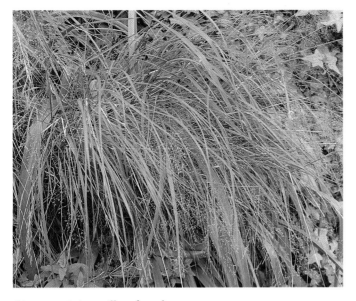

Stipa ramosissima, pillar of smoke.

LANDSCAPE USES: Whether used as a single specimen or planted in groups, pillar of smoke is an eye-catching accent. It is a good tall accent in the back of the border, and in pots or tubs. Its long, sturdy stems are every flower arranger's dream.

CULTURE AND PROPAGATION: Pillar of smoke prefers fertile, moist, well-drained soil in full sun. It will tolerate heavy, rocky, and sandy soils. Though drought-tolerant, it needs regular summer water to look its best. Since it will tolerate wind and exposed sites, it is good for coastal gardens.

Propagate by division or seed, although it is easiest to propagate from seed.

PESTS AND PROBLEMS: Pillar of smoke has no known pests or problems.

BOTANICAL NAME	*Stipa robusta*
PRONUNCIATION	STYE-pah roh-BUS-tah
COMMON NAME	Sleepy grass
USDA HARDINESS ZONE	7 to 9
ORIGIN	Arizona, New Mexico, Colorado
PREFERRED SITES	Plains, hills, open woods

DESCRIPTION: Native to the high plains, sleepy grass gets its common name from the narcotic effect it has on cattle and horses.

Large, clumping, cool-season sleepy grass has gray-green leaves ¼ to ⅜ inch wide and 2 to 3 feet tall borne in dense, arching tufts. Flowers form on tall upright culms 2 to 3 feet above the foliage. The flowers are showy, tan spikes ¾ inch wide and 8 to 12 inches long, with short ½- to 1-inch awns. The spikes flower in June and July. Although the short awns do not give this species of feather grass the light-catching quality typical of the genus, the flowers are showy and persistent on the plant.

LANDSCAPE USES: Sleepy grass makes an excellent accent and specimen grass for a tall background. It is good in mixed perennial borders and in dry gardens. Flowers are attractive in fresh and dried arrangements.

CULTURE AND PROPAGATION: Sleepy grass grows best in fertile, well-drained soil in full sun. Plants do not grow well in heavy wet soils and too much shade. Good drainage is essential. Sleepy grass will tolerate rocky and sandy soils and windy sites.

Propagate by seed or division, although propagation is easier from seed.

PESTS AND PROBLEMS: Sleepy grass has no known pests or problems.

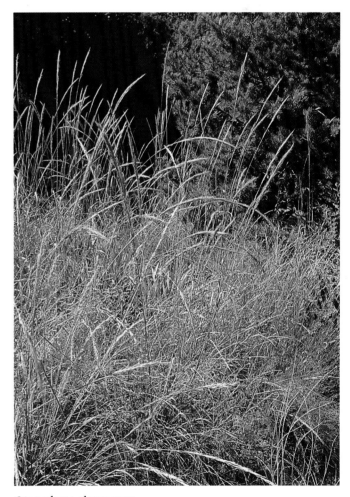

Stipa robusta, sleepy grass.

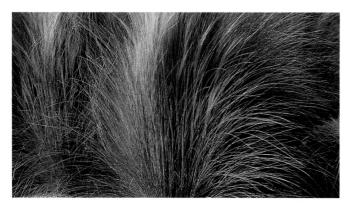

Stipa tenuissima, Mexican feather grass.

BOTANICAL NAME	**Stipa tenuissima**
PRONUNCIATION	STYE-pah ten-yoo-ISS-ih-mah
COMMON NAME	Mexican feather grass, fine-stem needle grass
USDA HARDINESS ZONE	7 to 10
ORIGIN	Texas, New Mexico, central Mexico
PREFERRED SITES	Open rocky slopes, 5,000 to 7,000 feet in elevation

DESCRIPTION: Fine-leaved, clumping Mexican feather grass has silky awns that appear to be like a flowing mane of blonde hair when mature. Needle-thin, flexible leaves form dense clumps 1½ feet tall and as wide. The bright green foliage is almost iridescent. Flowers bloom silky green in June and become golden at maturity. Although the awns are short, 1 to 2 inches long, they are numerous and make a spectacular sight when backlit. The flowers are showy from June to late fall.

LANDSCAPE USES: Mexican feather grass is striking planted alone or in large masses or drifts. A good slope cover, it provides excellent erosion control. It is also attractive in dry gardens, rock gardens, and coastal gardens. Bunches of Mexican feather grass make spectacular flower arrangements.

CULTURE AND PROPAGATION: Mexican feather grass prefers fertile, well-drained soil in full sun or partial shade. It tolerates a wide range of conditions, from heavy clay to sandy soils, as long as the soil dries out between waterings. It will tolerate light shade, coastal conditions, and windy sites, but does not like wet feet.

Propagate by seed; divisions are possible, but can be problematic.

PESTS AND PROBLEMS: This plant reseeds readily and can become somewhat invasive.

OTHER FEATHER GRASS SPECIES ARE:

Stipa comata (Needle-and-thread grass): a western U.S. native that grows 3 to 4 feet tall; extremely heat- and drought-tolerant.

Stipa extremorientale (Eastern feather grass): tall, showy flowers; grows 3 to 4 feet tall; good in cool-summer climates.

Stipa pennata (European feather grass): showy, pennantlike flowers distinguished by long, silky awns 8 to 12 inches long.

Stipa pulcherrima (Magnificent feather grass): European species with silky awns 12 to 18 inches long.

BOTANICAL NAME	**Themeda triandra 'Japonica'**
PRONUNCIATION	the-MEE-dah tri-AN-drah ja-PON-ih-kah
COMMON NAME	Japanese themeda
USDA HARDINESS ZONE	7 to 9
ORIGIN	China, Japan, Korea
PREFERRED SITES	Moist areas, streamsides

DESCRIPTION: Attractive, warm-season-growing Japanese themeda has soft, fuzzy foliage and showy flowers that are set off by a dazzling fall color. Rich, bright green leaves, ¼ to ½ inch wide, form an upright, arching clump 2½ to 3½ feet tall and as wide. The foliage has a delicate translucency that enhances its light-catching ability. The flowers appear on long, outwardly arching, curiously fuzzy stems in July and August. As they mature, the flowers become nodding panicles whose hairy bracts catch the light in the early morning and late afternoon. The flowers arch 1 to 2 feet above and beyond the foliage. In the fall, the flower stems and foliage become a blazing bright orange, continuing through shades of orange-red as the season progresses. The dormant foliage is an attractive red-brown or copper, providing continued interest well into winter.

LANDSCAPE USES: Japanese themeda, with its unusual habit, makes a unique architectural specimen in the garden. Give it plenty of room to best display its foliage and flowers. The plants look attractive in groups or masses in large gardens, parks, or golf courses, and along the water's edge. It is a fine choice for bringing fall color to the ground level of the garden. The flowers add color and texture to fresh and dried arrangements.

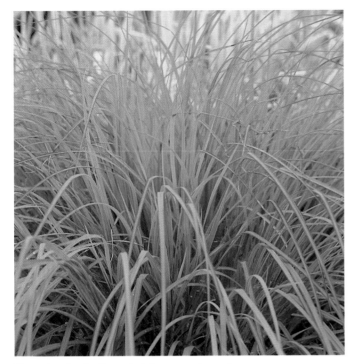

Themeda triandra 'Japonica', Japanese themeda.

CULTURE AND PROPAGATION: Japanese themeda prefers moist, fertile soil in full sun or light shade. Plants love the heat as long as moisture is present. Although drought-tolerant in Zones 7 and 8, plants grow poorly in hot, dry sites in arid western climates, where they should be kept in light shade or half-day sun. Plants need lots of heat to produce flowers. Japanese themeda tolerates coastal conditions, wind, and sandy soils.

Propagate by seed, or by division in spring or fall.

PESTS AND PROBLEMS: Japanese themeda has no known pests or problems.

BOTANICAL NAME	**Thysanoleana maxima**
PRONUNCIATION	THIH-san-oh-LEE-ah-nah MAX-ih-mah
COMMON NAME	Tiger grass
USDA HARDINESS ZONE	9 to 10
ORIGIN	Tropical Asia
PREFERRED SITES	Scrublands

DESCRIPTION: Large, subtropical, warm-season-growing tiger grass has bold bamboolike foliage and showy flowers. The broad, glossy, dark green leaves, 2 to 3 inches wide and tapering to a point, clothe sturdy stems ¼ to ½ inch thick. The stems and leaves reach 6 to 10 feet tall in upright, arching clumps. Mature specimens make a huge spreading mass of foliage 10 feet tall and almost as wide. The highly ornamental leaves give a unique sculptural quality to the garden, appearing lush and tropical. The flowers are borne in large, terminal, silky panicles 6 to 8 inches wide and 1 foot tall, emerging green and maturing to brown. The flowers begin to bloom in late summer and are showy into the winter. The foliage is damaged at temperatures below 40°F and freezes to the ground at 32°F, although plants have survived at 15°F for short periods of time.

LANDSCAPE USES: Tiger grass makes a bold tropical accent for subtropical and Mediterranean gardens, as a single specimen or in groups. It also makes a good screen or tall background, is dramatic along the water's edge near ponds and pools, and is an excellent tub and container subject. The foliage and flowers are striking in fresh and dried arrangements. Tiger grass is sometimes grown as a houseplant but must receive high levels of indirect light.

CULTURE AND PROPAGATION: Tiger grass prefers moist, fertile soil with good drainage and full sun or light shade. It tolerates a wide range of soils, from sandy to clay, as long as moisture is present. The leaf tips and margins will show signs of stress if moisture is insufficient. It is somewhat drought-tolerant in the shade. Plants also tolerate coastal conditions, but the leaves tatter in windy, exposed sites and need protection. Tiger grass tends to look yellowish in hot inland climates and will suffer in dry soils. In cold-winter climates, dig the plants well before the first chance of frost and overwinter them in a warm greenhouse.

Propagate by seed, or by division in late spring.

PESTS AND PROBLEMS: Tiger grass has no known pests or problems.

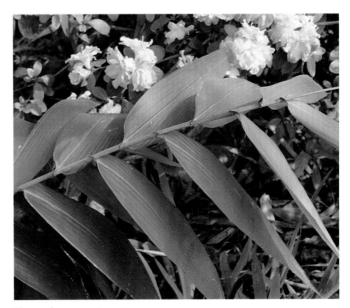

Thysanoleana maxima, tiger grass.

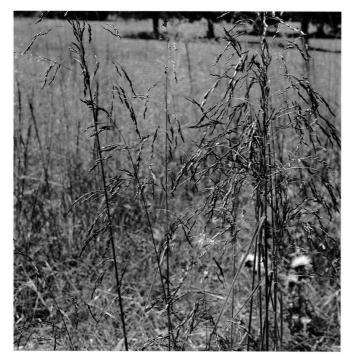

Tridens flavus, purple-top.

BOTANICAL NAME	***Tridens flavus***
PRONUNCIATION	TREYE-denz FLAH-vus
COMMON NAME	Purple-top
USDA HARDINESS ZONE	5 to 10
ORIGIN	North America: New Hampshire to Nebraska, south to Florida, west to Texas
PREFERRED SITES	Old fields, open woods

DESCRIPTION: A charming native eastern United States grass, purple-top has showy but delicate purple flowers that sway in the slightest breeze. Like many beautiful natives, this is considered a weed in many agricultural settings. In the proper place, however, it makes a fine ornamental grass. Its bright green leaves, ¼ to ½ inch wide, form upright clumps 1 to 1½ feet tall. A warm-season grass, purple-top begins flowering in late August and September. Its delicate, drooping panicles rise 4 to 4½ feet above the foliage, creating airy purple clouds of flowers. The flowers mature to golden brown and are mostly finished blooming by late fall. The plants become yellowish brown in the fall and straw-colored in the winter.

LANDSCAPE USES: Purple-top is excellent in large plantings and naturalized in meadows. The plants are attractive alone or in groups and are valued as a flowering accent. They are suitable for groundcover and slope plantings. The flowers are stunning in fresh and dried arrangements.

CULTURE AND PROPAGATION: Purple-top is an undemanding grass that tolerates a wide range of conditions and soils. It does best in moist, fertile soil in full sun. Plants are drought-tolerant once established but always look better with regular moisture. The grass tolerates medium shade but will not flower as heavily and may flop.

Propagate by seed, or by division in the spring or fall.

PESTS AND PROBLEMS: Purple-top's naturalizing tendencies can make it invasive in small gardens; still, it creates a fine meadow in Zones 7 to 9.

BOTANICAL NAME	***Tripsicum dactyloides***
PRONUNCIATION	TRIP-see-kum dak-til-OY-deez
COMMON NAME	Gamma grass, Eastern gammagrass
USDA HARDINESS ZONE	5 to 10
ORIGIN	North America: widespread from Massachusetts to Michigan, south to Florida, west to Texas
PREFERRED SITES	Wet ground; streamsides; moist, boggy sites

DESCRIPTION: Wide-ranging gamma grass is found throughout the eastern United States, though not usually in extensive stands. It is primarily noted for its luxurious foliage that forms lush masses of upright, arching leaves 4 to 6 feet tall and as wide. Medium to dark green, the leaves are ¾ to 1 inch wide and ½ to 3 feet long, forming a lush fountain. The flowers, though not particularly showy, are

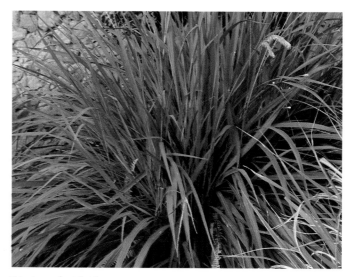

Tripsicum dactyloides, gamma grass.

unique. Long, upright, arching flower stems appear in July, rising slightly above the foliage. The flowers are borne in terminal racemes of three spikes with bright red anthers and brown pistils. The slender flower stalks move in the wind, adding grace and charm to the foliage. The plants are evergreen in subtropical climates. In mild climates, the foliage picks up red and brownish tints with the onset of fall. In cold climates, plants quickly freeze to the ground with the first hard frost.

LANDSCAPE USES: Gamma grass, with its lush foliage, makes a good background in subtropical plantings and is effective in groups. The luxuriant foliage contrasts against ferns and other shade-loving plants such as hellebores and bellflowers. Gamma grass is lovely as a single specimen, planted in groups near water, and in pots and tubs.

CULTURE AND PROPAGATION: Gamma grass prefers moist, fertile soil in full sun or partial shade. It tolerates a wide range of soil conditions, from sand to clay (as long as moisture is sufficient), windy coastal conditions, and considerable shade. Gamma grass will grow in all but the shadiest of gardens; in fact, the foliage tends to look richer in the shade. Under moist, warm conditions, this grass will naturalize readily.

Propagate by seed, or by division in spring. Propagation is easiest in spring.

PESTS AND PROBLEMS: Gamma grass has no known pests or problems.

BOTANICAL NAME	***Tripsicum floridana***
PRONUNCIATION	TRIP-see-kum flor-ih-DAH-nah
COMMON NAME	Florida gammagrass
USDA HARDINESS ZONE	7 to 10
ORIGIN	Southern Florida
PREFERRED SITES	Moist areas, ditches, low pinelands

DESCRIPTION: Clumping, warm-season-growing Florida gammagrass is similar to gamma grass (*Tripsicum dactyloides*) but has narrower leaves and is more compact. The glossy leaves are ¼ to ½ inch wide and 1½ to 2½ feet long, with a noticeable thin white stripe down the midrib. They form an upright, arching clump of foliage 2½ to 3½ feet tall and as wide. The plants are evergreen in warm and mild climates. In cold climates, the plants turn yellowish brown with the first freeze, becoming straw-colored in the winter.

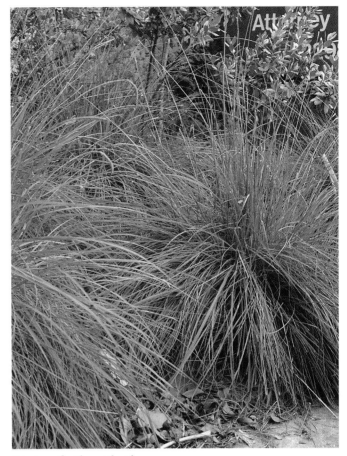

Tripsicum floridana, Florida gammagrass.

The flowers are borne on long, slender stalks that arch up and out from the plant 1 to 2 feet above the foliage. Noticeable but not particularly showy, the flowers do provide movement in the garden.

LANDSCAPE USES: Florida gammagrass provides excellent slope and bank cover when planted in masses or groups. Its foliage adds a stunning accent to subtropical gardens. Plants tolerate mucky and boggy soils and are good in or near water. Since it tolerates light to medium shade, this grass is effective in shady, moist sites and naturalizes well under a high canopy of trees.

CULTURE AND PROPAGATION: Florida gammagrass prefers moist, fertile soil in full sun or partial shade. Plants tolerate a wide range of soil conditions, from sand to clay, and are somewhat drought-tolerant when established; however, they will always look better with plenty of moisture. They also tolerate windy coastal conditions.

Propagation is easiest by seed, but the grass can be divided in spring.

PESTS AND PROBLEMS: Florida gammagrass reseeds readily in hot, moist climates. It may be invasive in small gardens.

163

TYPHA
CATTAILS

There are over 15 species of cattails, in their own family, Typhaceae. Members of this genus are found almost worldwide in both temperate and tropical climates. They usually grow in or near water or in moist sites. Cattails emerge from thick, creeping rhizomes and spread rapidly, colonizing large areas.

Their familiar flowers and seed heads form a brown, cigar-shaped spike that has delighted generations of children and adults worldwide. Cattails have been used for food, baskets, shelter, and transportation. Native Americans used cattails in arts and crafts as well. Recently, cattails have been used to clean and filter polluted water.

Cattails are mostly warm-season plants, going dormant in fall and winter. Interesting vertical foliage, distinctive flowers, and a range of heights from 6-inch miniatures to 8-foot giants make them versatile players in the garden. Often used in water gardens and containers, cattails are excellent in moist borders, too.

Some cattails are aggressive naturalizers, spreading rapidly from rhizomes and seeds. Plant aggressive species only if you have plenty of room or can confine them in sunken tubs or with deep root barriers. Once established, colonies of aggressive taller-growing cattails can be hard to remove from mucky or boggy sites.

BOTANICAL NAME	***Typha angustifolia***
PRONUNCIATION	TEYE-fah an-gus-tih-FOL-ee-ah
COMMON NAME	Narrow-leaved cattail
USDA HARDINESS ZONE	5 to 9
ORIGIN	North America, Europe; distributed worldwide
PREFERRED SITES	Moist areas, swamps, marshes

DESCRIPTION: Narrow-leaved cattail is a member of the cattail family, Typhaceae. It is a more refined version of the common cattail (*Typha latifolia*), its compact size and better-mannered growth making it a better choice for most gardens. The slender leaves, ½ to ¾ inch wide and 3 to 5 feet tall, are flat and sword-shaped. The foliage is a dull grayish green that turns yellow-brown in the fall. The flowers bloom in July or August and are typical cigar-shaped spikes ½ to ¾ inch wide and 4 to 12 inches long. The fall color is showy, and the plants provide interest into the winter.

LANDSCAPE USES: Narrow-leaved cattail is a good choice for the water's edge of ponds and pools. It is a good choice when naturalized to create wildlife habitats and reduce bankside erosion. It is also well-suited for tubs and water gardens. The flowers are striking in fresh and dried arrangements.

CULTURE AND PROPAGATION: Narrow-leaved cattail prefers fresh water 6 to 12 inches deep, fertile soil, and full sun. It tolerates a wide range of climatic conditions, including wind, heat, coastal conditions, and mildly saline and alkaline soils as long as moisture is present. It likes shade but flowers poorly and flops in too much shade.

Propagate by seed or division; division is easiest in the spring.

PESTS AND PROBLEMS: Narrow-leaved cattail can become invasive under ideal growing conditions. To control its spread, plant it in a root barrier sunk at least 2 feet deep.

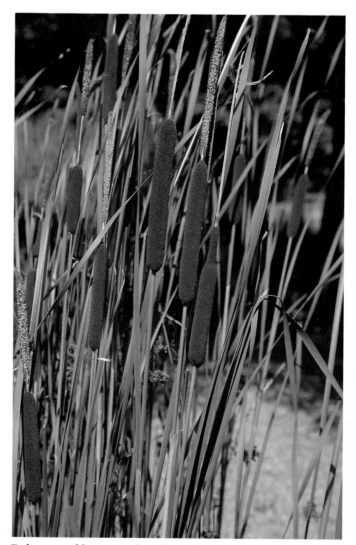

Typha angustifolia, narrow-leaved cattail.

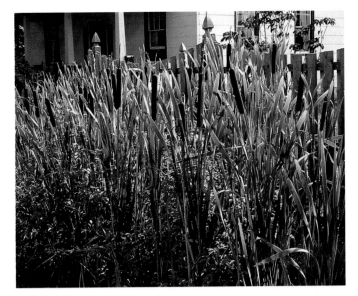

Typha latifolia, cattail.

BOTANICAL NAME	***Typha latifolia***
PRONUNCIATION	TEYE-fah lat-ih-FOL-ee-ah
COMMON NAME	Cattail, reed mace, bulrush
USDA HARDINESS ZONE	3 to 10
ORIGIN	Widely distributed: Europe, Asia, North America
PREFERRED SITES	Moist areas, swamps, marshes

DESCRIPTION: This is the familiar cattail known almost universally. A member of the cattail family, Typhaceae, this species forms typical brown spikelike flowers that shatter to reveal cottony seeds in the fall and winter. The spreading, warm-season plant forms huge colonies of vertical, flat-bladed leaves, ¾ to 1 inch wide and 6 to 10 feet tall. Leaves are topped by typical cigar-shaped flowers 1 to 1½ inches thick and 6 to 12 inches long. The flowers appear on sturdy stems 1 to 2 feet above the foliage from July through August, shattering from late fall into winter. The onset of cool temperatures brings yellow-brown fall color to the leaves, which are more showy some years than others. The leaves collapse in winter when the plant is dormant.

LANDSCAPE USES: This aquatic-growing cattail is an aggressive spreader best used in large gardens, parks, golf courses, and lakes. It can easily overrun a small pond or wet area; plant it in tubs to prevent it from spreading out of control. At its best in large areas, cattail creates wildlife habitat and shelter. If provided with plenty of moisture, it is a good pot and tub subject. Cattail provides an attractive backdrop for water lilies, and its flowers add interest to fresh and dried arrangements.

CULTURE AND PROPAGATION: Cattails prefer an aquatic habitat with fertile soil and water 6 to 12 inches deep. They tolerate brackish water and a wide variety of climates and soils, growing best in full sun or half-day shade.

Propagate by seed, or by division in the spring.

PESTS AND PROBLEMS: Cattails can easily get out of hand and need containment in small gardens.

BOTANICAL NAME	***Typha* sp. 'Miniature'**
PRONUNCIATION	TEYE-fah
COMMON NAME	'Miniature' cattail
USDA HARDINESS ZONE	5 to 6 (?); 7 to 9 (hardiness untested; may grow in Zones 5 and 6)
ORIGIN	Unknown; perhaps Japan or Siberia
PREFERRED SITES	Moist areas, shallow water

DESCRIPTION: This cattail is as yet unidentified and has not bloomed or fruited in cultivation. A member of the cattail family, Typhaceae, it was introduced from Japan but is reputed to be from Siberia. This warm-season-growing plant has typical cattaillike foliage that seldom reaches 8 inches tall. The plant forms a slowly spreading colony of foliage much like its giant cousins. The gray-green leaves grow ⅛ to ¼ inch wide and 4 to 6 inches tall. Neither the flowers nor the fruit have been observed in mild climates. The hardiness is untested in gardens north of Zone 7, but it is believed that the plant will tolerate, and perhaps even flower in, colder climates—to Zone 5. The foliage turns yellow-brown in the fall with the onset of cool temperatures.

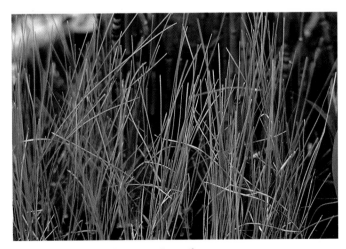

Typha sp. 'Miniature', 'Miniature' cattail.

LANDSCAPE USES: 'Miniature' cattail is ideal for small water gardens and pots. Its diminutive size makes it interesting as a bonsai specimen and for rock gardens. It is a good low groundcover and filler between stepping stones in moist or wet areas.

CULTURE AND PROPAGATION: 'Miniature' cattail prefers fertile moist or wet soil in full sun. It grows in shallow water 2 to 3 inches deep, and can grow in deeper water with age. It tolerates a wide range of soil conditions and wind, heat, and coastal conditions, as long as moisture is present. It also tolerates light shade, but grows best in full sun. In hot, arid desert climates, however, it needs half-day shade. Although it is spreading, plants are rarely, if ever, invasive.
   Propagate by division only, in spring.

PESTS AND PROBLEMS: 'Miniature' cattail has no known pests or problems.

BOTANICAL NAME	*Typha minima*
PRONUNCIATION	TEYE-fah MIN-ih-mah
COMMON NAME	Dwarf Japanese cattail
USDA HARDINESS ZONE	4 to 9
ORIGIN	Japan, Eurasia
PREFERRED SITES	Moist areas, swamps, marshes

DESCRIPTION: A curious miniature that resembles the common cattail (*Typha latifolia*), dwarf Japanese cattail is a member of the cattail family, Typhaceae. It is distinguished by short, narrow leaves and showy, fattened spikes. This spreading, warm-season plant has delicate light gray-green leaves, ¼ to ½ inch wide and 1 to 2 feet tall. The leaves are topped by reddish brown barrel-shaped flower spikes, 1 to 2 inches wide and 3 to 4 inches long. The flowers bloom from May through June, growing 6 to 12 inches above the foliage and shattering by late summer. The foliage turns an attractive yellow-brown in the fall. The form and color of the foliage provide winter interest.

LANDSCAPE USES: Dwarf Japanese cattail is suitable for small pools, ponds, and moist areas where other cattails are too tall or too invasive. It is a good pot and tub subject that makes a fine patio specimen. The plants are also effective in moist borders and wet, boggy soil. This is the best cattail selection for small gardens and ponds. Truly a fine plant for borders, it is underused in moist perennial borders. The foliage and flowers provide interest almost year-round and are beautiful in fresh and dried arrangements.

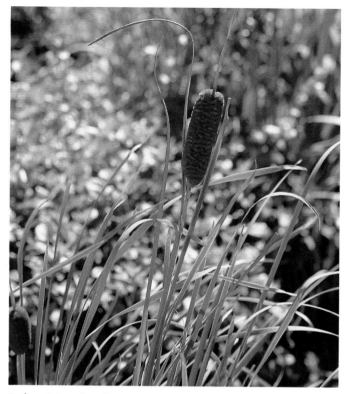

Typha minima, dwarf Japanese cattail.

CULTURE AND PROPAGATION: Dwarf Japanese cattail prefers rich, moist, fertile soil and shallow water in full sun, although it tolerates light shade. It will grow in water 6 to 12 inches deep. It tolerates coastal conditions, wind, and heat, if sufficient moisture is present.
   Propagate by seed or division; division is easiest in the spring.

PESTS AND PROBLEMS: Dwarf Japanese cattail has no known pests or problems.

BOTANICAL NAME	*Uncinia egmontiana*
PRONUNCIATION	un-SIN-ee-ah eg-mon-tee-AN-nah
COMMON NAME	Orange hook sedge
USDA HARDINESS ZONE	8 to 9
ORIGIN	New Zealand
PREFERRED SITES	Streamsides, moist edges

DESCRIPTION: Orange hook sedge, a member of the sedge family, Cyperaceae, is sought after for its brilliant orange-red foliage. A clumping, cool-season grass, it forms a neat mound of arching foliage 6 to 12 inches tall. The foliage is evergreen in mild climates, but in cooler zones, its thin, glossy leaves, ⅛ to ¼ inch wide and 8 to 12 inches long, are a dazzling bright orange. The leaves are fine-textured and weep outward, becoming a fountain of orange. The flowers are typical, insignificant sedge-type flowers. A small hooked flower head gives this sedge its name.

LANDSCAPE USES: Orange hook sedge's handsome foliage is an effective accent when blended with red, brown, or burgundy foliage, such as that of 'Palace Purple' heuchera (*Heuchera micrantha* 'Palace Purple') or cardinal flower (*Lobelia cardinalis*). It is a good plant near ponds and pools and in tubs and pots. Orange hook sedge looks its best spilling over rocks on slopes near streams and is a fine rock garden specimen.

CULTURE AND PROPAGATION: Orange hook sedge prefers moist, well-drained, rich soil in full sun or partial shade. Plants must have constant moisture and good drainage to look their best. In hot inland climates they need half-day sun. They tolerate coastal conditions if moisture is sufficient. This plant loves a cool root run and may be difficult to grow in hot, arid southwestern gardens.

   Propagate by seed, or by division in the spring or fall.

PESTS AND PROBLEMS: Orange hook sedge has no known pests or problems.

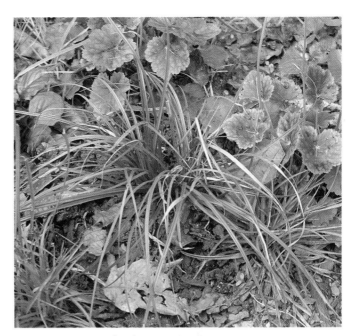

Uncinia unciniata, red sedge.

BOTANICAL NAME	***Uncinia unciniata***
PRONUNCIATION	un-SIN-ee-ah un-sin-ee-AH-tah
COMMON NAME	Red sedge, red hook sedge
USDA HARDINESS ZONE	8 to 9
ORIGIN	New Zealand
PREFERRED SITES	Moist edges, streamsides

DESCRIPTION: Red sedge, a member of the sedge family, Cyperaceae, is admired for its rich, reddish mahogany-colored leaves. A clumping, cool-season grass, it forms a neat mound of foliage 16 to 18 inches tall and as wide. The glossy leaves, ¼ to ⅜ inch wide and 6 to 10 inches long, arch up and out from the base. The foliage is evergreen in mild climates. The flowers are insignificant and have somewhat typical sedge-type flower heads.

LANDSCAPE USES: Red sedge makes a fine accent alone or in groups. Its rich red-brown color provides an effective contrast to yellow-green foliage and blends beautifully with silver foliage. It is a good choice for shady borders, the areas near ponds and pools, pots and tubs, and rock gardens.

CULTURE AND PROPAGATION: Red sedge prefers moist, well-drained, rich soil in full sun or light shade. The plants must have moisture, or they tend to look shabby. They will tolerate coastal conditions if moisture is sufficient. Good drainage is also essential for healthy growth. In hot, inland climates, the plants grow best with half-day sun or light shade.

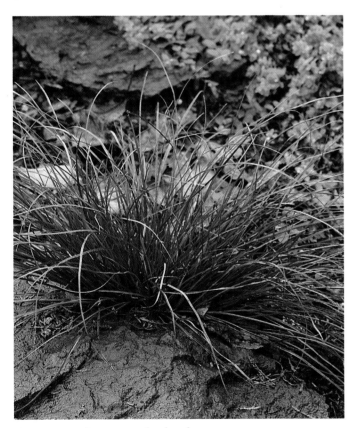

Uncinia egmontiana, orange hook sedge.

Propagate by seed, or by division in spring or fall. The plants may be somewhat variable by seed, showing various degrees of reddish foliage. Propagate by division to preserve attractively colored forms.

PESTS AND PROBLEMS: Red sedge has no known pests or problems.

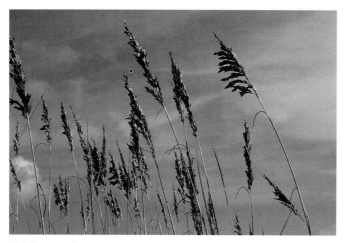

Uniola paniculata, sea oats.

BOTANICAL NAME	***Uniola paniculata***
PRONUNCIATION	yoo-nee-OH-lah pan-ih-kyoo-LAH-tah
COMMON NAME	Sea oats, spike grass
USDA HARDINESS ZONE	7 to 10
ORIGIN	Virginia to Florida, west to Texas, eastern Mexico
PREFERRED SITES	Sand dunes

DESCRIPTION: Upright, arching, rhizomatous sea oats is an endangered species protected by law in most areas. It is one of the prettiest native coastal dune grasses. Its arching, gray-green, 3- to 8-foot-tall foliage forms dense colonies in the sand. The leaves, ¼ to ½ inch wide, are somewhat sharp-edged. A warm-season grass, it is evergreen in subtropical climates. The flowers, long arching stems topped by showy brown panicles, occur throughout the growing season. They are persistent and look good well into the winter. The plants turn brown in the fall, going dormant in winter in colder climates.

LANDSCAPE USES: Sea oats is ideal for stabilizing dunes, controlling erosion, and providing habitat for birds and other animals. It grows well in coastal gardens. Its flowers are lovely in fresh and dried arrangements.

CULTURE AND PROPAGATION: Sea oats prefers well-drained, sandy soil in full sun or partial shade. It tolerates wind, salt spray, and heat. The plants form deeply penetrating rhizomes and are somewhat drought-tolerant once established.

Propagate by division only; the seed is usually sterile.

PESTS AND PROBLEMS: The same laws that protect often endanger already-endangered plants. Sea oats may be difficult to obtain legally, forcing the use of non-native grasses. Since collection of these plants is illegal in most states, it is important to contact your local agricultural extension office for a list of legal sources.

BOTANICAL NAME	***Vetiver zizanioides* (also known as *Vetiveria zizanioides*)**
PRONUNCIATION	VET-ih-ver zih-ZAN-ee-OY-deez
COMMON NAME	Vetiver, khus-khus, khas-khas
USDA HARDINESS ZONE	9 to 10
ORIGIN	India, Asia, northern Africa
PREFERRED SITES	Moist areas, river banks

DESCRIPTION: Tall, clumping, warm-season-growing vetiver has been cultivated for centuries for its sweet aromatic roots, used to make baskets, furniture, and screens, which become fragrant when wet. This feature is no doubt a plus in tropical climates. Vetiver oil, derived from the roots, has long been a source of perfume.

A robust grower, vetiver forms a tight vertical clump of foliage 2 to 4 feet wide and 4 to 8 feet tall. The glossy bronze-green leaves, ¼ to ¾ inch wide, are V-shaped and have the curious habit of folding over 1 to 2 feet from the tip. The leaves become a rich purple-red at the fold. The foliage is evergreen in subtropical climates and blushes purple-red where winter temperatures drop into the 30s and 40s. Although the foliage freezes to the ground below 30°F, the plants have survived short periods at 15°F. The flowers are showy spikes that grow 2 to 3 feet above the foliage. The flowers, 3 to 4 inches wide and 1 to 1½ feet long, form fluffy plumes from August through September.

LANDSCAPE USES: Vetiver makes a fine hedge or screen in subtropical and mild climates. It is a good screen and background plant in tropical gardens. It tolerates coastal conditions and is effective as a windbreak. The bent leaf tips add an interesting air to the plant: They move in the wind while most of the foliage stands solidly at attention. The flowers are beautiful in fresh and dried arrangements.

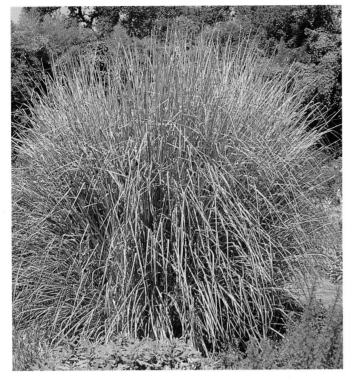

Vetiver zizanioides, vetiver.

CULTURE AND PROPAGATION: Vetiver prefers moist, rich soil in full sun or partial shade. It is extremely tolerant of a wide range of conditions from heavy clay to dune sand. It also tolerates boggy soils, yet is quite drought-tolerant when established. Vetiver tolerates windy coastal conditions. The plants grow in light shade but flop if the shade is too deep. Unlike most *Miscanthus* or other tall deciduous grasses, vetiver remains evergreen in mild climates. In cold climates, dig the plants and overwinter them in a greenhouse at 40°F or above.

Propagate by seed, or by division in late spring.

PESTS AND PROBLEMS: Vetiver has no known pests or problems.

BOTANICAL NAME	***Zea perennis***
PRONUNCIATION	ZEE-ah per-REN-is
COMMON NAME	Perennial corn
USDA HARDINESS ZONE	9 to 10
ORIGIN	Mexico
PREFERRED SITES	Tropical grasslands

DESCRIPTION: Clumping perennial corn is the first cousin to edible corn. Its lustrous, cornlike leaves clothe thick stems to make a large, sprawling clump up to 12 feet tall. Thick red canes, ½ to ¾ inch wide, are covered by gray-green leaves, ½ to 1 inch wide and 6 to 12 inches long. The leaves become stained red with the cool temperatures of fall. The flowers are typical cornlike tassels, more interesting than showy. Actual small ears of corn will form, but they are not edible. This subtropical grass is capable of 8 feet of growth in one season. The foliage increasingly reddens with cold weather, and the stems become redder as the season progresses. Tender to frost, perennial corn is evergreen in mild climates, but freezes to the ground if temperatures dip below 30°F.

LANDSCAPE USES: Perennial corn is best used as a tall, tropical-looking accent. It makes a suitable screen, and its sprawling habit adds to its wild tropical character. It is good in pots or tubs. Its interesting foliage is sometimes used in fresh or dried arrangements.

CULTURE AND PROPAGATION: Perennial corn prefers fertile, moist soil in full sun or light shade. It resents wind and dry conditions. Though this grass will tolerate some drought, it tends to look shabby when subjected to hot, dry situations. It tolerates wet and heavy soils.

Propagate by division, seed, or cuttings of mature canes.

PESTS AND PROBLEMS: Staking may be necessary as plants tend to flop.

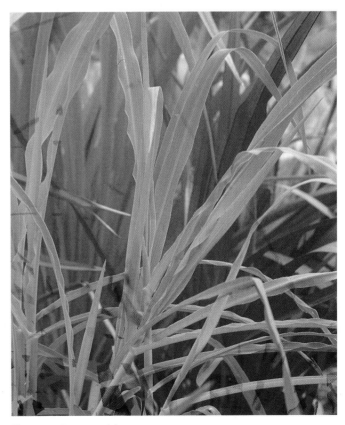

Zea perennis, perennial corn.

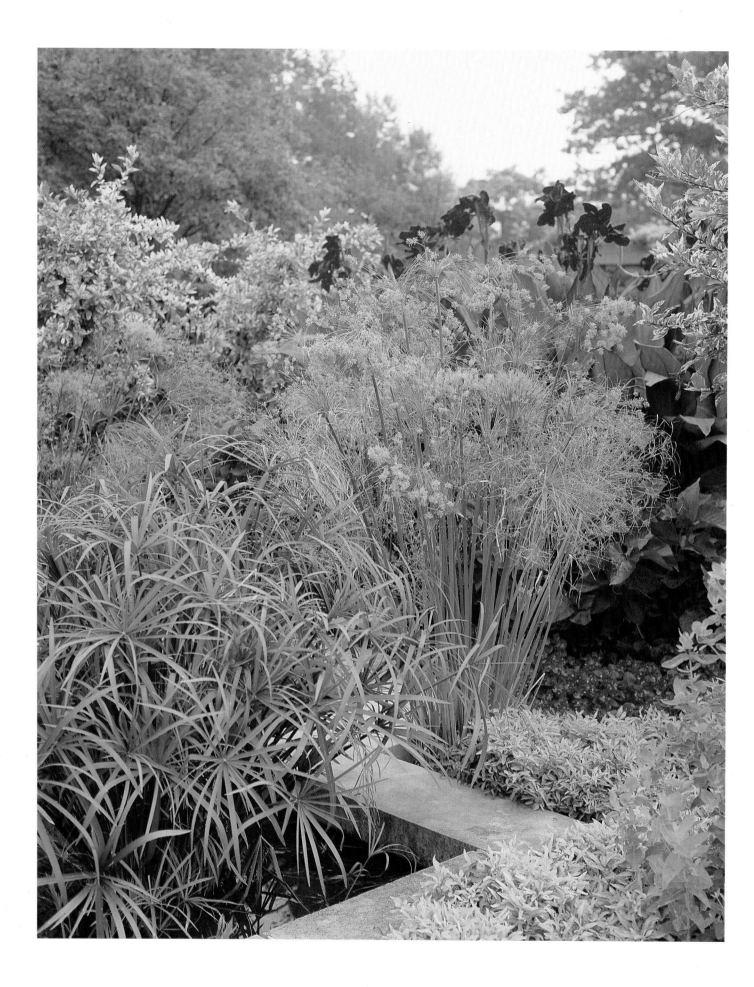

PART III

DESIGNING WITH ORNAMENTAL GRASSES

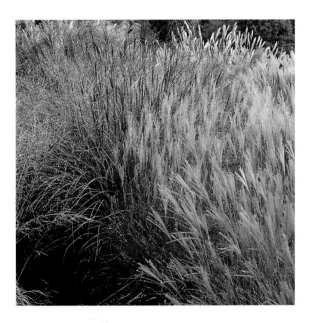

Opposite: The umbrella plant, *Cyperus alternifolius*, in the pond is flanked by Egyptian papyrus, *Cyperus papyrus*. Both of these sedges make fine accents because of the contrast between their lush foliage and the textures of the surrounding plants. Above: A fine sampling of some of the best *Miscanthus* cultivars currently available. From right foreground to upper left-hand corner: *Miscanthus sinensis* 'Yaku Jima'; *M. sinensis* 'Purpurascens', with red-orange foliage; and *M. sinensis* 'Morning Light', with silvery foliage and bronze flowers.

GARDEN DESIGN WITH ORNAMENTAL GRASSES

The impact of ornamental grasses on American garden design is nothing short of phenomenal. Their great beauty and versatility have brought them to the center of the design stage. Faced with literally hundreds of new choices, garden designers are just now beginning to realize the potential of ornamental grasses. There are grasses for every garden situation...big or small, sunny or shady, formal or informal.

There are no specific rules for how to use grasses in garden design. Tall grasses can provide screening or shade. Miniatures make excellent groundcovers. Flowering grasses can be used as accents, either alone or in groups. Apply the same principles you'd use when selecting other garden plants. The most important rule is to know the plants' likes and dislikes and always consider your local conditions. The best choices for Miami may not be appropriate in Maine or Vancouver. Experiment until you find the grasses that look and grow best in your garden.

The next pages offer some sample plans created by several noted American designers who are using ornamental grasses in their gardens. The designs cover typical garden situations—a foundation planting, a shady area under trees, a sunny meadow area (the prairie garden), and a sunny border site. Feel free to work with and adapt their plans—they are presented for inspiration, with the thought that perhaps the best new American gardens are still to come.

Cutting Gardens for Sun and Shade

Because grasses come in all colors, shapes, and sizes, they lend themselves to many types and styles of floral arrangements. Ranging from delicate miniatures to bold giants, grasses can be stars or supporting players in arrangements of every size, style, and season. They can be used fresh, dried, or even dyed. Properly picked, most grasses are extremely long-lasting. Their light-catching qualities and subtle colors make them invaluable in cut arrangements.

Don't limit yourself to using only the grass flowers—the foliage, stems, and seedheads are just as useful. The smooth burgundy canes of 'Pele's Smoke' sugarcane (*Saccharum officinarum* 'Pele's Smoke') add a beautiful richness to arrangements. The bright cadmium-colored seeds of crimson seed sedge (*Carex baccans*) look delightful combined with other seeds or pods. Many grasses, such as prairie cord grass (*Spartina pectinata*), have attractive leaves that can add vertical, horizontal, or arching lines to arrangements.

The best time to cut grasses for use in fresh arrangements is just as the flowers are emerging from the foliage. If you wait until the flowers have completely emerged, some grasses will shatter soon after picking. Cut grasses in midafternoon, after the dew has dried but before the dampness of evening arrives. Place cut foliage and flowers to be used fresh in a bucket of water, or keep them damp until you can arrange them. If you're cutting grasses for dried arrangements, hang them upside down until needed

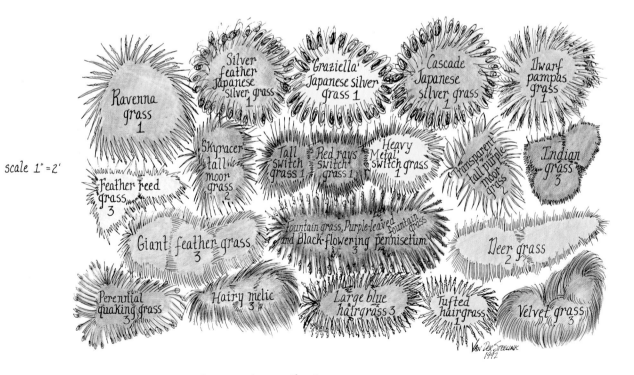

A Cutting Garden for Sunny Locations by John Greenlee

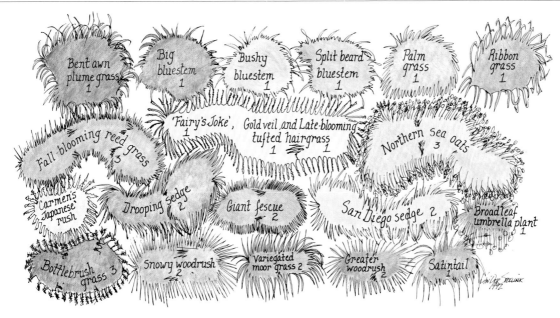

A Cutting Garden for Lightly Shady Locations by John Greenlee

or stand them in a vase in a cool, dry, darkened room. If you're planning to dry grasses, don't keep them in water.

These cutting gardens are designed to provide grass flowers for arrangements and displays. The grasses included will give you cutting material all year, whether you have a sunny or shady location.

Grasses for Sun

Briza media (Perennial quaking grass)

Calamagrostis acutiflora 'Stricta' (Feather reed grass)

Cortaderia selloana 'Pumila' (Dwarf pampas grass)

Deschampsia caespitosa (Tufted hairgrass)

Erianthus ravennae (Ravenna grass)

Holcus lanatus (Velvet grass)

Koeleria glauca (Large blue hairgrass)

Melica ciliata (Hairy melic)

Miscanthus sinensis 'Silberfeder' (Silver feather Japanese silver grass)

Miscanthus sinensis 'Graziella' ('Graziella' Japanese silver grass)

Miscanthus sinensis 'Kaskade' (Cascade Japanese silver grass)

Molinia caerulea subsp. *arundinacea* 'Skyracer' ('Skyracer' tall moor grass)

Molinia caerulea subsp. *arundinacea* 'Transparent' ('Transparent' tall moor grass)

Muhlenbergia rigens (Deer grass)

Panicum virgatum 'Strictum' (Tall switch grass)

Panicum virgatum 'Heavy Metal' ('Heavy Metal' switch grass)

Panicum virgatum 'Rotstrahlbusch' (Red rays switch grass)

Pennisetum alopecuroides (Fountain grass)

Pennisetum alopecuroides 'Moudry' (Black-flowering pennisetum)

Pennisetum setaceum 'Rubrum' (Purple-leaved fountain grass)

Sorghastrum nutans (Indian grass)

Stipa gigantea (Giant feather grass)

Grasses for Light to Medium Shade

Andropogon gerardii (Big bluestem)

Andropogon glomeratus (Bushy bluestem)

Andropogon ternarius (Split beard bluestem)

Calamagrostis arundinacea var. *brachytricha* (Fall-blooming reed grass)

Carex pendula (Drooping sedge)

Carex spissa (San Diego sedge)

Chasmanthium latifolium (Northern sea oats)

Cyperus albostriatus (Broadleaf umbrella plant)

Deschampsia caespitosa 'Fairy's Joke' ('Fairy's Joke' tufted hairgrass)

Deschampsia caespitosa 'Goldschleier' (Gold veil tufted hairgrass)

Deschampsia caespitosa 'Tardiflora' (Late-blooming tufted hairgrass)

Erianthus contortus (Bent awn plume grass)

Festuca gigantea (Giant fescue)

Hystrix patula (Bottlebrush grass)

Imperata brevifolia (Satintail)

Juncus 'Carmen's Japanese' ('Carmen's Japanese' rush)

Luzula nivea (Snowy woodrush)

Luzula sylvatica (Greater woodrush)

Molinia caerulea subsp. *caerulea* 'Variegata' (Variegated moor grass)

Phalaris arundinacea var. *picta* (Ribbon grass)

Setaria palmifolia (Palm grass)

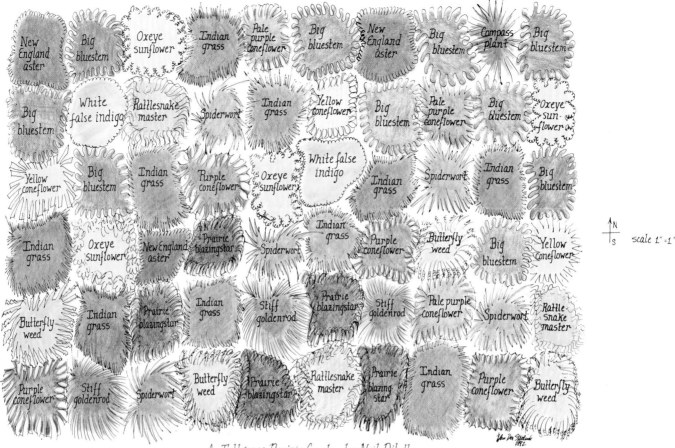

A Tallgrass Prairie Garden by Neil Diboll

A Tallgrass Prairie Garden

This is a simple meadow garden composed of native American prairie wildflowers and grasses. The garden is strongly vertical with plants up to 8 feet tall. It looks best planted against a background of tall shrubs or as a focal point at a distance.

If you want to make a larger garden, link two or three of these plans end to end to form a border planting. You can also curve the rectangular form to fit a given space or design requirement. If you combine this prairie garden with berry-producing shrubs, you can create excellent habitat for butterflies and songbirds. The shrubs provide nesting sites, cover, and food, and the prairie plants are unsurpassed nectar sources. Many of the prairie flowers and grasses also produce highly nutritious seeds that are relished by birds.

The prairie wildflowers provide an ever-changing palette of color in this garden throughout the summer. When the first hard frosts of fall hit, the grasses put on their autumnal golds, bronzes, and auburns to continue the garden show well into the winter months.

Prairie plants are known for their durability, drought tolerance, and low maintenance requirements. Their dense root systems squeeze out weeds and protect the soil from erosion. You'll have to weed and water this garden until the plants are established. But once established, the only care this prairie garden needs is to burn off the previous year's growth in spring or rake off and compost the garden debris.

Andropogon gerardii (Big bluestem)
Aster novae-angliae (New England aster)
Asclepias tuberosa (Butterfly weed)
Baptisia leucantha (White false indigo)
Echinacea pallida (Pale purple coneflower)
Echinacea purpurea (Purple coneflower)
Eryngium yuccifolium (Rattlesnake master)
Heliopsis helianthoides (Oxeye sunflower)
Liatris pycnostachya (Prairie blazingstar)
Ratibida pinnata (Yellow coneflower)
Silphium laciniatum (Compass plant)
Solidago rigida (Stiff goldenrod)
Sorghastrum nutans (Indian grass)
Tradescantia ohiensis (Spiderwort)

Neil Diboll is owner of and consulting ecologist for Prairie Nursery in Westfield, Wisconsin. Neil designs native landscapes and lectures on prairie gardening across North America.

174

A Shady Grass Garden

This shaded garden under two large, multistemmed white birches combines 12 grasses and grasslike plants with perennials that like a semi-shaded spot with moist, humus-rich soil. The background for this garden is formed by three large specimens of oakleaf hydrangea (*Hydrangea quercifolia*). The coarse texture of the hydrangeas shows off the finer texture of the grasses. Ferns serve as a background where the shrubs leave off and help to weave the garden together.

The predominant colors in this garden are white and yellow. The color display is created by flowers and foliage against a lush green background. Textures and forms vary and are combined to complement one another. The upright, arching forms of the ferns, northern sea oats (*Chasmanthium latifolium*), and drooping sedge (*Carex pendula*) create rhythm and provide continuity to the design. Interplant spring bulbs such as snowdrops, scillas, and daffodils in generous quantities for early spring interest.

C. Colston Burrell is a garden designer, writer, and photographer whose Minnesota-based design business, Native Landscapes, specializes in landscape restoration and the innovative use of native plants and perennials in garden design. Author of *Perennial Portraits 1991,* coauthor of *Rodale's Illustrated Encyclopedia of Perennials,* and contributor to *Rodale's All-New Encyclopedia of Organic Gardening,* Cole's articles and photographs have appeared in many gardening publications.

Adiantum pedatum (Maidenhair fern)

Asarum canadense or *A. europaeum* (Wild ginger)

Carex elata 'Bowles Golden' ('Bowles Golden' sedge)

Carex glauca (Blue sedge)

Carex morrowii 'Variegata' (Silver variegated Japanese sedge)

Carex pendula (Drooping sedge)

Carex plantaginea (Plantain-leaved sedge)

Carex siderostica 'Variegata' (Creeping variegated broad-leaved sedge)

Cimicifuga racemosa (Black snakeroot)

Chasmanthium latifolium (Northern sea oats)

Deschampsia caespitosa (Tufted hairgrass)

Dicentra spectabilis 'Alba' (White bleeding heart)

Digitalis grandiflora (Yellow foxglove)

Hakonechloa macra 'Aureola' (Golden variegated hakone grass)

Hosta 'Francee' ('Francee' hosta)

Hosta 'Frances Williams' ('Frances Williams' hosta)

Hydrangea quercifolia (Oakleaf hydrangea)

Hystrix patula (Bottlebrush grass)

Luzula nivea (Snowy woodrush)

Luzula sylvatica (Greater woodrush)

Osmunda claytoniana (Interrupted fern)

Pachysandra procumbens (Allegheny spurge)

Polygonum odoratum var. *thunbergii* 'Variegata' (Variegated Japanese Solomon's-seal)

Pulmonaria saccharata 'Janet Fisk' ('Janet Fisk' Bethlehem sage)

Rodgersia pinnata (Featherleaf rodgersia)

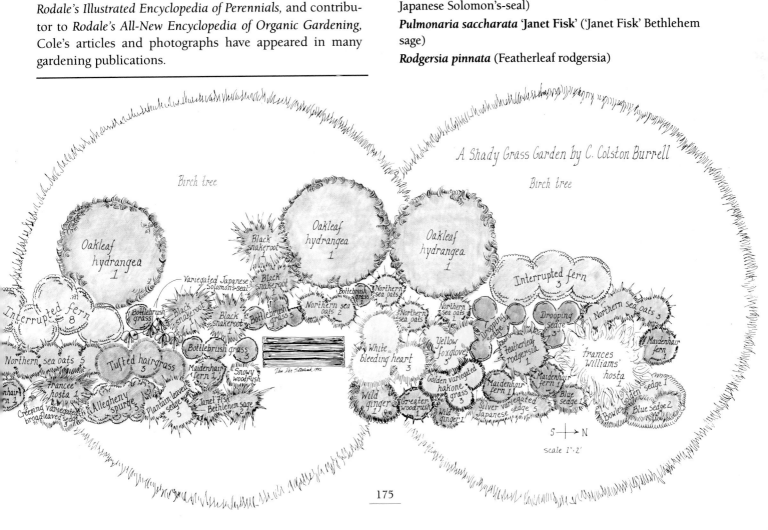

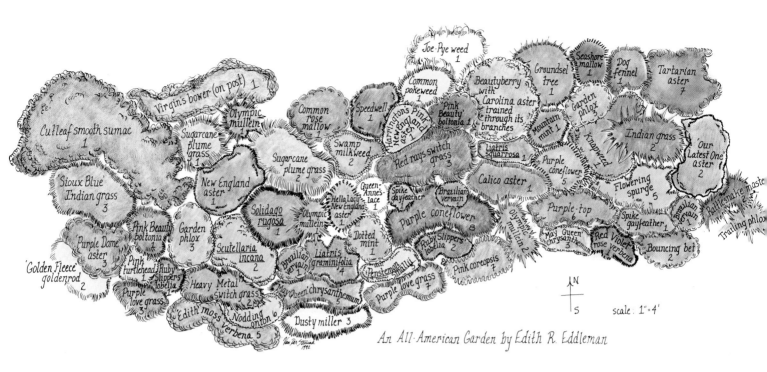

An All-American Garden by Edith R. Eddleman

scale: 1"=4'

An All-American Garden

This sunny south-facing border composed of native grasses and other long-flowering perennials is inspired by the tough and beautiful plants that inhabit the roadsides of eastern North America. The colors used are blue, pink, and purple, making the border a soft cloud of color accented by contrasting textures and forms.

Included are native grass cultivars such as the beautiful blue-leaved 'Heavy Metal' switch grass (*Panicum virgatum* 'Heavy Metal') and 'Sioux Blue' Indian grass (*Sorghastrum nutans* 'Sioux Blue'). A few non-native plants have been used: Brazilian vervain (*Verbena bonariensis*) and moss verbena (*Verbena tenuisecta*), which are South American but have naturalized alongside roads in the lower South.

Edith R. Eddleman is a garden designer, lecturer, photographer, and long-time plant enthusiast living in Durham, North Carolina. With Douglas Ruhren, she is volunteer coordinator and designer of the North Carolina State University Arboretum's flower garden.

Allium cernuum (Nodding onion)

Artemisia stellerana (Dusty miller)

Asclepias incarnata (Swamp milkweed)

Aster lateriflorus 'Horizontalis' (Calico aster)

Aster novae-angliae (New England aster)

Aster novae-angliae 'Harrington's Pink' ('Harrington's Pink' New England aster)

Aster novae-angliae 'Hella Lacy' ('Hella Lacy' New England aster)

Aster 'Our Latest One'

Aster 'Purple Dome'

Aster tataricus (Tartarian aster)

Baccharis halimifolia (Groundsel tree)

Boltonia asteroides 'Pink Beauty' ('Pink Beauty' boltonia)

Callicarpa americana (Beautyberry) with *Aster carolinianus* (Carolina aster) trained through its branches

Centaurea dealbata (Knapweed)

Chelone lyonii (Pink turtlehead)

Chrysanthemum 'May Queen'

Clematis virginiana (Virgin's bower) on post

Coreopsis rosea (Pink coreopsis)

Daucus carota var. *carota* (Queen-Anne's-lace)

Echinacea purpurea (Purple coneflower)

Eragrostis spectabilis (Purple love grass)

Erianthus giganteus (Sugarcane plume grass)

Eryngium yuccifolium (Rattlesnake master)

Eupatorium capillifolium (Dog fennel)

Eupatorium fistulosum (Joe-Pye weed)

Euphorbia corollata (Flowering spurge)

Hibiscus moscheutos (Common rose mallow)

Kosteletzkya virginica (Seashore mallow)

Liatris graminifolia

Liatris spicata (Spike gayfeather)

Liatris squarrosa

Lobelia 'Ruby Slippers'

Monarda punctata (Dotted mint)

Panicum virgatum 'Heavy Metal' ('Heavy Metal' switch grass)

Panicum virgatum 'Rotstrahlbusch' (Red rays switch grass)

Penstemon smallii

Phlox nivalis, white cultivar (Trailing phlox)

Phlox paniculata (Garden phlox)

Phytolacca americana (Common pokeweed)

Pycnanthemum incanum (Mountain mint)

Rhus glabra 'Laciniata' (Cutleaf smooth sumac)

Saponaria officinalis 'Rosea-Plena' (Bouncing bet)

Scutellaria incana

Solidago sphacelata 'Golden Fleece' ('Golden Fleece' golden-rod)

Solidago rugosa

Sorghastrum nutans 'Sioux Blue' ('Sioux Blue' Indian grass)

Tridens flavus (Purple-top)

Verbascum olympicum (Olympic mullein)

Verbena bonariensis (Brazilian vervain)

Verbena canadensis 'Red Violet' ('Red Violet' rose verbena)

Verbena tenuisecta 'Edith' ('Edith' moss verbena)

Veronica noveboracensis (Speedwell)

A Flowing Foundation Planting

This foundation planting is composed of soft, flowing drifts of grasses set among the spring and summer colors of hydrangeas and roses. It would be suitable for an east- or west-facing wall, or even a south-facing wall in the Pacific Northwest. The grasses form a groundcover beneath the shrubs and provide year-round interest. Beginning with the spring blossoms of the feather and moor grasses, the grasses provide flowering accents until late autumn. The strong winter colors of the grasses lighten and warm the garden under the typically gray winter skies where I garden.

Cynthia Woodyard is a photographer and garden designer in Portland, Oregon. Her own Portland garden has contained grasses for many years and is featured in *The American Woman's Garden Book.* Her horticultural photography has graced many magazines and books on both sides of the Atlantic.

Hydrangea quercifolia (Oakleaf hydrangea)

Imperata cylindrica 'Red Baron' ('Red Baron' blood grass)

Molinia caerulea 'Variegata' (Variegated moor grass)

Pennisetum alopecuroides (Fountain grass)

Rosa 'Betty Prior' ('Betty Prior' rose)

Stipa gigantea (Giant feather grass)

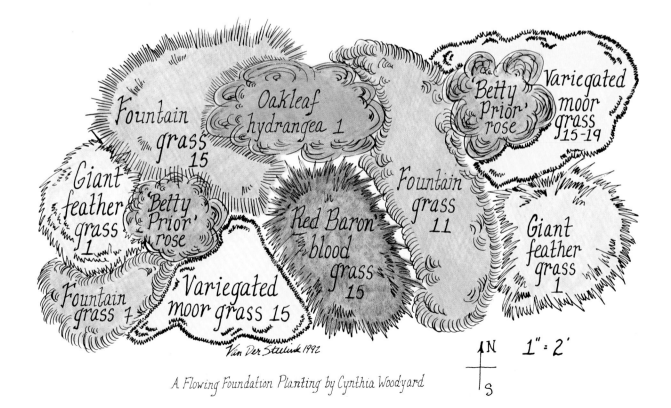

A Flowing Foundation Planting by Cynthia Woodyard

GLOSSARY

Annual   A plant that completes its lifecycle in a single growing season.

Anther   The pollen-bearing part of a stamen.

Auricle   An appendage of the leaf blade occasionally found in grasses usually at the blade base.

Awn   A slender, often silky, sometimes stiff bristle attached to the bracts of a grass flower.

Axil   The angle between a leaf and the stem to which it attaches.

Basal   At the base.

Biennial   A plant that completes its lifecycle in two growing seasons.

Blade   The usually flat part of the leaf, different from stem and sheath.

Bract   A modified, often reduced leaf, usually situated near a flower or inflorescence.

Bunch grass   A grass that grows as a clump.

Calcareous   Calcium-rich soil.

Cane   Thickened culm, or stem, of a grass.

Clumping   Growing in tufts or bunches. A clumping grass does not run or creep.

Collar   A membranous or hairy appendage at the base of the leaf where it connects to the sheath.

Colony   A group, or stand, of plants.

Cool-season grass   A grass that grows mostly in the cooler seasons of fall, winter, and/or spring. It grows best between 60° and 75°F and tends to be evergreen.

Crown   The base of the plant arising from the soil line.

Culm   The stem of a grass, sedge, or rush.

Cyme   An inflorescence with central flowers maturing first. Typical of sedges.

Deciduous   Not persistent; dying back to the ground each year. Foliage that does not remain evergreen.

Dioecious   Having separate male and female plants.

Herbaceous   Not woody. Applied to a plant whose aboveground parts do not form hard wood.

Inflorescence   The flowering structure of a grass; the arrangement of the flowers on a stem.

Internode   The part of an above- or underground stem between two nodes.

Lemma   The outer or upper scalelike bract in the spikelet.

Ligule   A small, membranous projection occasionally present at the top of the sheath or the base of the blade.

Linear   Leaves that are longer than wide.

Lodicule   A specialized structure in grasses found between the lemma and the palea; it serves to open and close the flower.

Mediterranean climate   Climate characterized by mild, rainy winters; dry, hot summers; and a moderating coastal influence.

Naturalize   To colonize an area naturally, by seed or stolons.

Node   A joint on the stem at which leaves, bracts, or branches are produced.

Ovary   The structure that bears the seed after fertilization.

Palea   The inner or upper scalelike bract in the spikelet.

Panicle   The flower head of a grass, or, in particular, a branched flower head with a main axis and divided branches with stalked spikelets.

Perennial   A plant that lives for more than two growing seasons.

Pistil   The female part of a flower, composed of ovary, stigma, and style; the fertilized ovary becomes the seed.

Prairie   Vegetation consisting mainly of grass, like the great interior grasslands of North America.

Raceme   An inflorescence with stalked spikelets borne along a single axis.

Rhizome   An underground stem from which roots and shoots emerge along the internodes.

Root   The part of the plant below ground that takes up water and nutrients from the soil. Grass roots are usually fibrous.

Runner   An aboveground stem that creeps along the ground, and from which roots and shoots emerge at the nodes. Also called *stolon*.

Running grass   A grass that spreads from stolons or rhizomes.

Scree   A coarse, stony soil found naturally on alpine slopes. Rock and trough gardeners imitate scree with a soil mix composed of coarse sand, grit, or coarse gravel, and leaf mold or peat.

Sheath   The basal part of the leaf that wraps around the stem and holds it in place.

Siliceous   Containing silica, which adds a rough texture and strength to foliage and stems. *Equisetum* spp. are siliceous.

Sod-forming grass   A grass that spreads from stolons and/or rhizomes to form a dense mat.

Specimen   A plant grown singly as an accent.

Spicate   Bearing single or multiple leaves.

Spike   An inflorescence composed of stalkless flowers arranged on a single axis; also, a general term for grass flowers.

Spikelet   An individual grass flower. Most inflorescences are composed of many spikelets.

Stamen   The male organ of a flower, composed of anther and filament.

Stem   The smooth, usually cylindrical structure that holds the leaves and inflorescence of a grass; also called *culm*.

Stigma   The structure that receives the pollen.

Stolon   An aboveground stem that creeps along the ground, producing roots and new plants at the nodes. Also called a *runner*.

Stoloniferous   Having stolons.

Stratification Treatment of seeds to speed or induce germination; may involve exposure to heat or cold, soaking, or other treatment of the seed.
Terminal At the tip of a branch or stem.

Umbel An inflorescence in which all the flower spikes arise from the same point.
Variegated Marked with colors in spots or streaks. Variegated grasses are green with white, gold, or yellow.

Viviparous Producing new plantlets on the mother plant, often on or instead of flowers. These plantlets, which will grow into new plants, may be removed or left to fall to the ground.

Warm-season grass A grass that grows best at temperatures between 80° and 95°F. Usually deciduous, they become dormant in the fall and winter and begin actively growing in spring.

BIBLIOGRAPHY

Beetle, Alan A. *Distribution Of The Native Grasses Of California.* California Agricultural Experiment Station, 1947.

Brooklyn Botanic Garden Record. *Plants & Gardens: Ornamental Grasses.* Brooklyn: Brooklyn Botanic Garden, Inc., 1988.

Brown, Lauren. *Grasses: An Identification Guide.* Boston: Houghton Mifflin Company, 1979.

Cornell University. Staff of the Liberty Hyde Bailey Hortorium. *Hortus Third: A Concise Dictionary of Plants Cultivated in the United States and Canada.* New York: Macmillan Publishing Co., Inc., 1976.

Crampton, Beecher. *Grasses In California.* Berkeley, Calif.: University of California Press, 1974.

Farrelly, David. *The Book Of Bamboo.* San Francisco: Sierra Club Books, 1984.

Gould, Frank W. *Grasses Of The Southwestern United States.* Tucson, Ariz.: The University of Arizona Press, 1951.

——. *The Grasses Of Texas.* College Station, Tex.: Texas A & M University Press, 1975.

Grounds, Roger. *Ornamental Grasses.* London: Christopher Helm Ltd, 1989.

Hahlenberg, Mary Hunt, and Mark Schwartz. *A Book About Grass: Its Beauty and Uses.* New York: E. P. Dutton, Inc., 1983.

Hitchcock, A. S. *Manual Of The Grasses Of The United States,* Volumes One and Two, second edition. New York: Dover Publications, Inc., 1971.

Jelitto, Leo, and Wilhelm Schacht. *Hardy Herbaceous Perennials,* Volume I (A-K) and Volume II (L-Z). Portland, Oreg.: Timber Press, 1990.

Karel, Leonard. *Dried Grasses, Grains, Gourds, Pods and Cones.* Metuchen, N.J.: The Scarecrow Press, Inc., 1975.

Loewer, H. Peter. *Growing And Decorating With Grasses.* New York: Walker and Company, 1977.

Madson, John. *Where The Sky Began: Land Of The Tallgrass Prairie.* Boston: Houghton Mifflin Company, 1982.

Munz, Philip A. *A Flora Of Southern California.* Berkeley, Calif.: University of California Press, 1974.

Munz, Philip A., and David D. Keck. *A California Flora with Supplement.* Berkeley, Calif.: University of California Press, 1959 (Supplement 1968).

Oakes, A. J. *Ornamental Grasses and Grasslike Plants.* New York: Van Nostrand Reinhold, 1990.

Ottesen, Carole. *Ornamental Grasses: The Amber Wave.* New York: McGraw-Hill Inc., 1989.

Reinhardt, Thomas A., Marina Reinhardt, and Mark Moskowitz. *Ornamental Grass Gardening: Design Ideas, Functions And Effects.* Los Angeles: HP Books, a division of Price Stern Sloan Inc., 1989.

Rotar, Peter P. *Grasses Of Hawaii.* Honolulu: University of Hawaii Press, 1968.

Sunset Books and Sunset Magazine Editors. *Sunset New Western Garden Book.* Menlo Park, Calif.: Lane Publishing Co., 1979.

Warnock, Barton H. *Wildflowers Of The Big Bend Country, Texas.* Alpine, Tex.: Sul Ross State University, 1970.

——. *Wildflowers Of The Davis Mountains And Marathon Basin, Texas.* Alpine, Tex.: Sul Ross State University, 1977.

Wasowski, Sally, and Julie Ryan. *Landscaping With Native Texas Plants.* Austin, Tex.: Texas Monthly Press, Inc., 1985.

Welch, William C. *Perennial Garden Color.* Dallas: Taylor Publishing Company, 1989.

MAIL-ORDER SOURCES

Ornamental Grasses

Baylands Nursery
2835 Temple Court
East Palo Alto, CA 94303

Kurt Bluemel, Inc., Nurseries
2740 Greene Lane
Baldwin, MD 21013

Carroll Gardens, Inc.
Box 310
444 East Main Street
Westminster, MD 21157

Coastal Gardens & Nursery
4611 Socastee Boulevard
Myrtle Beach, SC 29575

Endangered Species
Box 1830
Tustin, CA 92681-1830

Garden Place
P.O. Box 388
6780 Heisley Road
Mentor, OH 44060

Greenlee Nursery
301 E. Franklin Avenue
Pomona, CA 91766

Holbrook Farm and Nursery
115 Lance Road
P.O. Box 368
Fletcher, NC 28732

Limerock Ornamental Grasses
R.D. 1, Box 111-C
Port Matilda, PA 16870

Logee's Greenhouses
141 North Street
Danielson, CT 06239

Mellingers
2310 W. South Range Road
North Lima, OH 44452

Neufeld Nursery
1865 California Street
Oceanside, CA 92054

Niche Gardens
1111 Dawson Road
Chapel Hill, NC 27516

Pacific Coast Seed
7074-D Commerce Circle
Pleasanton, CA 94566

Paradise Gardens
14 May Street
Whitman, MA 02382

Park Seed Co., Inc.
P.O. Box 31
Greenwood, SC 29648

Prairie Nursery
P.O. Box 306
Westfield, WI 53964

Rice Creek Gardens
11506 Highway 65
Blaine, MN 55434

S & S Seeds
P.O. Box 1275
Carpinteria, CA 93013

Siskiyou Rare Plant Nursery
2825 Cummings Road
Medford, OR 97501

Springbrook Gardens, Inc.
P.O. Box 388
6776 Heisley Road
Mentor, OH 44061-0388

Sunlight Gardens
Route 1, Box 600A
Hillvale Road
Andersonville, TN 37705

Sunnybrook Farms Nursery
P.O. Box 6
9448 Mayfield Road
Chesterland, OH 44026

William Tricker, Inc.
7125 Tanglewood Drive
Independence, OH 44131

Van Ness Water Gardens
2460 N. Euclid Avenue
Upland, CA 91786

Andre Viette Farm and Nursery
Route 1, Box 16
Fishersville, VA 22939

Wayside Gardens
1 Garden Lane
Hodges, SC 29696-0001

White Flower Farm
P.O. Box 50
Litchfield, CT 06759

Wildlife Nurseries
P.O. Box 2724
Oshkosh, WI 54903

Wildwood Nursery
3975 Emerald Avenue
LaVerne, CA 91750

Ya-Ka-Ama Nursery
6215 Eastside road
Forestville, CA 95436

Ornamental and Native Grass Plants and Seeds

Abundant Life Seed Foundation
P.O. Box 772
Port Townsend, WA

Applewood Seed Company
5380 Vivian Street
Arvada, CO 80215

Bamert Seed Co.
Rt.3, Box 1120
Muleshoe, TX 79347

W. Atlee Burpee & Co.
300 Park Avenue
Warminster, PA 18974

Ernst Crownvetch Farms
R.D. 5, Box 806
Meadville, PA 16335

G. S. Grimes Seed Co.
Box 398
201 Main Street
Smethport, PA 16749

High Altitude Gardens
P.O. Box 4238
Ketchum, ID 83340

Larner Seeds
P.O. Box 407
235 Fern Road
Bolinas, CA 94924

Milaeger's Gardens
4838 Douglas Avenue
Racine, WI 53402-2498

Missouri Wildflowers Nursery
9814 Pleasant Hill Road
Jefferson City, MO 65109

Native Gardens
5737 Fisher Lane
Greenback, TN 37742

Native American Seed
3400 Long Prairie Road
Flower Mound, TX 75028

Northplan Seed Producers
P.O. Box 9107
Moscow, ID 83843

Park Seed Co., Inc.
P.O. Box 31
Greenwood, SC 29648

Plants of the Southwest
Route 6, Box 11-A
Santa Fe, NM 87501

Plants of the Wild
Box 866
Tekoa, WA 99033

Prairie Moon Nursery
Route 3, Box 163
Winona, MN 55987

Prairie Nursery
P.O. Box 306
Westfield, WI 53964

Prairie Ridge Nursery
R.R. 2
9738 Overland Road
Mount Horeb, WI 53572-2832

Redwood City Seed Co.
P.O. Box 361
Redwood City, CA 94064

Stock Seed Farms, Inc.
28008 Mill Road
Murdock, NE 68407-2350

Thompson and Morgan
P.O. Box 1308
Jackson, NJ 08527

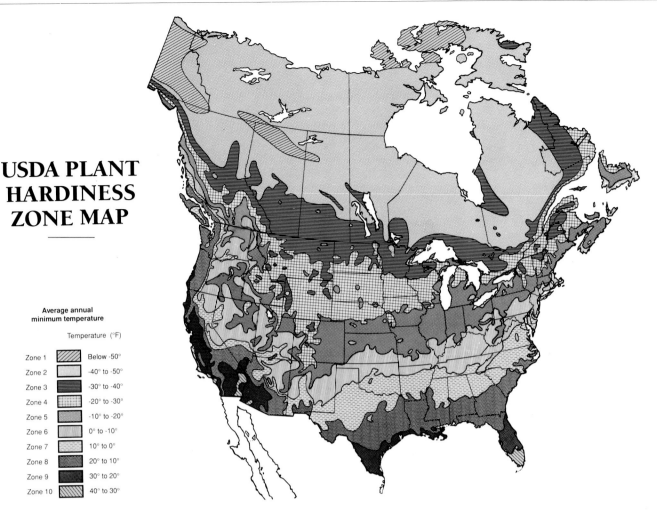

USDA PLANT HARDINESS ZONE MAP

Average annual minimum temperature

Temperature (°F)

Zone 1		Below -50°
Zone 2		-40° to -50°
Zone 3		-30° to -40°
Zone 4		-20° to -30°
Zone 5		-10° to -20°
Zone 6		0° to -10°
Zone 7		10° to 0°
Zone 8		20° to 10°
Zone 9		30° to 20°
Zone 10		40° to 30°

COMMON TO BOTANICAL NAMES INDEX

A 'Adagio' Japanese silver grass *Miscanthus sinenthis* 'Adagio'
African love grass *Eragrostis curvula*
Alkali dropseed *Sporobolus airoides*
Alkali sacaton *Sporobolus airoides*
Alpine bluegrass *Poa alpina* var. *vivipara*
'Anderson' wild rye *Elymus glaucus* 'Anderson'
April green fescue *Festuca amethystina* 'April Gruen'
'Arabesque' Japanese silver grass *Miscanthus sinenthis* 'Arabesque'
Arrow reed *Arundo pliniana*
Atlas fescue *Festuca mairei*
Australian blue grass *Poa costineata*
Australian silver rush *Juncus polyanthemus*
'Autumn Fire' Japanese silver grass *Miscanthus sinensis* 'Herbstfeuer'
'Autumn Light' Japanese silver grass *Miscanthus sinensis* 'Autumn Light'
Autumn moor grass *Sesleria autumnalis*
Autumn sorcery fountain grass *Pennisetum alopecuroides* 'Herbstzauber'
Azure blue fescue *Festuca cinerea* 'Azurit'

B Bamboo muhly grass *Muhlenbergia dumosa*
Banded bulrush *Schoenplectus tabernaemontana* 'Zebrinus'
Beardless wild rye *Elymus tritichoides*
Bear grass *Xerophyllum tinax*
Bearskin fescue *Festuca scoparia*
'Beatles' sedge *Carex* × 'The Beatles'
'Bend' love grass *Eragrostis trichoides* 'Bend'

Bent awn plume grass *Erianthus contortus*
'Berkeley Hills' rye *Elymus glaucus* 'Berkeley hills'
Berkeley sedge *Carex tumulicola*
Bermuda grass *Cynodon dactylon*
Big bluestem *Andropogon gerardii*
Black-flowering sedge *Carex nigra*
Black pampas grass *Cortaderia richardii*
'Blaze' little bluestem *Schizachyrium scoparium* 'Blaza'
Blue fescue *Festuca cinerea*
Bluefinch fescue *Festuca cinerea* 'Blaufink'
Blue fox fescue *Festuca cinerea* 'Blaufuchs'
Blue gramma *Bouteloua gracilis*
Blue hairgrass *Koeleria brevis; K. glauca*
Blue lyme grass *Elymus arenarius* 'Glaucus'
Blue moor grass *Sesleria caerulea*
Blue oat grass *Helictotrichon sempervirens*
Blue sedge *Carex glauca*
Blue sheep's fescue *Festuca amethystina* 'Superba'; *F. cinerea*
Blue-silver fescue *Festuca cinerea* 'Blausilber'
Blue wheat grass *Agropyron magellanicum*
Blue wild rye *Elymus glaucus*
Bottlerush grass *Hystrix patula*
'Bowles Golden' sedge *Carex elata* 'Bowles Golden'
Broadleaf umbrella plant *Cyperus alternifolius*
Bronze luster fescue *Festuca amethystina* 'Bronzeglanz'
'Bronze' New Zealand hair sedge *Carex comans* 'Bronze'
Bronze veil tufted hairgrass *Deschampsia caespitosa* 'Bronzeschleier'

'Bronze Veil' tufted hairgrass *Deschampsia caespitosa* 'Bronze Veil'
Broom sedge *Schyzachyrium scoparium*
Buffalo grass *Buchloe dactyloides*
Bulbous oat grass *Arrhenatherum elatius*
Bulrush *Scirpus lacustris; Typha latifolia*
'Burgundy Giant' fountain grass *Pennisetum* 'Burgundy Giant'
Bushy bluestem *Andropogon glomeratus*

C 'Cabaret' Japanese silver grass *Miscanthis sinensis* 'Cabaret'
California black-flowering sedge *Carex nudata*
California fescue *Fescue californica*
California gray rush *Juncus patens*
California meadow sedge *Carex pansa*
Canada wild rye *Elymus canadensis*
Cane bluestem *Bothriochloa barbinoides*
'Canyon Prince' wild rye *Elymus canadensis* 'Canyon Prince'
'Carmen's Japanese' rush *Juncus* 'Carmen's Japanese'
Cascade Japanese silver grass *Miscanthus sinensis* 'Kaskade'
Cassian fountain grass *Pennisetum alopecuroides* 'Cassian'
Catlin sedge *Carex texensis*
Cattail *Typha latifolia*
'Champ' big bluestem *Andropogon gerardii* 'Champ'
Chinese silver grass *Miscanthus giganteus*
Christ's tears *Coix lacryma-jobi*
Common reed *Phragmites australis*

Spring blue fescue *Festuca cinerea* 'Fruehlingsblau'
'Squaw' red switch grass *Panicum virgatum* 'Squaw'
Squirreltail *Hordeum jubatum*
'Staefa' tall moor grass *Molinia caerulea* subsp. *arundinacea* 'Staefa'
'Stanislaus 5000' wild rye *Elymus glaucus* 'Stanislaus 5000'
'Stanislaus 2000' wild rye *Elymus glaucus* 'Stanislaus 2000'
Strawberries and cream ribbon grass *Phalaris arundinacea* 'Feesey's Form'
Striped giant reed *Arundo donax* 'Variegata'
Sugarcane *Saccharum officinarum*
Sugarcane plume grass *Erianthus giganteus*
'Sunningdale Silver' pampas grass *Cortaderia selloana* 'Sunningdale Silver'
'Sun Stripe' pampas grass *Cortaderia selloana* 'Sun Stripe'
Sweet vernal grass *Anthoxanthum adoratum*
Switch grass *Panicum virgatum*
Sylvan sedge *Carex sylvatica*
Sylvan woodrush *Luzula sylvatica*

T Tall purple moor grass *Molinia caerulea* subsp. *arundinacea*
Tall switch grass *Panicum virgatum* 'Strictum'
'Tanomanoyuki' sweet flag *Acorus gramineus* 'Tanomanoyuki'
'Tauern Pass' *Luzula sylvatica* 'Tauern Pass'
Tear grass *Coix lacryma-jobi*
Tender fountain grass *Pennisetum setaceum*
Texas sedge *Carex texensis*
'Texoka' buffalo grass *Buchloe dactyloides* 'Texoka'
Tiger grass *Thysanolena maxima*
Toe toe *Cortaderia fulvida*

Tom Thumb fescue *Festuca cinerea* 'Daeumling'
'Transparent' moor grass *Molinia caerulea* subsp. *arundinacea* 'Transparent'
Tufted hairgrass *Deschampsia caespitosa*
Turkey foot *Andropogon gerardii*

U Umbrella palm *Cyperus alternifolius*
Umbrella plant *Cyperus alternifolius*
'Undine' Japanese *Miscanthus sinensis* 'Undine'

V Variegated bird's foot sedge *Carex ornithopoda* 'Variegata'
Variegated broadleaf umbrella plant *Cyperus albostriatus* 'Variegatus'
Variegated calamus *Acorus calamus* 'Variegatus'
Variegated cocksfoot grass *Dactylis glomerata* 'Variegata'
Variegated Japanese sedge *Carex hachioensis* 'Evergold'
Variegated Japanese silver grass *Miscanthus sinensis* 'Variegatus'
Variegrated manna grass *Glyceria maxima* 'Variegata'
Variegated moor grass *Molinia caerulea* 'Variegata'
Variegated orchard grass *Dactylis glomerata* 'Variegata'
Variegated palm grass *Setaria palmifolia* 'Variegata'
Variegated St. Augustinegrass *Stenotaphrum secondatum* 'Variegatum'
Variegated sweet flag *Acorus calamus* 'Variegatus'
Variegated umbrella plant *Cyperus alternifolius* 'Variegatus'
Variegated velvet grass *Holcus lanatus* 'Variegatus'

Velebit sedge *Carex speciosa*
Velvet grass *Holcus lanatus*
Virginia wild rye *Elymus virginicus*
Volga wild rye *Elymus racemosus* 'Glaucus'

W 'Warrior' switch grass *Panicum virgatum* 'Warrior'
Wavy hairgrass *Deschampsia flexuosa*
Weather vane silver grass *Miscanthus sinensis* 'Wetterfane'
Weeping brown New Zealand sedge *Carex flagelifera*
Weeping love grass *Eragrostis trichoides* 'Bend'
'Weserbergland' fountain grass *Pennisetum alopecuroides* 'Weserbergland'
White-flowering fountain grass *Pennisetum caudatum; Pennisatum villosum*
White-striped bulrush *Schoenplectus tabernaemontana* 'Albescens'
White-striped Japanese sweet flag *Acorus gramineus* 'Variegatus'
Wild barley *Hordeum* spp.
Wild oats *Chasmanthium latifolium*
Wild rice *Zizania aquatice*
Wild rye *Elymus*
Willis fescue *Festuca valesiaca* 'Glaucantha'
Windplay tall moor grass *Molinia caerulea* subsp. *arundinacea* 'Windspiel'

Y 'Yaku Jima' Japanese silver grass *Miscanthus sinensis* 'Yaku Jima'
Yellow foxtail grass *Alopecurus pratensis*
Yellow sedge *Carex elata* 'Bowles Golden'
'Yodonoyuki' sweet flag *Acorus gramineus* 'Yodonoyuki'
Yorkshire fog *Holcus lanatus*

Z Zebra grass *Miscanthus sinensis* 'Zebrinus'
Zebra rush *Schoenplectus tabernaemontana* 'Zebrinus'

INDEX